Plastic and Reconstructive Surgery of the Face and Neck

Proceedings of the Second International Symposium

Plastic and Reconstructive Surgery of the Face and Neck

Proceedings of the Second International Symposium

Volume 1: Aesthetic Surgery

Edited by
George A. Sisson, M.D.
M. Eugene Tardy, Jr., M.D.

GRUNE & STRATTON

A Subsidiary of Harcourt Brace Jovanovich, Publishers

New York San Francisco London

Library of Congress Cataloging in Publication Data

International Symposium on Plastic and Reconstructive
Surgery of the Face and Neck, 2d, Chicago, 1975.
Plastic and reconstructive surgery of the face and
neck.

Sponsored by the American Academy of Facial Plastic
and Reconstructive Surgery.
Includes bibliographical references and indexes.
CONTENTS: v. 1. Aesthetic surgery.—v. 2. Rehabilitative surgery.
1. Surgery, Plastic—Congresses. 2. Face—Surgery—Congresses. 3. Neck—Surgery—Congresses. I. Sisson,
George A. II. Tardy, Medney Eugene, 1934–
III. American Academy of Facial Plastic and Reconstructive Surgery. IV. Title. [DNLM: 1. Neck—Surgery—Congresses. 2. Face—Congresses. 3. Surgery, Plastic—Congresses. WE705 P713]
RD118.A1I6 1975 617′.52 76-57989
ISBN 0-8089-0941-X (v. 1)
ISBN 0-8089-0956-8 (v. 2)

Grune & Stratton, Inc.
111 Fifth Avenue
New York, New York 10003

Distributed in the United Kingdom by
Academic Press, Inc. (London) Ltd.
24/28 Oval Road, London NW 1

Library of Congress Catalog Number 76-57989
International Standard Book Number 0-8089-0941-X

Printed in the United States of America

Table of Contents

Preface

"Medicine is the only world wide profession, following everywhere the same methods, actuated by the same ambitions, and pursuing the same ends. This homogeneity, its most characteristic feature, is not shared by the law, and not by the church, certainly not in the same degree. While in antiquity the law rivals medicine, there is not in it that extraordinary solidarity which makes the physician at home in any country, any place where two or three sons of men are gathered together . . . . A powerful stimulus in promoting this wide organic unity is our great international gatherings . . . . "I may say to you that one of the distressing bewilderments of the layman who only desires the working out of a broad plan is the extraordinary bitterness of professional jealousy between not only schoolmen and nonschoolmen but between schoolmen themselves, and the reflections which are cast on one another as belonging to that clique, which makes it exceedingly difficult for the layman to understand what way there is out of these squabbles."

Sir William Osler
Unity, Peace, and Concord
in Aequanimitas, 1905

In his farewell address to the medical profession seventy years ago, Sir William Osler outlined several truths still inherent in the practice of medicine. Perhaps now, more than ever before, these precepts should be reiterated and recognized as important strengths, since presently our profession is subjected to the greatest scrutiny ever by both the consumer and the lawmaker. Today, it is imperative that the various disciplines of medicine be united. We must not be drawn into jurisdictional disputes which would blur our public image and weaken our position in any political action. Cooperation becomes essential for a favorable future base. The free interchange of information and ideas and the sharing of experiences will help to better gird all specialities so medicine's obligation to the consumer can be well met and its responsibilities to the legislative process intelligently fulfilled.

It was our hope that the Second International Symposium on Plastic and Reconstructive Surgery of the Face and Neck would provide a forum whereby its members, in consortium with its many friends in general surgery, oral surgery, and general plastic surgery could hold a meeting in the continued search for excellence in the teaching and practice of their surgical art.

The Symposium was more than a success. It was gratifying to see the various disciplines sit down for one week and share new concepts, techniques and philosophies without rancor or built-in prejudices.

The multidisiplinary attendance was apparent as was the international flavor, with over twenty countries represented. Approximately 100 papers, 15 panels, 45 instructional courses, and 40 cine-clinics were presented. The true interchange of philosophies and information continued late into the evening social functions.

The mixed background of the 1000 attendees provided a built-in flexibility rather than the traditional rigidities often prominent in the smaller and "select" society meetings. Those in attendance were well aware of the difficulties encountered in gaining new information in this most exacting and complex region. No one man nor one medical specialty can expect to be expert in all the new techniques rapidly developing in the region of the head and neck.

It was apparent early that the American Academy of Facial Plastic and Reconstructive Surgery, host of the Second International Symposium, was obligated to publish these scientific proceedings. A natural division of the presentations into aesthetic and reparative attitudes makes possible the publication of these two volumes. This work should provide ready reference for the attendees as well as make possible further dissemination of this information for those unable to attend. As these volumes take their place in the continuum of medicine, only history can judge their true value.

Today, we can say this international meeting, conceived for the continuing search for excellence, reflected well on the medical profession by demonstrating "unity, peace, and concord."

George A. Sisson, M.D.
General Chairman
and
M. Eugene Tardy, Jr. M.D.
Program Chairman

Second International Symposium
on Plastic and Reconstructive
Surgery of the Face and Neck

Contributors

Jack Anderson, M.D. New Orleans, Louisiana

Jacob S. Aronoff, M.D. New York, New York

Richard W. Babin, M.D. Los Angeles, California

Crowell Beard, M.D. San Jose, California

G. Jan Beekhuis, M.D. Detroit, Michigan

William H. Bell, M.D. Dallas, Texas

Walter E. Berman, M.D. Beverly Hills, California

David Bernstein, M.D. New York, New York

Eugene Bortnick, M.D. Kansas City, Kansas

Rinaldo F. Canalis, M.D. Los Angeles, California

Bernard H. Cohen, M.D. Miami, Florida

Jorge de Autueno, M.D. Buenos Aires, Argentina

Hans Denecke, M.D. Heidelberg, West Germany

Howard Diamond, M.D. New York, New York

Ralph L. Dicker, M.D. New York, New York

Richard T. Farrior, M.D. Tampa, Florida

Willard E. Fee, Jr., M.D. Stanford, California

Sidney S. Feuerstein, M.D. New York, New York

Irving J. Fine, M.D. Perth Amboy, New Jersey

Pierre F. Fournier, M.D. Paris, France

William H. Friedman, M.D. New York, New York

Richard L. Goode, M.D. Stanford, California

Jack P. Gunter, M.D. Dallas, Texas

John R. Hilger, M.D. Tacoma, Washington

Kenneth H. Hinderer, M.D. Pittsburgh, Pennsylvania

Donald J. Huttner, M.D. Denver, Colorado

Carlos Juri, M.D. Buenos Aires, Argentina

Jose Juri, M.D. Buenos Aires, Argentina

Frank M. Kamer, M.D. Los Angeles, California

Harold J. Kaplan, M.D. Los Angeles, California

Jack D. Kerth, M.D. Chicago, Illinois

Mark E. Krugman, M.D. Los Angeles, California

Leonard A. Lewis, M.D. Miami, Florida

Jean-Paul Lintilhac, M.D. Paris, France

E. Gaylon McCollough, M.D. Birmingham, Alabama

Michael L. Merrin, M.D. Los Angeles, California

Rodolphe Meyer, M.D. Lausanne, Switzerland

Charles M. Monell, M.D. Beverly Hills, California

Julius Newman, M.D. Upper Darby, Pennsylvania

Alberto Gonzalez Otharan, Buenos Aires, Argentina

Morey L. Parkes, M.D. Los Angeles, California

Carl N. Patterson, M.D. Durham, North Carolina

Lionello Ponti, M.D. Rome, Italy

Donald G. Powell, M.D. Durham, North Carolina

F. Mark Rafaty, M.D. Palo Alto, California

Sorrel S. Resnick, M.D. Miami, Florida

Robert L. Simons, M.D. North Miami Beach, Florida

Trent W. Smith, M.D. Columbus, Ohio

V. P. Sood, M.D. New Delhi, India

D. Bluford Stough III, M.D. Hot Springs, Arkansas

Ronald W. Strahan, M.D. Los Angeles, California

Fred J. Stucker, M.D. Philadelphia, Pennsylvania

Victor R. Syracuse, M.D. New York, New York

M. Eugene Tardy, Jr., M.D. Chicago, Illinois

William K. Wright, M.D. Houston, Texas

Plastic and Reconstructive Surgery of the Face and Neck

Proceedings of the Second International Symposium

Nose

Rhinoplasty Tip Procedures (Panel)

Robert L. Simons:

The session in Rhinoplasty Tip Procedures developed as an informal clinic in nasal analysis and preferred method of treatment. Four patients were presented with two of the panel members discussing each case.

Case I

The first patient (Fig. 1 A–E) was analyzed by Dr. Jack Anderson and Dr. Hans Denecke.

Dr. Anderson's comments follow:

"From the frontal view (Fig. 1A), this young lady's nose is (1) too wide in the mid-third, (2) thick with acneiform, oily skin, (3) slightly dependent in the tip region with the presence of a hanging columella, and (4) too fat and bulbous in the tip. There is asymmetry of the face with slanting of the lips and unequal position of the eyes.

In the right lateral view (Fig. 1B) there is an obvious dorsal hump and hanging columella. The tip is inadequately projected with the dorsum too long for this face. The columella angle is approximately 90°. The soft tissue triangles (facets) are enlarged with a "pseudo-notching" of the alae due to the hanging columella. The chin is slightly receeding with a more marked lack of projection over the mid-third, malar region of the face.

On the smiling view (Fig. 1C), there is little additional information. I rarely use smiling views.

Left profile (Fig. 1D) again emphasizes the hanging columella and "pseudo-notching" of the alae.

On the basal view (Fig. 1E) the mesial crura fill no more than two-thirds of the columella. The soft tissue triangles are large and there is evidence of retraction at the base of the columella. The actual width and triangularity of the lobule is satisfactory.

To correct this problem of insufficient tip projection, I would do a high cartilage-splitting incision three-fifths of the way up the cartilage. I would carry this incision laterally cutting through the cartilage past the midpoint of the alae. The transfixion incision would be carried deep down to the nasal spine because of the lack of tip projection.

The cartilaginous dorsum would then be lowered without cutting the upper laterals away from the septum, followed by an intramucosal hump removal. Due to the high length of the dorsal hump, medial osteotomies would not be necessary.

I would then do a submucous resection, which I perform in 85 to 90 percent of my cases to ensure more leverage for infracturing of the nasal bones. The lateral osteotomies would be performed through an internal approach.

A rim incision on the columella would then be made to excise the hanging columella. To correct the supratip fullness, I would remove soft tissue and then possibly score in a cross-hatching fashion the subdermal tissue to allow the skin to drape more easily.

Finally, I would use a cartilage strut between the short mesial crura to help ensure better tip projection."

Dr. Denecke's approach to this same patient was as follows:

"I would first correct the bony structures and then adapt the cartilaginous nose to the new bony shape. Following decollément of the dorsum, the bony hump would be removed and the pyramid narrowed in the routine manner.

The lower lateral cartilages would be approached through the eversion method with resection of the upper portion of the lower lateral cartilages.

The wide columella must be narrowed by removing soft tissue from between the mesial crura. To correct the nasolabial angle it would be necessary to remove a small strip of cartilage from the caudal septum.

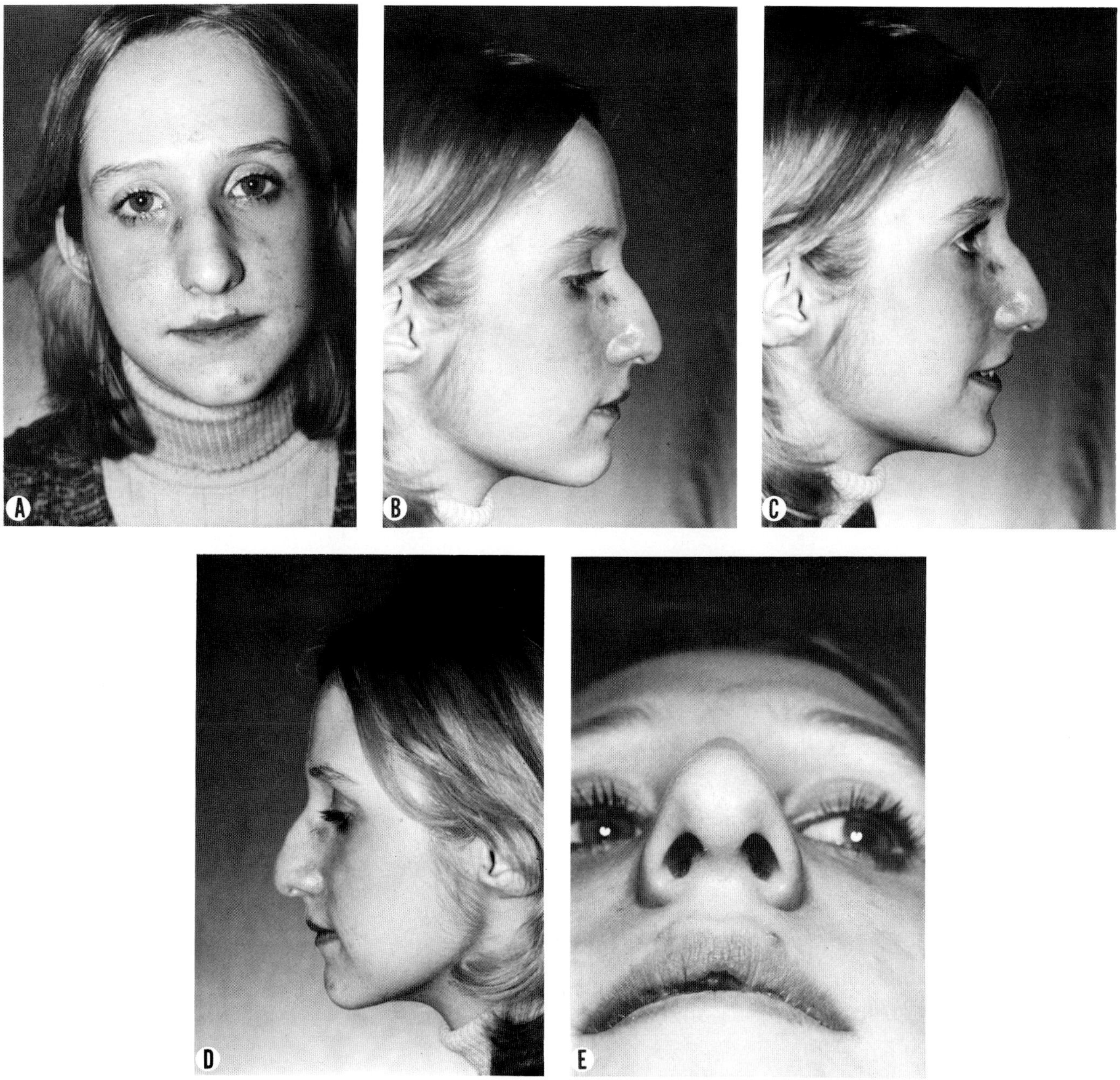

Fig. 1. (A) Frontal. (B) Right lateral. (C) Right lateral smiling. (D) Left lateral. (E) Base.

Correct suturing of the transfixion incision will help hold the nasal tip angle in its new, desired position."

Dr. Anderson added a final note on his reasons for doing the tip first—primarily, to guard against excessive hump removal by initially fixing the two points between the tip of the nose and the nasal frontal angle, and secondarily, because of the desirability of doing the more delicate work earlier in the procedure.

Case II

The discussants of the second case were again Dr. Anderson and Dr. Denecke.

Dr. Anderson began the analysis.

"The frontal view (Fig. 2A) shows the obvious facial asymmetry, with the right side more concave than the left. There is a slanted position of the lips and uneven eyebrows. There is widening of the bony nose in the mid-third with deviation of the lower bony and cartilaginous portion suggesting an old fracture. There is an interesting concavity of the right alar cartilage. The columella is retracted with a long upper lip and suggestion of notching of the right alae. There is also a tendency toward widening of the nasal base.

The right lateral view (Fig. 2B) shows a moderately shallow nasofrontal angle with a bony hump and a retracted columella. The nasolabial angle is approximately 90° and there is good chin projection.

The dorsal length of the nose is a little too long in relationship to the facial plane of the nose. One again notes the concavity of the right ala with notching of the alar margin.

The left lateral view (Fig. 2C) appears similar to the right view.

The basal view (Fig. 2D) shows good triangularity with asymmetry of the nostrils due to dislocation and deviation of the caudal septum. Again there is the problem of short mesial crura.

My approach to this case would again be with high cartilage splitting incisions through which the undermining of the nose would follow. A hemitransfixion incision is used as a preference for approach to correction of caudal septal deflections. After lowering the cartilaginous dorsum the bony hump would be removed intramucosally. In removing the bony hump I would attempt to deepen the nasofrontal angle at this time. I would then do a submucous resection and reconstruction. The medial osteotomies would be carried up only to the tip of the frontal spine. Internal lateral osteotomies would follow.

Straightening of the nasal spine might then be necessary. A cartilage strut would be placed between the medial crura to maintain and possibly increase the tip projection.

I prefer handling the dimpling or concavity of the alar cartilage by making a small rim incision and inserting a piece of crushed cartilage as an onlay graft."

Dr. Denecke's comments on the same case then followed.

"This is a deflected nose in the bony and cartilaginous portion with a subluxation of the septum.

First one should correct the bony pyramid, attempting not to make a straight dorsum because of the prominent chin.

The deviated septum is approached through the transfixion incision. Once mobilized and medially positioned, it is stabilized with sutures and packing. Bringing it forward with the columella will help to alleviate the retracted columella.

The tip is modeled through the eversion technique, possibly resecting more cartilage on the left than the right. One might also cross hatch the subdermal tissue on the left to encourage inward draping to match the concavity on the right."

In response to direct questioning, Dr. Anderson added that in such a short nose, one does not want to cause marked rotation by breaking the spring of the alar cartilage laterally. Rather a slight trimming of the cephalic border of the lower lateral cartilage, along with insertion of a cartilaginous strut to bring the columella down would be preferable treatment in this case.

Dr. Smith suggested that an alternative approach to filling in the alar depression might be the breaking of the cartilaginous spring at the dome to allow the cartilages to flare out.

Dr. Diamond expressed his preference for resecting cartilage from the left ala to match the relative depression on the right rather than using fillers or cartilage reversals.

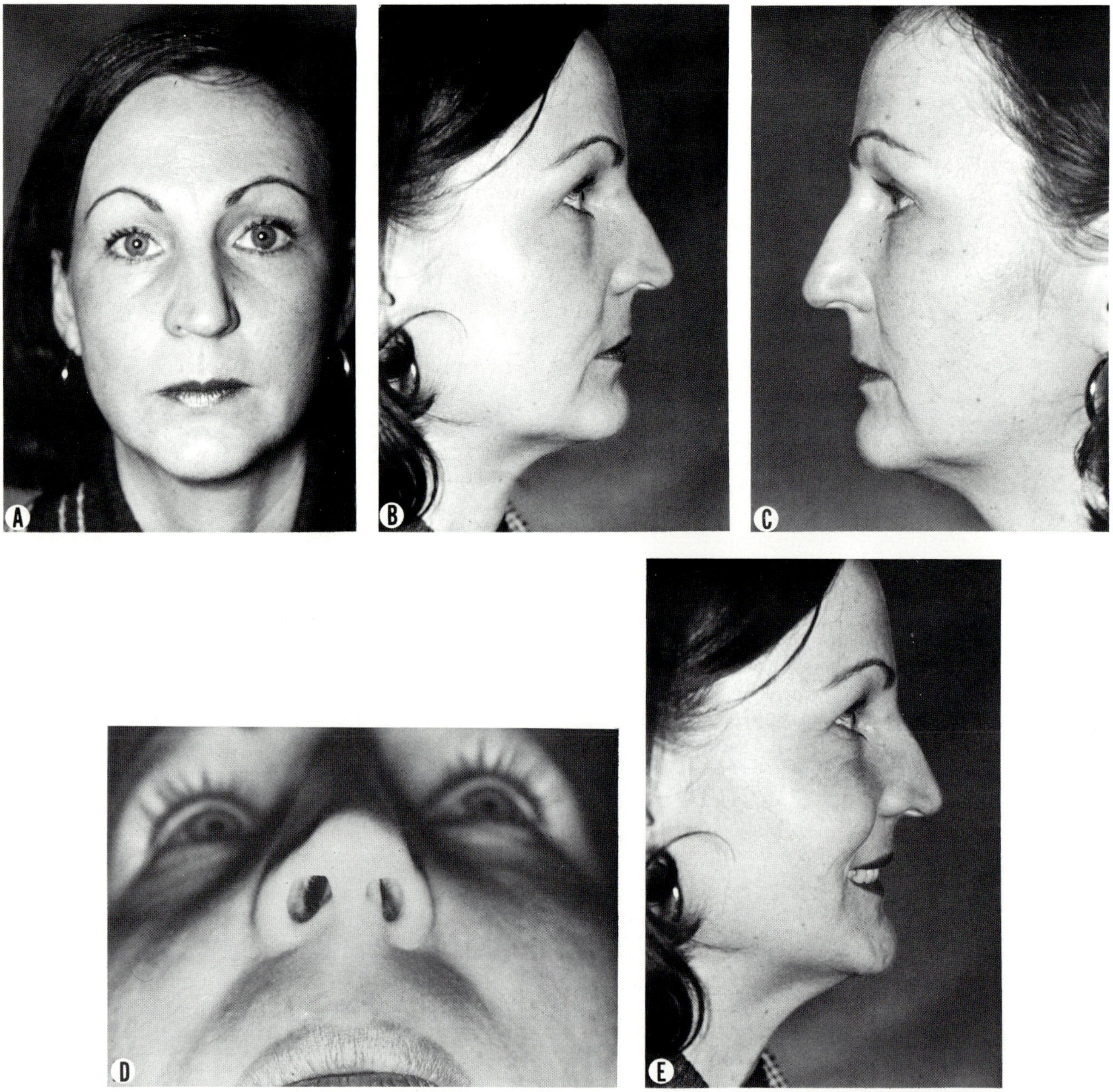

Fig. 2. (A) Frontal. (B) Right lateral. (C) Left lateral. (D) Base. (E) Right lateral smiling.

Case III

The third case was reviewed by Dr. Howard Diamond and Dr. Gene Tardy.

Dr. Diamond's comments follow.

"In general one should strive for simplicity and control in rhinoplasty. An analysis of the nose must be in relationship to the rest of the face. Patients do not like changes in their basic facial characteristics and therefore I seldom do base resections or Weir procedures.

The frontal view (Fig. 3A) in this case shows a slightly wide bony bridge and a mild bulbosity of the tip. The length of the upper lip is acceptable.

The right lateral view (Fig. 3B) emphasizes the prominent bulbousness of the tip with the mild dorsal hump. The columella is slightly hanging but would not be objectionable if the nose was rotated into its proper position.

One can see projection of the nasal spine on the smiling view (Fig. 3C), and there is slight foreshortening of the upper lip. The smiling view also shows increased rounding of the tip.

My approach to this case would be with my routine procedure. After mobilization of the soft tissues I would first model the nasal tip. The intracartilaginous incision must be reversed above and backward from the angle of the dome to maintain tip projection. Cutting near the angle will depress the tip.

Following the tip modeling, one can clearly see the amount of hump to remove. A slight dorsal hump is frequently preferable to an overly smooth, operated appearance."

Dr. Tardy's analysis of the same case was as follows.

"The rounded, amorphous tip suggests soft, underdeveloped alar cartilages that do not provide good tip support. This nose needs minimal change and a very conservative approach. The tip should be rotated slightly without lowering the profile.

The basal view (Fig. 3D) shows fullness at the base of the columella and attractive vertical nostrils.

The surgical approach to this problem would be through intercartilaginous incisions and a partial transfixion incision.

The resection of the alar cartilages would be limited medially and laterally to maintain good tip support and projection. I would do medial and lateral osteotomies, but do not wish to effect any sizable change in the profile."

Dr. Smith expressed the opinion that this third case actually represented a slightly projecting nose which required procedures to reduce the overall projection.

In response to a question regarding projecting noses, Dr. Diamond made the point that a nose is projecting only in relationship to a relatively short upper lip. The upper lip can be lengthened by removal of portions of the nasal spine and rotation of part of the base of the medial crura into the upper lip. Resection of tip cartilages carried well into the angle can further reduce tip projection.

Dr. Anderson raised the question of this patient having a short nose, not requiring any rotation.

Dr. Diamond responded by pointing out the acute relationship between the angle of the nostrils and position of the upper lip. He added that in females, it was at times necessary to seemingly over-rotate to correct the effect of plunging nostrils in a short nose.

Case IV

The final case was again discussed by Dr. Diamond and Dr. Tardy.

Dr. Diamond's analysis of Case IV follows.

"Here we see (Fig. 4A) a fairly attractive woman with a suggestion of slight bulbousness to the tip. The base of the nasal bones appear wider than desirable with a grooving of the nasal bridge and the nasal bones appearing to flare out to meet the maxilla.

On the right lateral view (Fig. 4B) there is a slight dorsal hump with a rounded nasal tip. Consideration must be given to the exact location of the angle of the medial and lateral crura so as not to lose projection in resection of these cartilages. The nostrils are in a greater than 90° relationship with the upper lip. There is a relatively shallow nasal frontal angle, which along with the firm chin must be considered in evaluating the amount of nasal hump to remove.

The base view (Fig. 4C) reveals no specific problems.

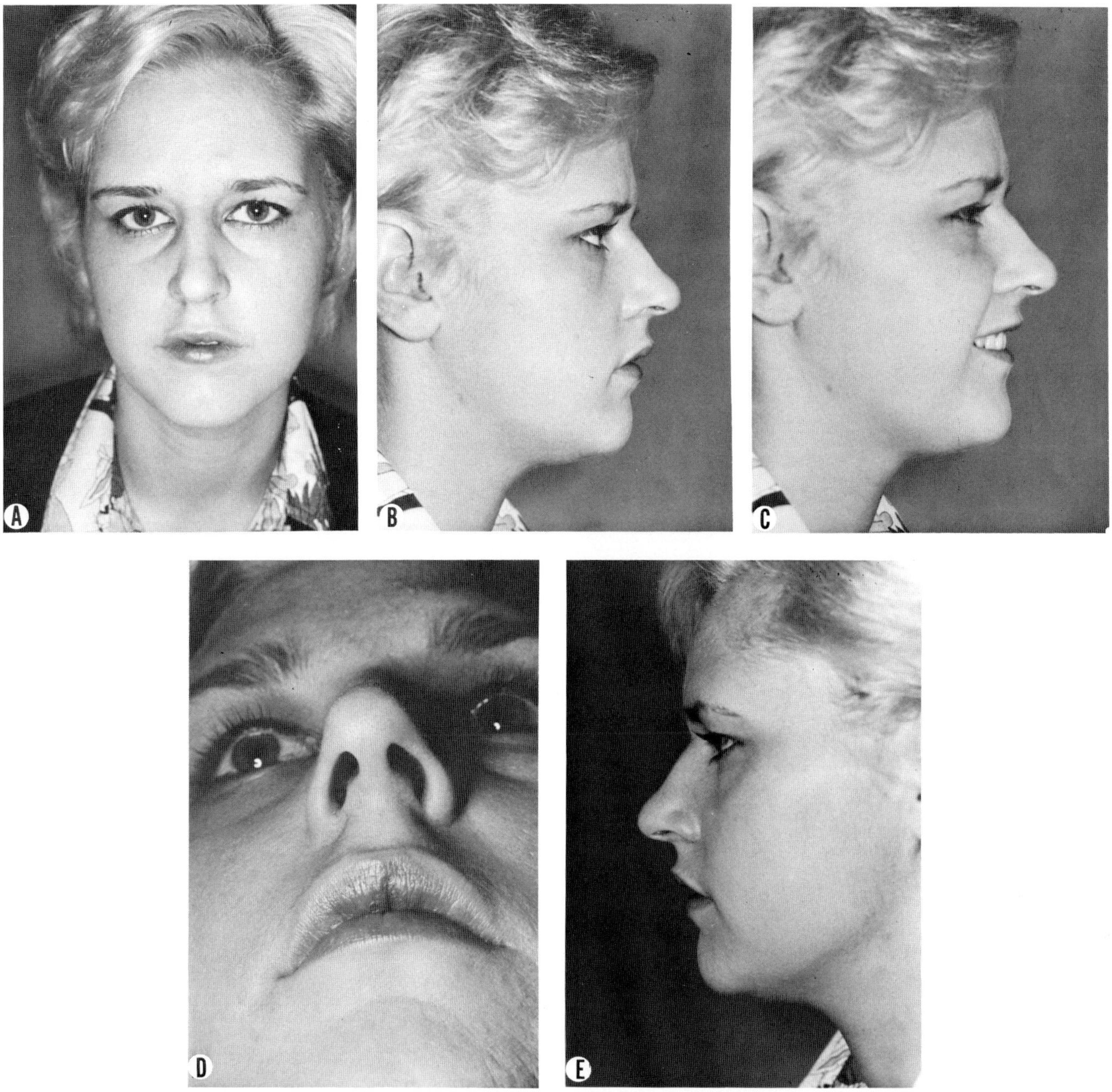

Fig. 3. *(A) Frontal. (B) Right lateral. (C) Right lateral smiling. (D) Base. (E) Left lateral.*

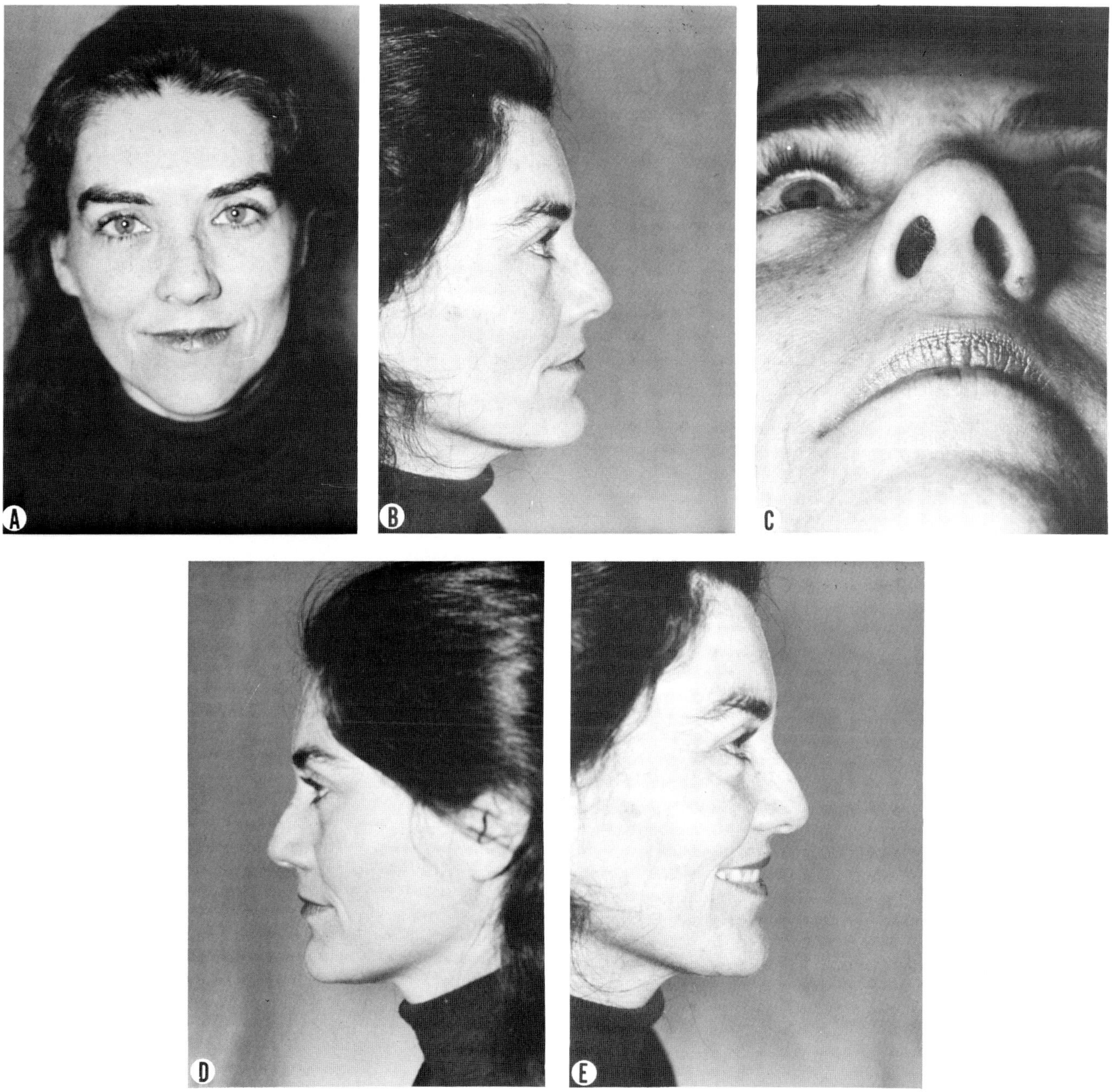

Fig. 4. (A) Frontal. (B) Right lateral. (C) Base. (D) Left lateral. (E) Right lateral smiling.

Again the nose in the lateral repose (Fig. 4D) shows the nostrils angling up in an obtuse relationship with the upper lip. The arch of the nostril on the left is slightly less prominent than the one on the right.

In this case one must be careful about changing the essential look with which the patient presents. Standard mobilization of the nose followed by the same tip approach as in the previous case would be followed. Because of the shallow naso-frontal angle I would remove very little of the nasal hump, with the resection being primarily of the cartilaginous dorsum. I would use a reverse angle resection of the tip cartilages and do nothing to shorten this nose.

Lateral osteotomies should be performed far laterally to prevent "the step-effect" in these wide nasal bones."

Dr. Tardy essentially agreed with Dr. Diamond's analysis restating that this woman had a basically attractive, small nose requiring conservative minimal changes.

The procedure he outlined involved a cartilage-splitting incision for removal of small portions of the cephalic border of the lower lateral cartilage to create little tip rotation.

He reemphasized the desirability of establishing the tip relationship first to prevent overzealous lowering of the dorsum in an essentially small nose. Dr. Tardy further suggested then lowering the cartilage in the supratip area prior to shaving the residual bony hump.

The session ended with the emphasis on conservatism in the general approach to rhinoplasty.

Rhinoplasty Complications (Panel)

Given good surgical technique, most complications in reduction rhinoplasty are basically caused by faulty surgical quantitation. A low cartilaginous hump called "pollybeak" results from: (1) too conservative lowering of the cartilaginous dorsum; (2) excess removal of the bony dorsum; (3) tip drop and inferior tip rotation secondary to resection of the cephalic lateral crus and posterior caudal septum, which are the main tip supports; or (4) soft tissue thickening in the supratip area. The soft tissue thickening is more likely in the presence of thick, oily skin and can sometimes be prevented by trimming the subcutaneous areolar tissues at the time of the original tip surgery or by injecting the supra tip area with Kenalog (triamcinolone acetonide) during the postoperative course. If secondary surgery is necessary, it should be postponed at least one year and should consist of rectifying the specific cause, such as lowering the cartilaginous dorsum and/or augmenting the bony dorsum by inserting cartilaginous grafts into a subcutaneous pocket. If scar tissue is present, it should be resected. If the tip has dropped, it should be freed from scar tissue and advanced relative to the caudal septum. This advancement must be supported. Berman and Smith prefer subcutaneous nylon sutures, attaching the medial crura to the caudal septum. Anderson prefers inserting a strong cartilage strut below and between the base of the medial crura. Webster and Wright have also used this method, but sometimes prefer inserting diced cartilage into this pocket to fill out the labial columellar angle.

Excessive resection of the cephalic lateral crura and the caudal upper lateral cartilages will cause raising of the nostril border. If the caudal septum has also been excessively shortened, the entire nose will be too short. Lengthening the nose can only be accomplished by increasing the length of the nasal skeleton. Meyer accomplishes this by intercartilaginous incisions and a transfixion. He then undermines the dorsal skin and applies traction to lengthen the nose. Since this traction also spreads the incisions, Meyer inserts composite conchal grafts into the cartilaginous incisions and a piece of inferior crus into the transfixion incision. This can also be accomplished by separating the upper lateral cartilages from the septum and also from the dorsal skin. The upper lateral cartilages are then detached from the undersurface of the nasal bone and the entire cartilaginous vault can be pulled downward and fixed in position with mattress sutures. The columella is brought caudally by inserting cartilaginous grafts into the membranous septum between the medial crura and the caudal septum and in front of and below the medial crura.

Sharp and often asymmetrical nasal tips are usually caused by cutting through the lower lateral cartilages near the dome, or by excessive resection of the cephalic portion of the dome area so that in healing, scar tissue will buckle one or both domes of the nasal tip. Anderson handles this deformity by making an alar rim incision, undermining the involved area and morcelizing the buckled dome. This is followed by placing a crushed on-lay cartilage graft over the involved area to strengthen it and prevent recurrent postoperative buckling.

Anderson handles bifid tip and columella by inserting crushed cartilage grafts; Berman prefers suturing the anterior medial crura together with a permanent mattress suture of nylon. The two medial crura are grasped just below their dome with a Brown-Adson forceps and then pulled down into view while a mattress suture of nylon is placed at the very tip of the Brown-Adson forceps. Webs of the nasal valves and stenosis of the nostrils result from excessive resection of vestibular lining. Correction involves intranasal incision, removal of scar tissue and replacement of lining by Z-plasties or composite conchal grafts. Z-plasties can also move tissue located lateral to the alae inside of the nostril border to correct stenosis.

Septum surgery is sometimes complicated by the appearance of a postoperative perforation. Berman feels that this complication can be almost entirely eliminated by conservatism in the original operation. He elevates only one septal flap. The other perichondrial flap is never elevated unless cartilage is to be resected in this area. Most of his septums are straightened by through and through incisions in the cartilage which create many septal blocks attached to the unelevated perichondrium. He then splints the septum in the straight position by sutures which simultaneously reattach the elevated perichondrial flap. Where perforations are already present, Wright closes them by rotation flaps from the inferior meatus and floor of the nose and pedicles the flaps posteriorly. Meyer prefers using a mucosal flap from the mouth, brought through in front of the nasal spine. All flap closures of septal perforations are improved by inserting cartilage or connective tissue between the septal flaps to thicken and strengthen the septum. These grafts have increased the success rate of septal perforation closure from 60 percent to more than 90 percent.

William K. Wright:

Closure of a perforated nasal septum is one of the most technically difficult of the intranasal operations. It is also one of the least appreciated by the patient. Because of this, it is probably not advisable to close a perforated septum unless the patient complains enough of bleeding, crusting, obstruction, whistling, etc., so that the surgeon is fairly sure that the patient will appreciate what has been accomplished. Etiology of these perforations come from:

1. Acute trauma
2. Infection
3. Various granulomas (Wegener's, luetic, etc.)
4. Caustic fumes such as chromic acid
5. Chronic trauma such as frequent cautery of the nose for epistaxis often associated with nose picking, removal of the crust
6. Atrophic rhinitis
7. Iatrogenic from surgery where there are opposing tears of the mucous membrane during a submucous resection.

Incidentally, if the perforation is a result of caustic fumes it is useless to close the perforation unless the patient intends to remove himself from the original cause. Otherwise, the perforation will soon recur.

Surgical techniques for closure of perforated septums consist of distant flaps from the mouth, turbinates, etc., or of local flaps from the adjacent septum, roof, and floor of the nose. All of these techniques were only 50 to 60 percent successful until a few years ago when we added to the flaps the replacement of the middle layer of the septum with connective tissue, using the same principles as were used in closing a perforated ear drum. This concept not only improved my percentage of results to approximately 90 percent, but it thickened and stiffened the septum so that the longterm results were much better. Without the middle layer, the closed septums were thin and had a tendency toward atrophic rhinitis with crusting and some danger of reperforation. Fairbanks has used dessicated epicranium for the middle layer; I prefer mastoid periosteum with the attached superficial areolar tissue. This is a living graft and I put in a piece that is thick enough so that it completely plugs the perforation and expands underneath the mucous membrane on both sides of the septum, creating a septum that is slightly thicker than normal which results in some tendency for stuffiness postoperatively. This decreases the old postoperative tendency to atrophic rhinitis. If stuffiness is a persisting problem, the submucosal connective tissue can later be thinned with an injection of Kenalog. By the use of these large, thick, living connective tissue grafts, and by swinging mucosal flaps down from the roof of the nose and from the floor and inferior meatus, I have been able to confidently expect to close a perforation 2.5 to 3 cm. If I am not able to close the mucous membrane on both sides, I try to avoid having the same area of mucous membrane on both sides of the nose; that is, I might expose the top portion of the graft on the left side and the bottom portion of the graft on the right side. The raw area of the graft will epithelize with mucous membrane over a six to eight week period.

One final way of handling very large perforations is to plug them with silastic buttons that are inserted into the perforation and grooved so that they do not tend to slip out on either side. This method was first described a good many years ago by one of our panelists, Dr. Rudolph Meyer, and I shall leave its discussion to him. Although I have not personally used this method, I have observed with considerable interest four or five doctors that have used it, and they tell me that their patients have tolerated these buttons extremely well, some over a year, and that the patients like the buttons and do not want them removed.

Walter Berman:

Clarifying the complications of rhinoplastic surgery is vital to a more complete understanding of nasal surgery. The mechanics of why various postoperative problems develop, and their subsequent treatment is the crux of nasal plastic surgery.

Nasal nomenclature has long been a process of misunderstanding. To this end Dr. Richard Webster, Dr. Jack Anderson and myself have evolved a simplified terminology.

Wide and/or Irregular Nasal Tip

Little is new in life or the nose. Our discussion is more of an evolvement of prior techniques. We have had good results utilizing a delivery, or crural rim technique. The only incisions are between the upper and lower cartilages and at the inferior aspect of the lateral, dome and medial crural cartilages.

Excessive superior cartilage of the lower lateral cartilages is removed. An intact 5 mm inferior rim of the lower lateral cartilage is left. No incisions are made in the dome area. Any fibrofatty tissues are then removed between the domes, and a thorough morselization of the cartilaginous side performed. This morselization is of the domes and adjacent crural cartilages.

A Brown-Adson forceps is used to hold the two domes in their new position, while a 4–0 clear nylon horizontal matress suture is applied.

The suture is cut on the knot which probably accounts for some retraction and the lack of having to remove any of these dome sutures that have been placed through the vestibular skin. This technique has been used a few hundred times in the past several years.

During the tip delivery method, various other deformities may be treated. Sharp edges at the dome may be trimmed and/or morselized, scar tissue removed and inequalities equalized.

If further reduction of tip projection is desired, a section of the anterior portion of the medial columnellar cartilage is removed. The prior dome and adjacent cartilages would be morselized and a new dome formed. I would strongly suggest not to remove any vestibular skin. This skin does contract and helps to hold the cartilages in better position.

Contraction of the Internal Nasal Valve

This iatrogenic problem is most often associated with mucosal and cartilaginous incisions and removal of tissues at the junction of the septum and upper lateral cartilages.

We have found a simplified technique of utilizing this contracted scar tissue. A laterally based sliding flap rotates one to one and one half centimeter of septal mucosa into the previous contracture site. The denuded area of the septum will re-epithelialize spontaneously. If this is a bilateral condition, the following options are possible.

The first and safest is staging the second side after epithelialization has occurred on the first side. A flap from a noncorresponding portion of the septum is transposed to cover the donor site of the original flap. The later, and least probable, is a replacement graft.

Iatrogenic problems of rhinoplastic surgery will not cease. With meticulous preservation of nasal lining and cartilaginous supports, we hope to see fewer necessities of secondary nasal surgeries.

As some future rhinologist descendant of Isaac Newton may say, "For every incision and removal of support, there is a corresponding contraction and collapse of the nasal framework."

R. Meyer:

Unfortunately there is still no rhinologic surgeon who has not to admit that a certain number of his rhinoplasties become imperfect and unsatisfactory for the patient (or perhaps only for the operator), even when the result on the operating table was entirely blameless.

Since this fascinating but difficult surgery seems to be easy in the hand of the skilled and experienced surgeon, more and more young operators perform rhinoplasties with too much audacity and thus the number of badly operated noses is not yet decreasing.

The larger proportion of perfect results by the experienced operator is attributable to more skill in the operating technique, to the selection of cases and adaption of the particular methods, to the preoperative shape of the nose and to the newly created shape ensuring the maintenance of the achieved result.

In spite of the improvement in technical ability of the operators the rhinoplastic intervention has not become shorter in duration because today we add an important refining work to the basic maneuvers such as marginal and basal resection in selected cases, insertion of struts and battens for perfecting the angles of the tip and columella and careful suturing of all incisions.

The most frequent complications in corrective rhinoplasty are the typical pathognomonic supratip protrusion (*parrot beak*), *irregularities of the bony contour* and *asymmetries of the cartilaginous framework* with eventual *twisting or buckling* of the tip as well as a *loss of tip projection.* These sequelae of an imperfect work are usually easy to correct in a secondary intervention which should not be undertaken before the tenth month after the primary operation.

The parrot beak due to contracture of hyperplastic corrective tissue (Safian)[1] is secondarily corrected by a slightly exaggerated removal of subcutaneous scar tissue in the supratip region approaching from a small intracartilaginous incision (Fig. 1).

Irregular bony contours are corrected by means of a raspatory or a fine chisel while in cases of evident asymmetry the osteotomies have to be repeated (Figs. 2 and 3). In those cases we usually perform a complete secondary rhinoplasty refining at the same time the tip of the nose. An osteotomy line and the lower edge of the nasal bones can be visible, both faults due to the fact that too much subcutaneous tissue has been removed at that level.

To straighten a crooked dorsum of the nose with twisted tip it is particularly important to dissect free the antero-inferior part of the septum not only extramucously but extraperichondrally. Thus the asymmetric insertion of the upper lateral cartilage can be severed and brought into a better position. Fragments of the septum and the lower lateral cartilages can be resected and repositioned into the tip in order to achieve a perfect symmetry of the tip.

Sometimes cases of pinched noses caused by too much resection in the lateral crus of the alar cartilages and of the corresponding vestibular skin

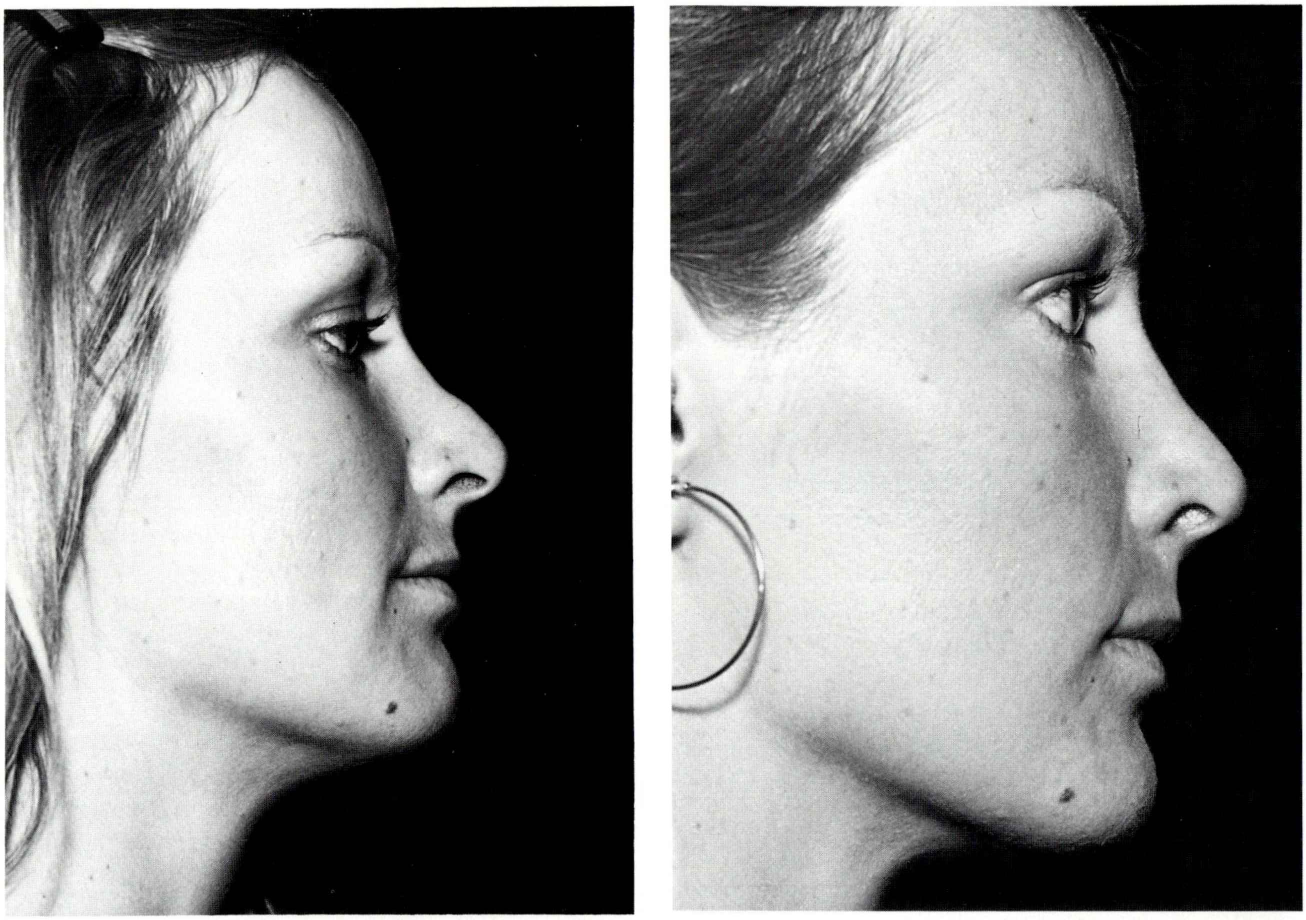

Fig. 1. Supratip protrusion before and after secondary correction.

present difficult secondary corrective problems and may necessitate autogenous cartilage grafting from the ear or from the septum (Figs. 2 and 4).

Less frequent are retracted columella (Fig. 5) or a too short tip of the nose (Fig. 6) as a result of too generous resections at the septal cartilage or at the upper lateral and lower lateral cartilages. Because of the important amount of subcutaneous and submucous scar tissue, of the loss of internal lining of the nostril and of the scar retraction of the membraneous septum, secondary lengthening of the tip of the nose and of the anterior part of the septum can prove to be very difficult. It necessitates the extramucous dissection at the level of the upper lateral cartilages and eventually the lining with composite grafts at the level of the intercartilaginous incision or of the transfixion or both.

The French authors Pollet[2] and Jost[3] have deepened the study of freeing the dorsum of the septum from the mucosal vault at the level of the upper lateral cartilage by cutting the paramedian insertion of the latter at the septum bilaterally. This procedure was advocated by Fomon for special cases of correction of the crooked septal border.

The importance of this vault preservation in the lengthening procedure has been emphasized especially by Pollet.[2] The freed vault can be brought downward together with the upper lateral cartilage and has then to be fixed in the new position by means of several mattress sutures (Figs. 6 and 7).

Correction of secondary cases with loss of tip projection can be achieved by inclusion of cartilage battens or struts into the columella or/and into the membraneous septum.[4–6] At the same time we correct a hidden columella by these supports which are introduced at different levels into different subcutaneous pockets (Fig. 5). For 8 years we have made in nearly every rhinoplasty and particularly in secondary rhinoplasties a very superficial pocket

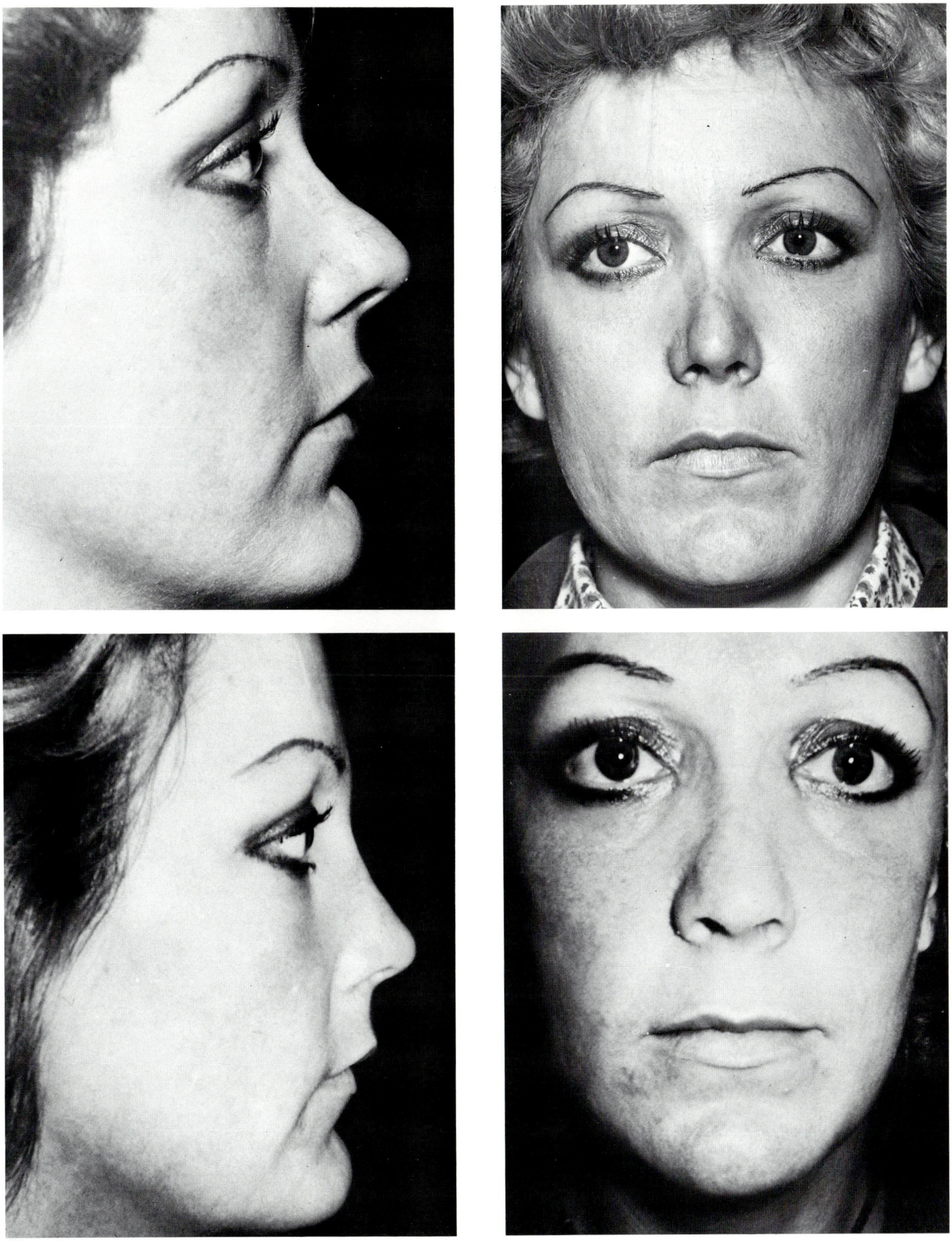

Fig. 2. Irregular bony contour and straight columella before and after secondary correction.

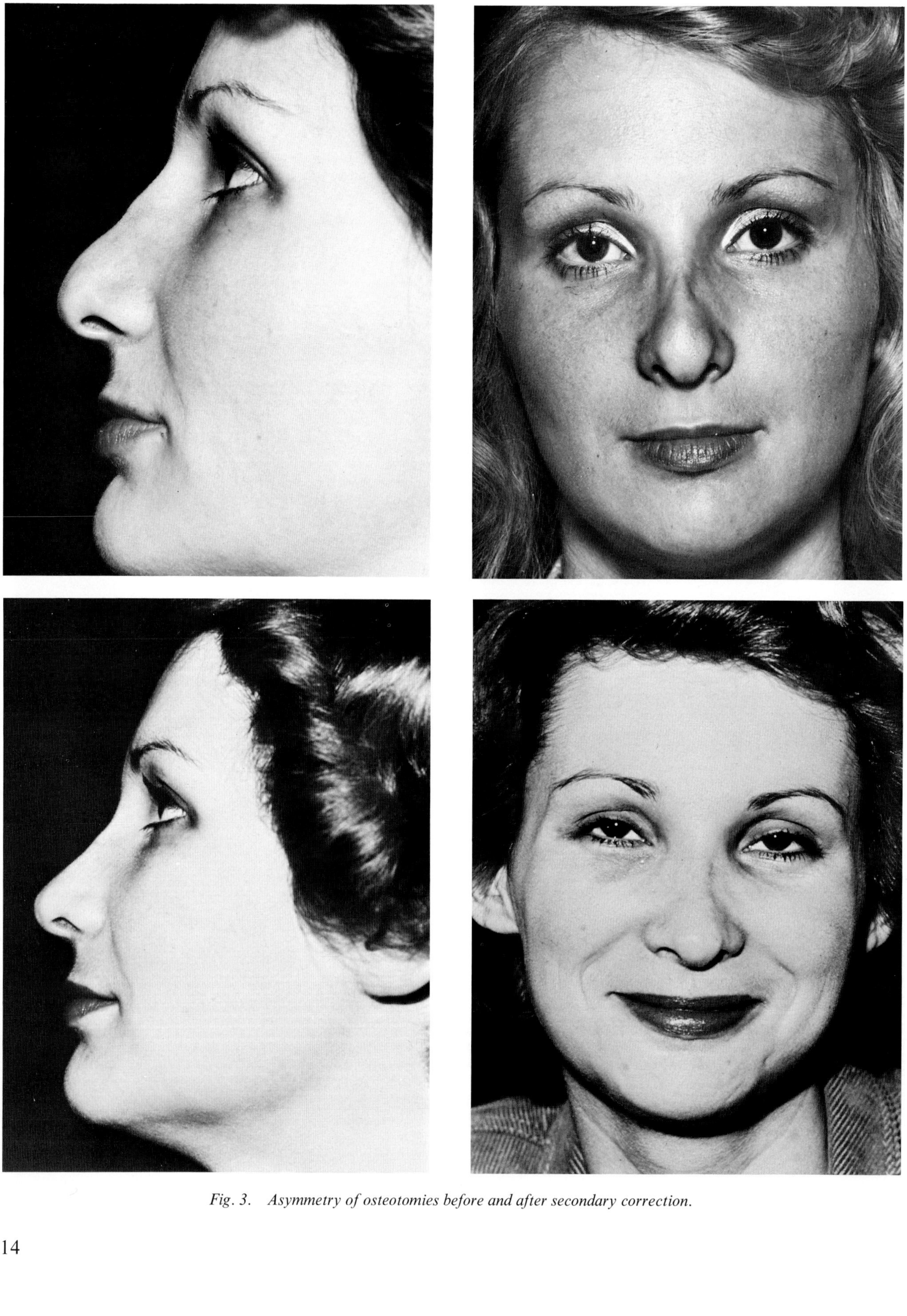

Fig. 3. Asymmetry of osteotomies before and after secondary correction.

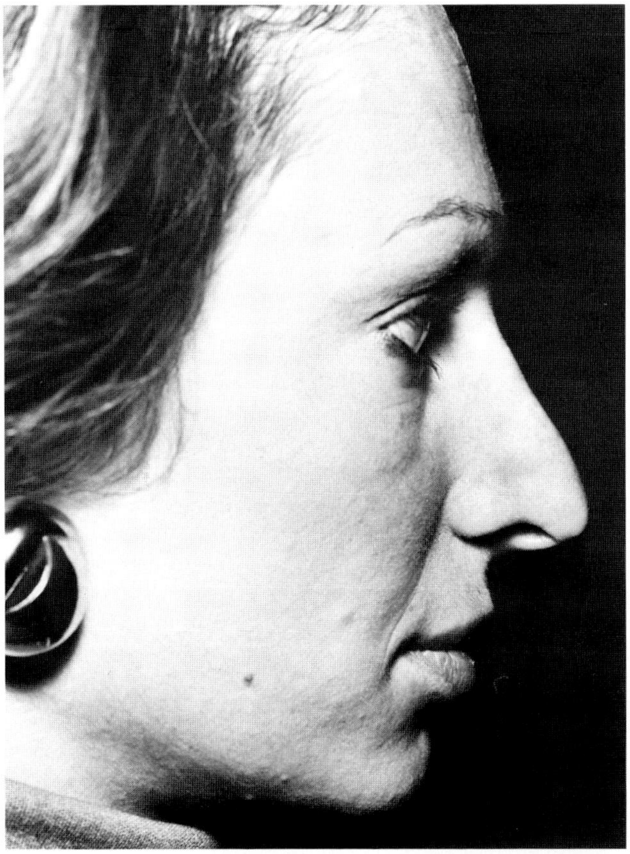

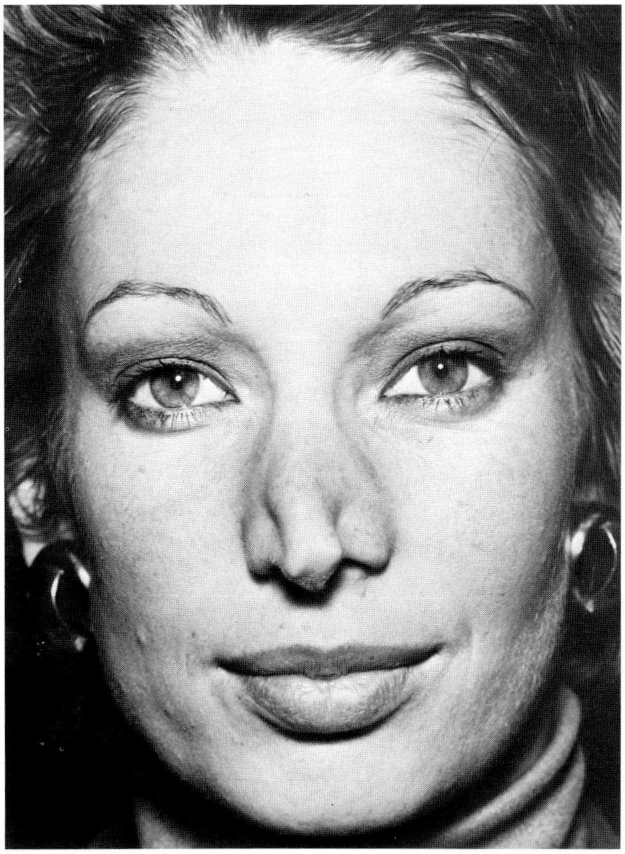

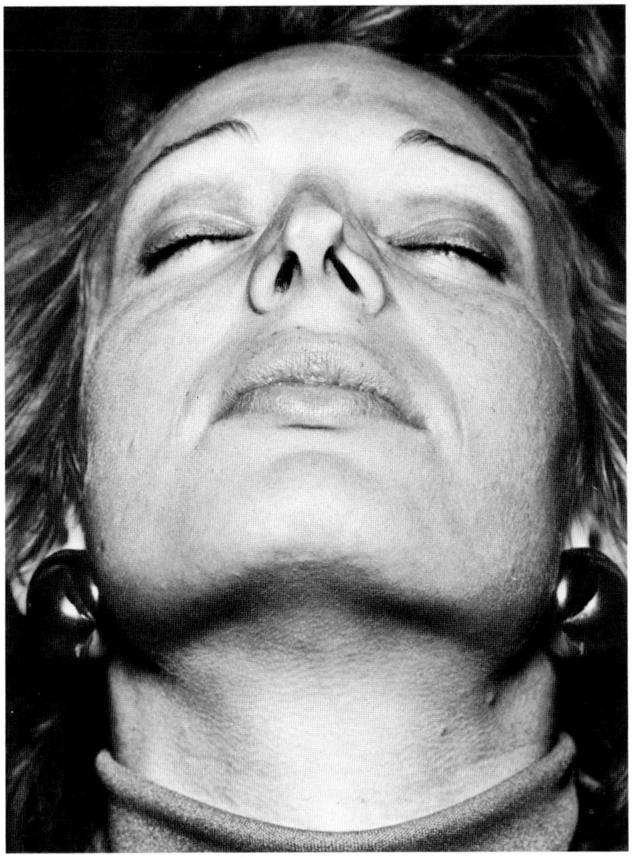

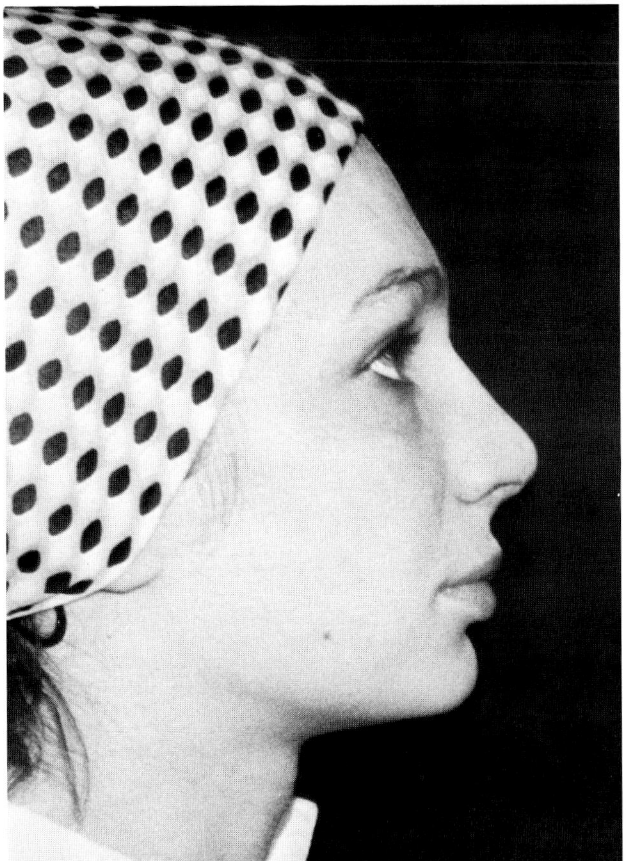

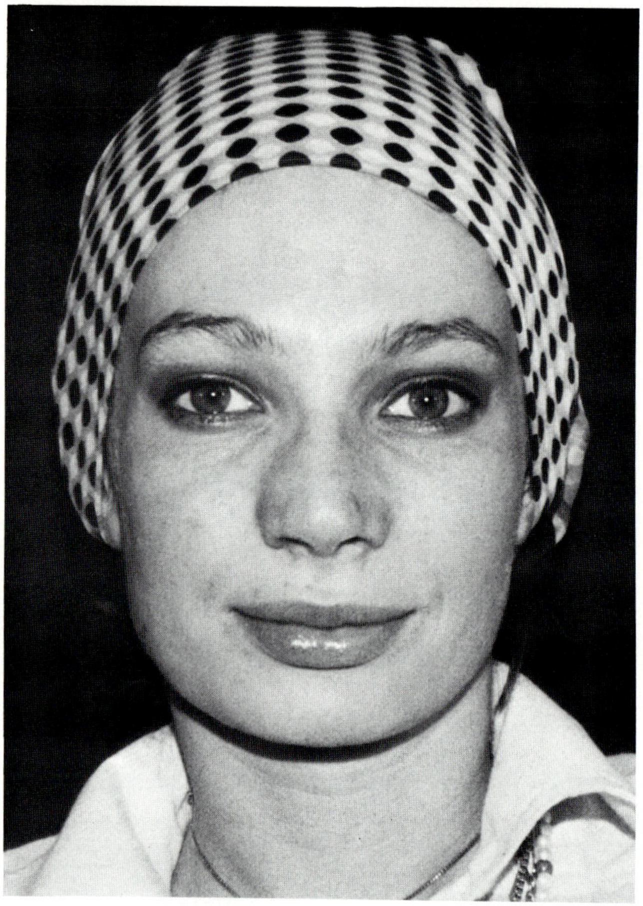

Fig. 4. Pinched nose with twisted tip before and after correction with septum and alar cartilage grafts.

in the two anterior thirds of the columella from a small marginal incision and we fill it with one, two or three battens of cartilage in order to emphasize the protrusion of the tip and the double angle in the tip columella line (Figs. 2, 6, and 8). This problem has been reviewed by Jost[3] and Pollet[2] too. They use complex constructions composed of two or more cartilage grafts fixed with nonabsorbable thread to one or both medial crura and with steel wire to the nasal spine in order to avoid upward displacement. We feel that such constructions can still move secondarily in the big pocket made in the columella and membraneous septum and we prefer to put several struts and battens in different noncommunicating pockets.[7]

Webs of the valve may occur resulting from too long intercartilaginous incisions or from cutting off too much vestibular skin. They have to be eliminated secondarily by resection, Z-plasties, or transposition of small skin flaps. The secondary problem becomes more difficult if the incorrect primary operation has produced a stenosis of the nostril which is usually resulting from too long an intercartilaginous incision or from excision of the vestibular skin at the level of the lower lateral cartilage. To restore the airway in the secondary correction of such cases we have to excise the fibrous subcutaneous and submucous tissue of the vestibule and fix the vestibular skin border and the margin of the mucosa by mattress sutures tied over a splint of plastic sheet.

Several techniques have been described in order to eliminate vestibular stenosis. For 8 years we[8] have been using a sickle-shaped full thickness island flap from the alar groove which is moved to the floor of the newly-built vestibule. This maneuver pulls the ala outward, widens the vestibule, and prevents new stenosis. We combine this technique with a composite graft in order to cover the raw surface of the lateral wall. It is preferable to combine several techniques, adapting them to the different vestibule stenosis.

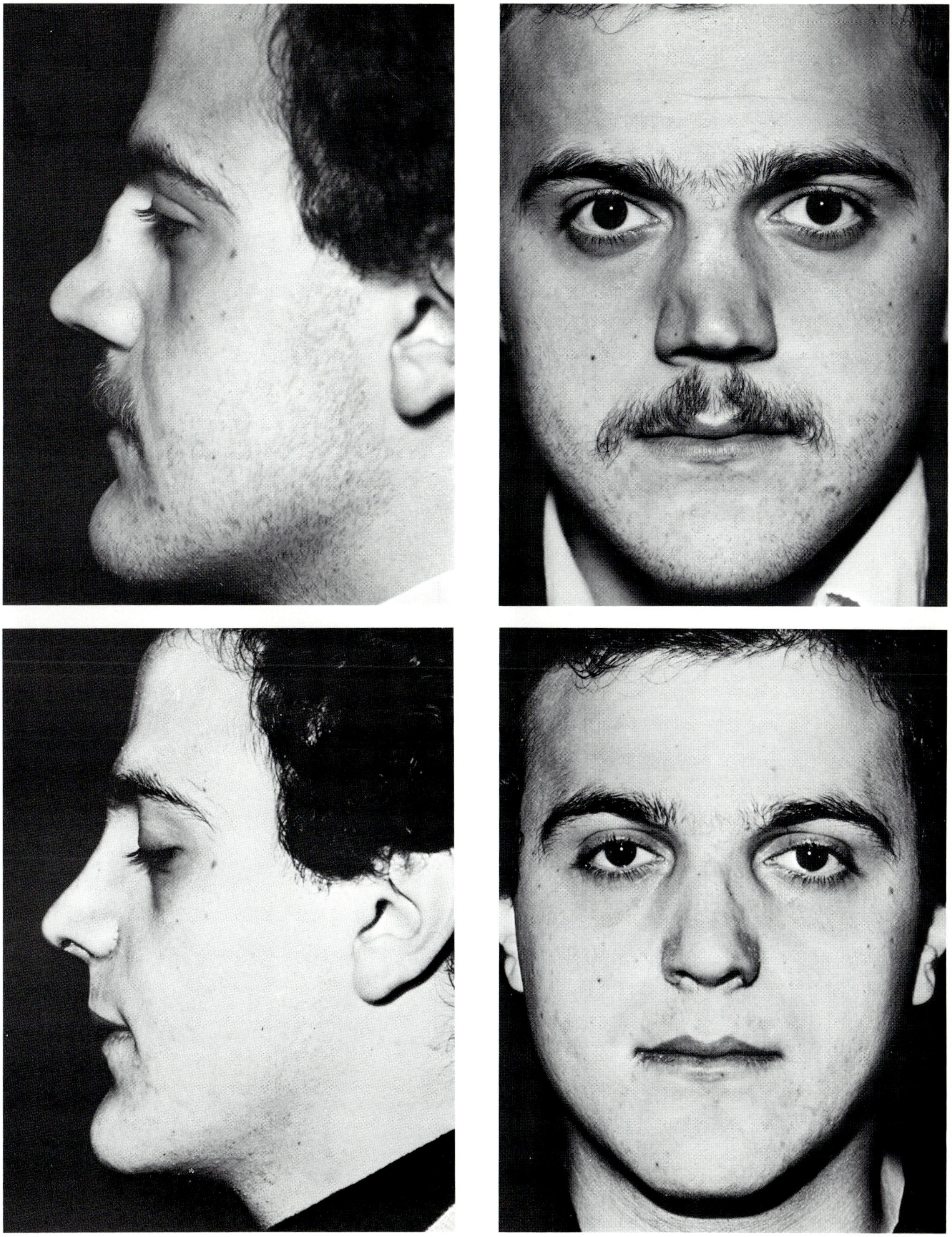

Fig. 5. Retracted columella and depressed tip before and after correction with septum cartilage grafts.

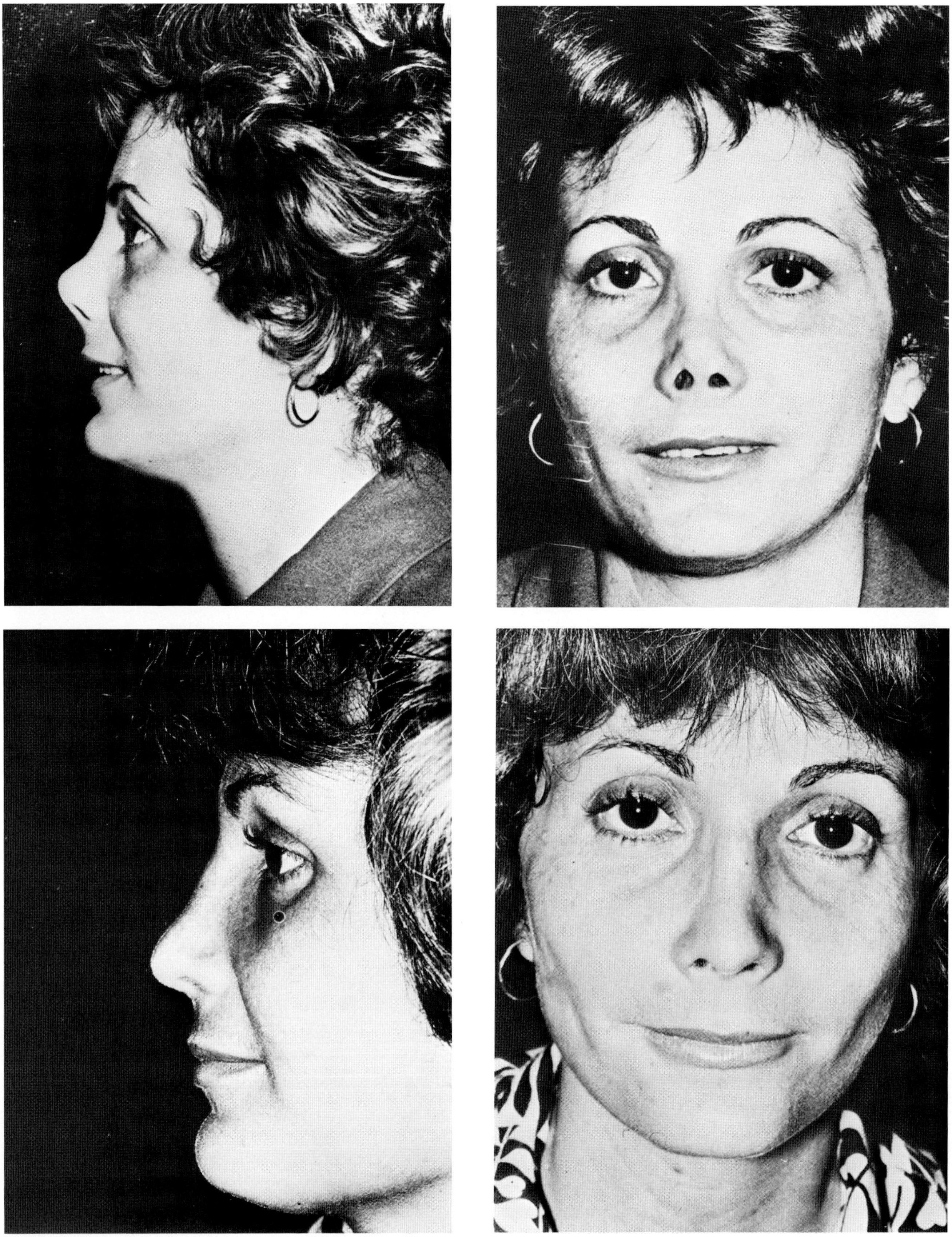

Fig. 6. Too short nose before and after secondary lengthening of the tip by extramucous dissection and sliding technique.

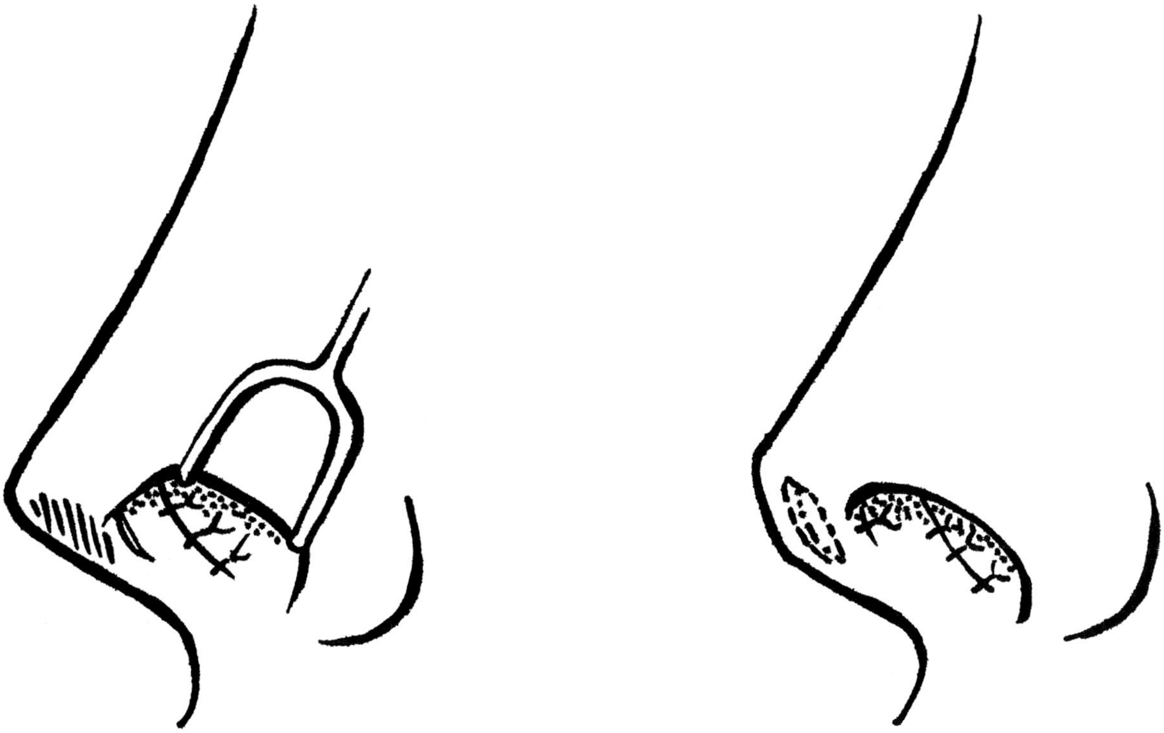

Fig. 7. Correction of a too straight columella line by means of insertion of cartilage struts into the anterior part of the columella.

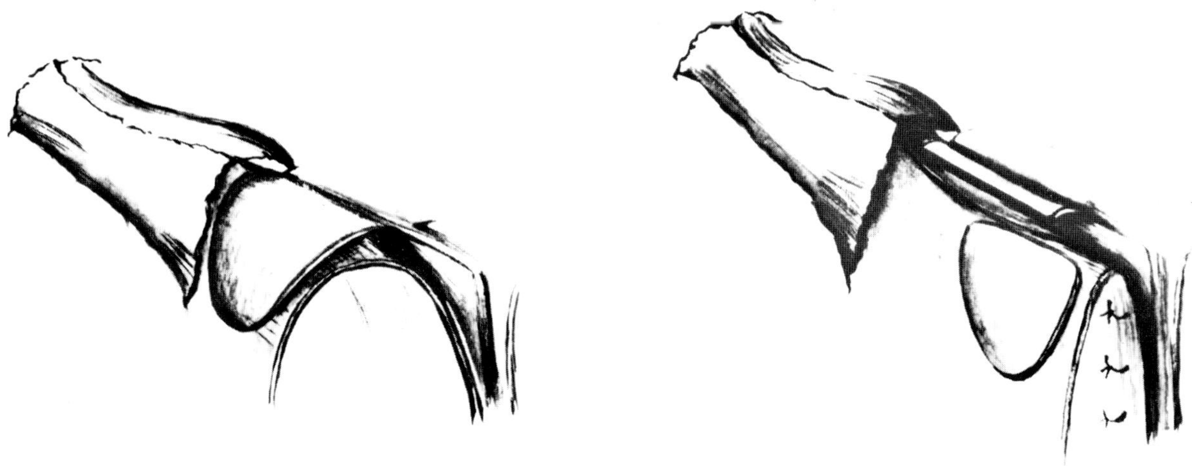

Fig. 8. Extramucous technique for lengthening of the nose at the level of the upper lateral cartilages. (Illustration with kind permission of Springer Verlag Berlin-Heidelberg-New York.)

References

1. Safian J: Fact and fallacy in rhinoplastic surgery. Brit J Plast Surg 11:45, 1958
2. Pollet J: Utilisation des exérèses ostéo-cartilagineuses au cours de la rhinoplastie. Ann Chir Plast 17:90, 1972
3. Jost G: Correction du défaut de projection de la pointe du nez. Ann Chir Plast 17:245, 1972
4. Meyer R: Pitfalls and complications in rhinoplasty. In: Plastic surgery of head and neck, Vol I, p 445. Denecke H-J, Meyer R, Springer Heidelberg, New York, 1966
5. Meyer R: Correction of rhinoplasty complications. Transactions of the 5th International Congress of Plastic and Reconstructive Surgery, p 1153, Butterworths, Australia, 1971
6. Meyer R: What is new in rhinoplasty. Int Microform J, New York, 1974
7. Meyer R, Novoselac N: Neue Aspekte in der korrigierenden Nasenplastik. HNO 22, 154, 1974 (Springer Heidelberg)
8. Meyer R: Nasal-septal perforation and nostril stenosis. In: The unfavorable result in plastic surgery, p 321. M. Goldwyn. Little, Brown & Co, Boston, 1972

Surgery of the Aging Nose

Carl N. Patterson, Durham, N.C.

The purpose of this paper is to present the changes that occur in the nose with aging, to show how these changes in many cases produce obstruction to the nasal airway, and to show how these changes may make the entire face appear older. By recognizing some of the basic weak factors in nasal anatomy and by planning for the future in your surgery, you will be able to present your patient with an improved physiological as well as an improved cosmetic result.

The signs of aging are more manifest in the nose and face (Fig. 1) than in most other parts of the body. These signs begin in the middle teen years, but do not really progress until the "ripe old age" of twenty-five. In the young individual the skin is taut on the face and body but it hangs loosely on older people, with folds, wrinkles, wattles, bags, and droopy noses, all accentuating the appearance of age.

General Factors

In order to appreciate the changes that occur in the nose as a part of the aging process, one must first understand the general changes that occur in the skin, fat, connective tissue, muscle, and bone.

The epidermis is the interface between the internal structures of the body and the outside world. This effective skin barrier protects us from external irritants and controls the amount of water which passes outward from the dermis. With aging, loss of internal moisture causes a loss of flexibility of the skin. There is a regressive change in the cellular structure in addition to an increase of degenerative over the regenerative changes. Cellular division and repair are retarded.

Loss of hydration also occurs in the subcutaneous tissue of the skin. Each layer decreases in thickness. The dermis shows a loss in the number of elastic fibers, and atrophy of the collagen fibers. The subcutaneous tissue shows a gradual absorption of the adipose tissue, with increased fragility and sclerosis of the blood vessels.

There is slow muscle atrophy resulting in a loss in muscle mass and consequently loss of muscle tone. Again there is a decrease in layer thickness along with loss of hydration. There is absorption of the bone mass due to the atrophic changes in this layer.

Considering all these changes, we can see that with aging we have an atrophic skin layer which has become stretched now covering a total surface area that has decreased significantly in size.

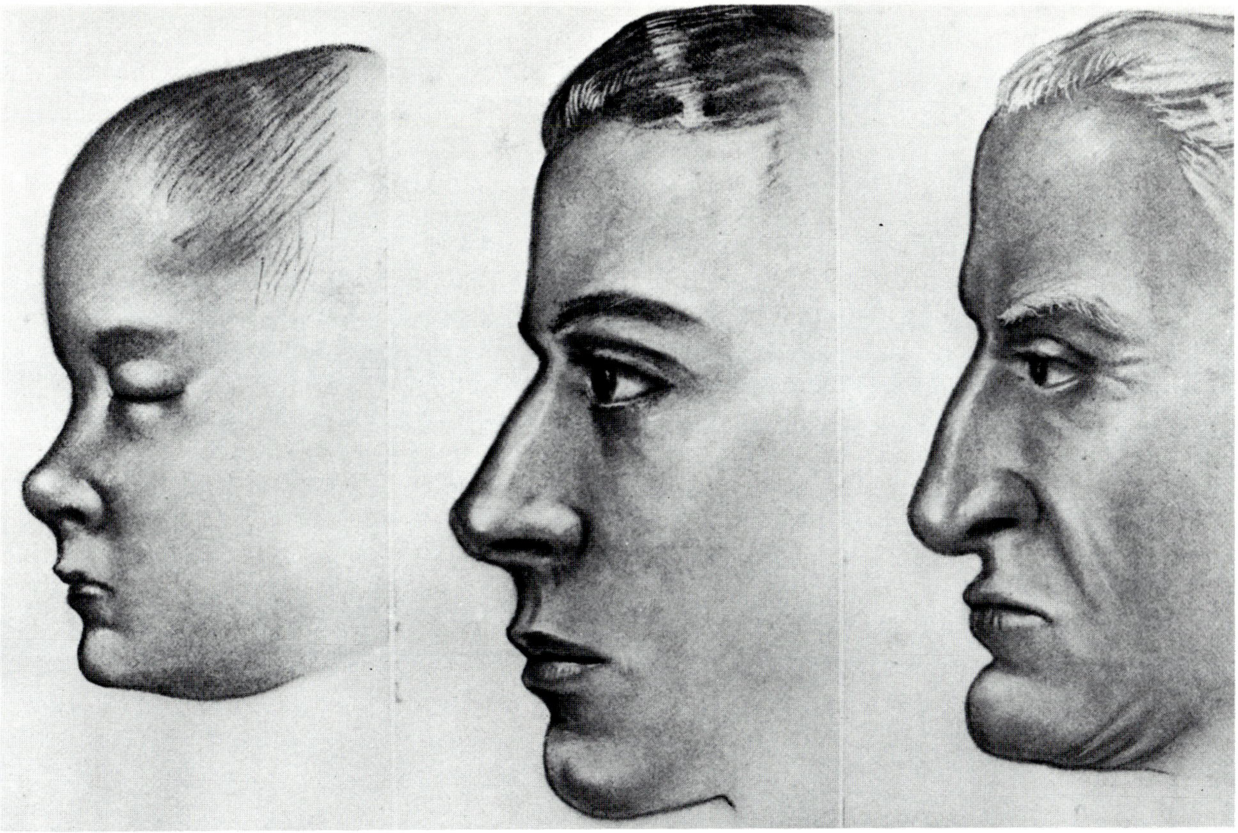

Fig. 1. Note change from a concave to a convex nasal dorsum, downward rotation of the lobule, columellar retraction, and consequent apparent shortening of the upper lip. (Seltzer, A. P. Plastic Surgery of the Nose. J. B. Lippincott, 1949.)

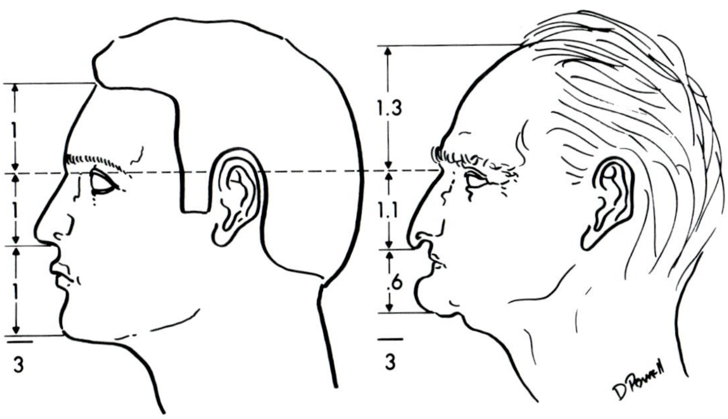

Fig. 2. Note the changes in the proportions of the three vertical dimensions of the face. The nose is actually as well as relatively longer.

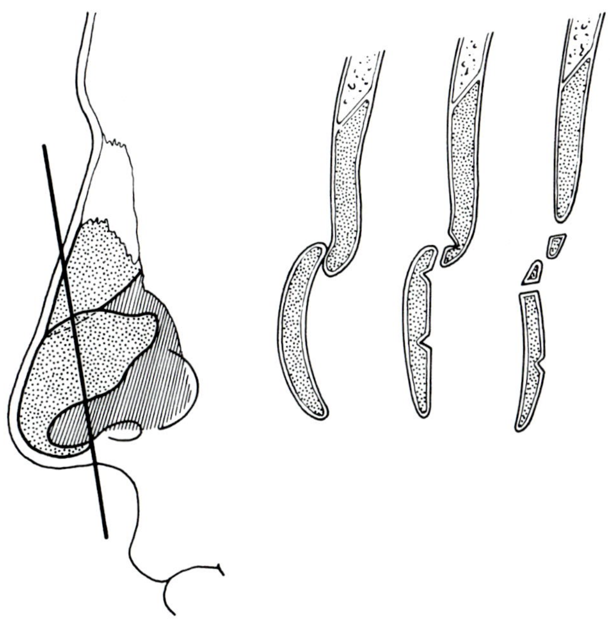

Fig. 3. Note separation and finally fragmentation of this cartilage relationship. (Aging Changes of the Form and Infrastructure of the External Nose. Jelena Krmptic-Nemanic, Ivica, Kostovic, and Pavao Rudan, Zagreb, Yugoslavia; Plastic and Reconstructive Surgery of the Face and Neck, Vol. 1, 1970.)

Local Factors

As aging progresses, the upper third of the face changes (Fig. 2). The hair becomes thinner and the hairline recedes. Vertical frown lines appear.

The vertical dimension of the lower third of the face decreases with aging, as noted by several factors. The muscle mass of the orbicularis oris decreases. The teeth are ground down with usage. Some teeth are lost and subsequent shifting of the remaining teeth results in a changed bite. The occlusal surfaces of the incisor teeth deviate anteriorly. Many times all of the teeth are lost. There is some absorption of the maxilla and mandible.

The middle third of the face appears longer in the vertical dimension because of the actual as well as relative lengthening of the nose in the process of aging.

The fixed or upper two-fifths of the nose is made up of the nasal bones, the nasal processes of the frontal and maxillary bones, the ethmoid plate and vomer. The cartilaginous nose is made up of the upper and lower lateral cartilages, covered with muscle, connective tissue, and skin. The quadrilateral cartilage contributes to the support of this portion of the nose.

As the nose ages, the most significant changes occur in the cartilages. In the young person, the caudal border of the upper lateral is curved outward (Fig. 3) while the cephalic border of the lower lateral is curved inward. These cartilages are held together by firm connective tissue. As the process of aging progresses in the skin, soft tissue,

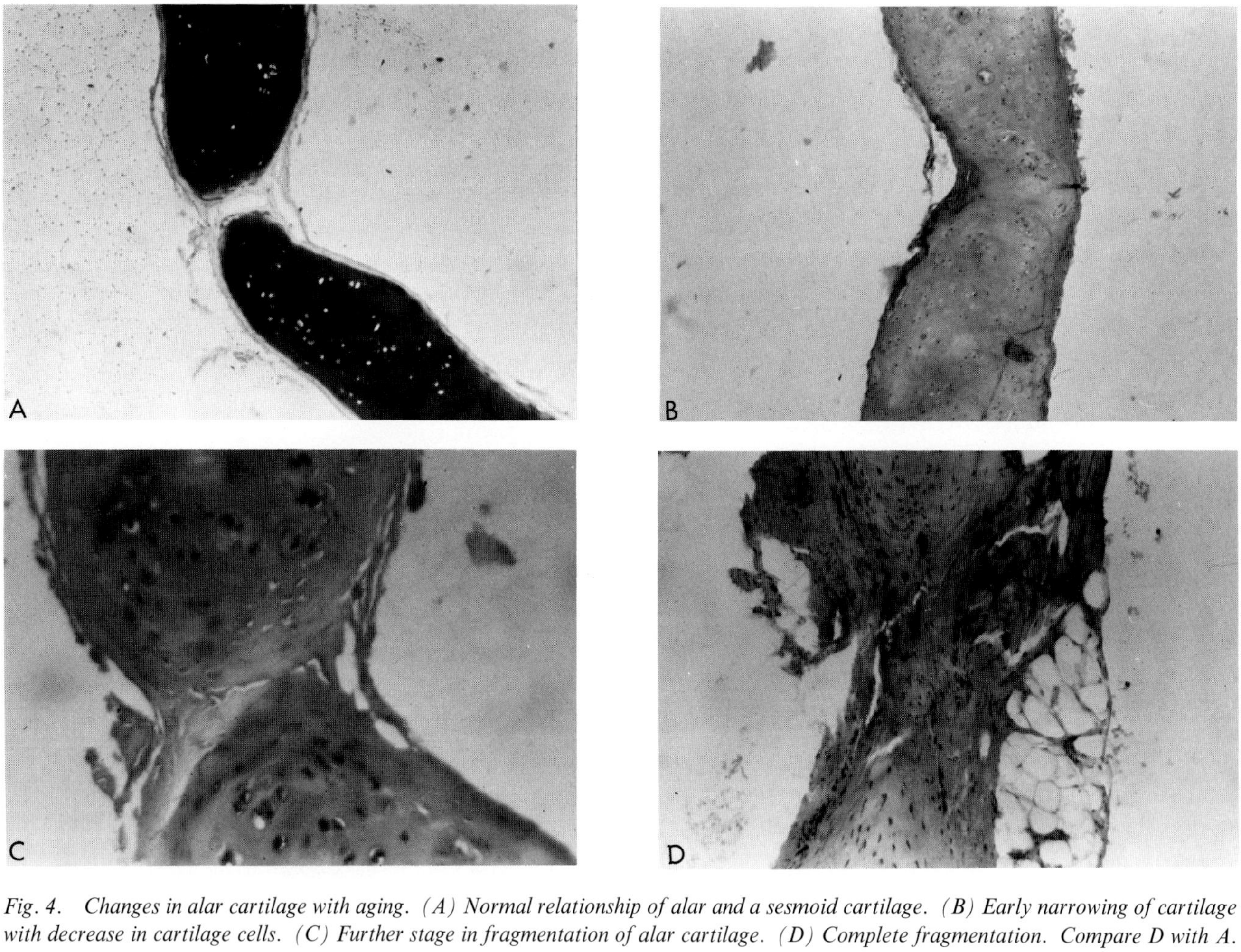

Fig. 4. Changes in alar cartilage with aging. (A) Normal relationship of alar and a sesmoid cartilage. (B) Early narrowing of cartilage with decrease in cartilage cells. (C) Further stage in fragmentation of alar cartilage. (D) Complete fragmentation. Compare D with A.

cartilage, and connective tissue, this most important relationship changes. The cartilages slowly separate, and they actually fragment (Fig. 4A–D). This picture is accentuated by the force of gravity, plus the decrease in the size of the fat pad in front of the anterior nasal spine. All of these factors produce an elongation of this mobile portion of the nose.

Along with this change in anatomical position of the mobile portion of the nose, there occurs a retraction of the columella and a divergence of the feet of the medial crura, which further shortens the columella and allows additional downward rotation of this portion of the nose. Thus, the nose is actually longer, as well as appearing relatively longer due to the shortening of the vertical dimension of the lower third of the face.

A face is said to look youthful (Fig. 5), in balance, and artistically appealing when the three vertical dimensions are equal. Therefore to make the face appear youthful, the problems of the elongated mobile portion of the nose must be corrected.

The downward rotation of the cartilaginous nose (Fig. 6A,B) changes the pathway of the inspiratory air currents producing varying degrees of obstruction to the nasal airway regardless of the position of the nasal septum. Unfortunately most older patients have some septal problems which

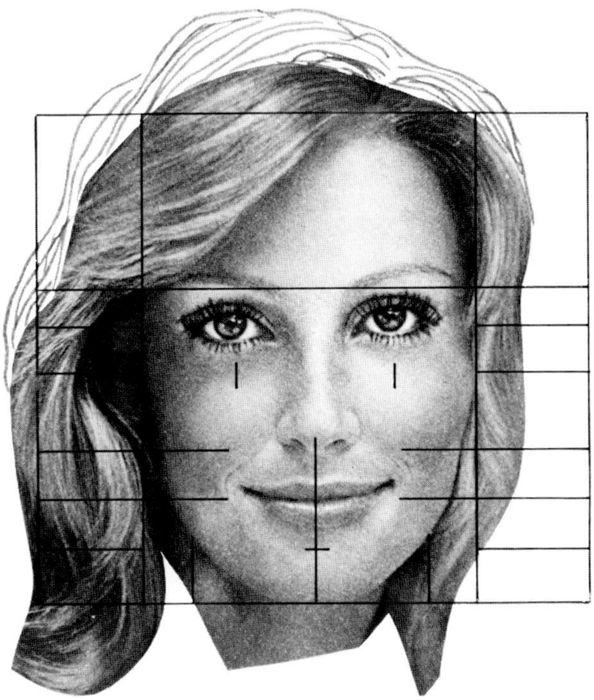

Fig. 5. The face is divided into equal thirds. The face appears balanced.

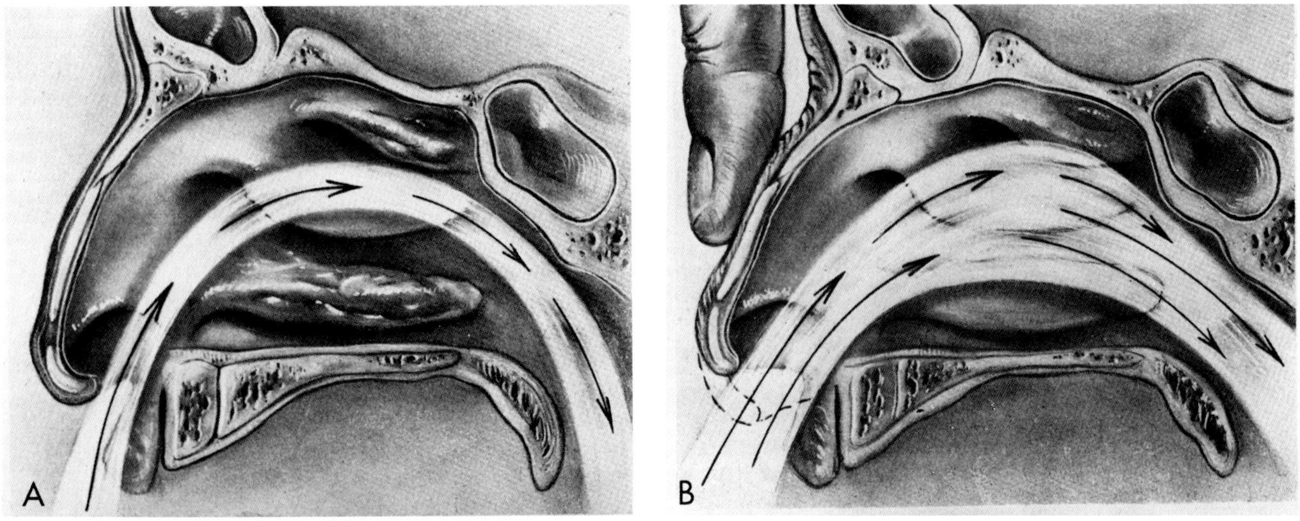

Fig. 6. (A) The downward rotation of the lobule alters the inspiratory air current. (B) Note change in inspiratory air currents by elevation of the mobile nose. (Seltzer, A. P.: Plastic Surgery of the Nose. J. P. Lippincott, 1949)

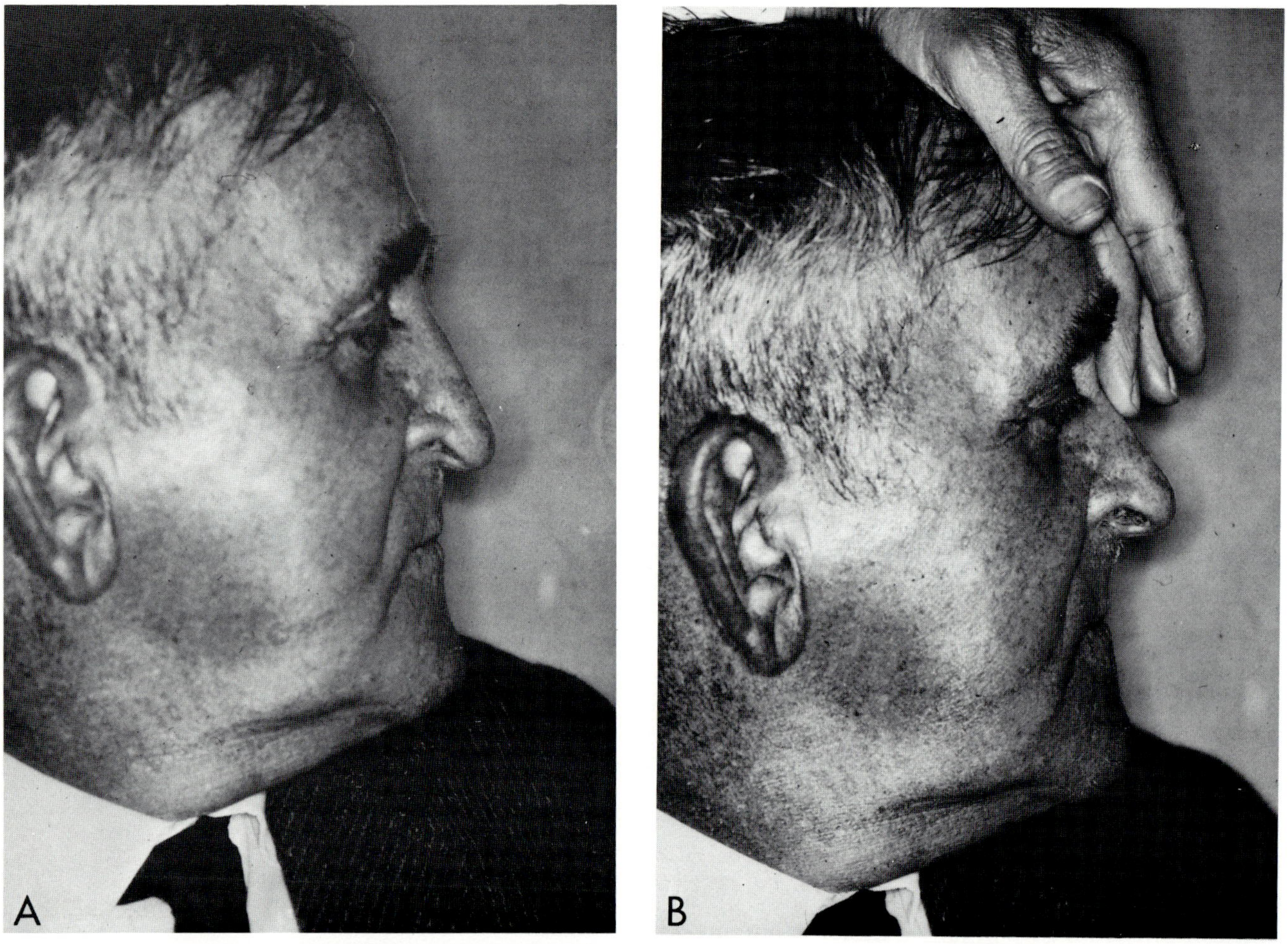

Fig. 7. (A) Note downward rotation of lobule and retraction of the columella which alters the inspiratory air current. (B) Note change in nostril direction and columella retraction by simple elevation of the tip.

have produced only minimal symptoms of nasal obstruction in earlier life, but when the effects of aging are superimposed (Fig. 7A,B) these people really have nasal problems. Since most of these people are 50 plus years of age, many are not desirous of having much or any alteration of their appearance; however, it behooves the surgeon to recognize all of the deformities causing nasal obstruction, point them out to the patient and correct them.

The correction of these deformities is accomplished by increasing the stability while maintaining the flexibility of the nose. This is accomplished by a septoplasty which preserves most of the cartilaginous septum and by a cartilaginous rhinoplasty. It is necessary to shorten the length of the cartilaginous nose. This is accomplished by resection of a 2 to 4 mm portion of the cephalic border of each lateral crus of the lower lateral cartilage and resection of a strip of cartilage from the anterior caudal border of the septum, or by a high transfixion resection (Fig. 8A,B). Interposed soft tissue is removed from the divergent feet of the medial crura so they may be moved toward their normal relationship with the septum. Two or three autogenous pieces of septal cartilage are placed in front of the medial crura and anterior nasal spine. This changed angle of the columella plus upward rotation of the lower lateral cartilage establishes a firm tripod relationship. Thus the nose has had its stability increased and yet has maintained its flexibility.

At times, it is necessary to perform surgery on the external bony pyramid; however, this should be kept at a minimum. The bony hump that was apparent when the cartilaginous nose was rotated

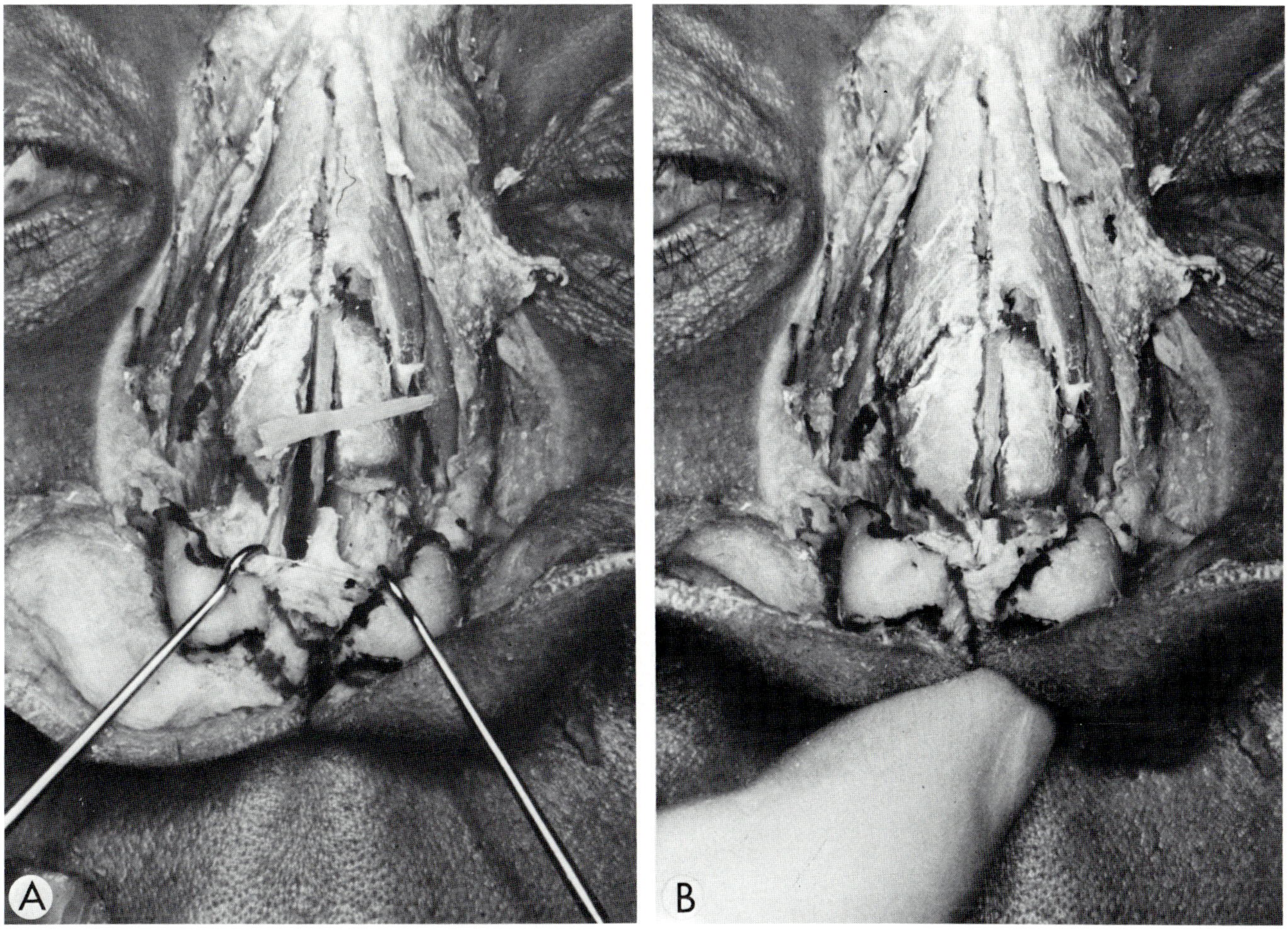

Fig. 8. (A) Anatomical dissection showing high transfixion incision. (B) Anatomical dissection showing elevation of the tip with minimal disturbance of the interdomal connective tissue.

downward is most often corrected to some degree when the shortening and elevation (Fig. 9) is complete. At times a small mastoid rongeur is used to greenstick fracture the nasal bones and to correct some of the wideness or irregularities.

Wide undermining of the skin is necessary in the correction of the aging nose. It is to some degree like a face lift. At times resection of some of the fibrous tissue and muscle from the under surface of the skin helps achieve reduction in the mass of the lobule. Reposition of the skin in the shortened and aged nose is extremely important. The skin should be manipulated toward the nasion and held in this position by careful taping and splinting. By maintaining these structures in position for 10 to 12 days, the skin readapts quite well. I want to emphasize at this point that these procedures are primarily to improve function. The improvement in cosmesis is secondary.

Typical Case Presentations

Case I

This 55-year-old white male (Fig. 10A–D) had experienced nasal obstruction since adolescence but his symptoms had markedly increased in the past 10 years so that comfortable nasal breathing was not possible unless he manually raised the tip of his nose. On occasions he would tape his nose up at night in order to fall asleep. Correction was obtained by a septoplasty and a cartilaginous rhinoplasty. Note the shortening of the nose and the change in the direction of the naris opening.

Case II

This 25-year-old white male (Fig. 11A–C) had noticed increasing nasal obstruction for the past

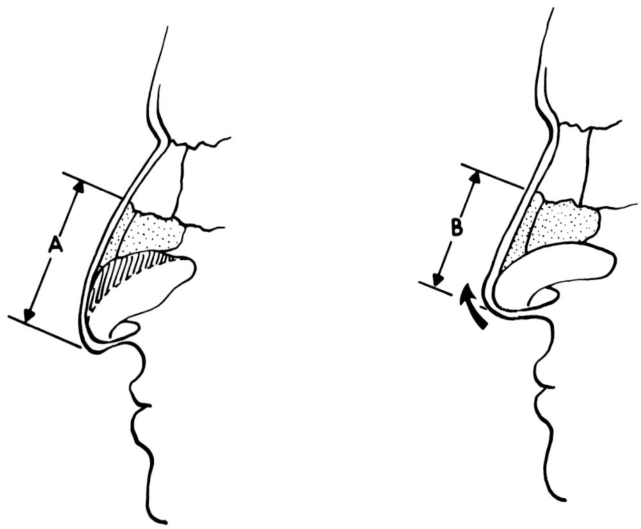

Fig. 9. Shortening of the nose often obliterates the hump and makes the upper lip appear longer.

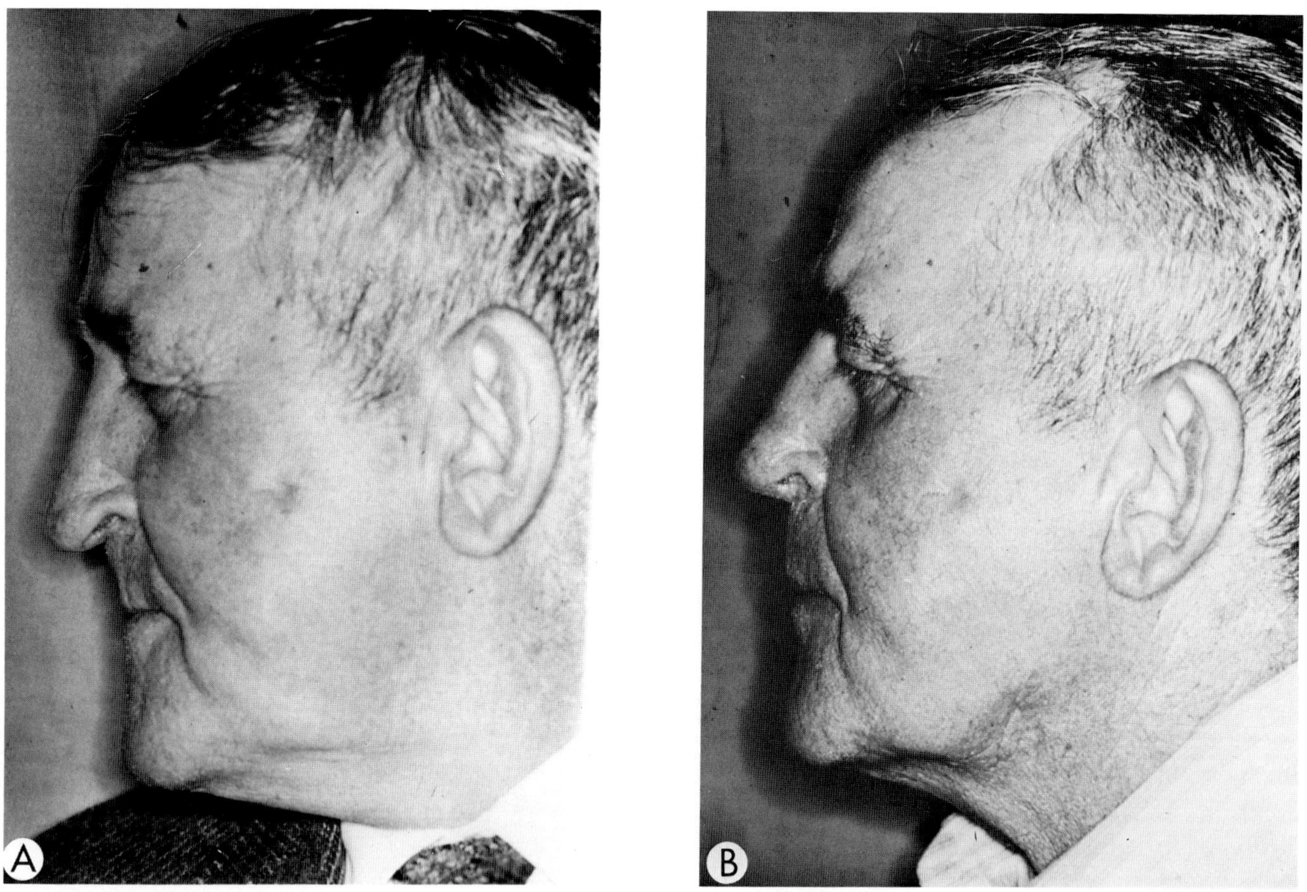

Fig. 10. (A) Case I. Preoperative view shows angle between upper lip and columella to be less than 40 degrees. (B) Postoperative view shows columellar lip angle increased to about 90 degrees. The length of the nose is decreased.

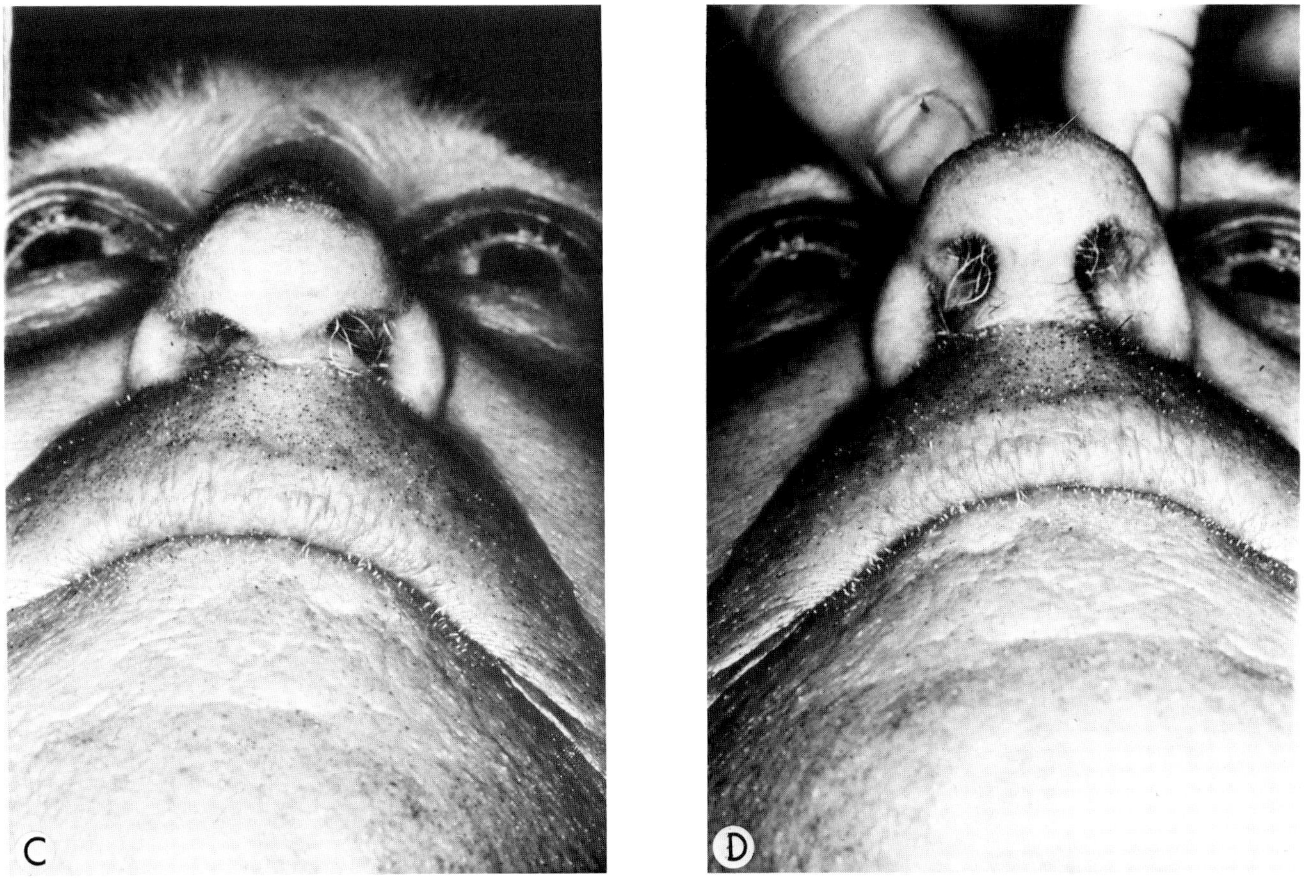

Fig. 10. continued (C) Base view shows marked downward rotation of the lobule. Note naris slits. (D) Note change in direction of naris slits by elevation of lobule.

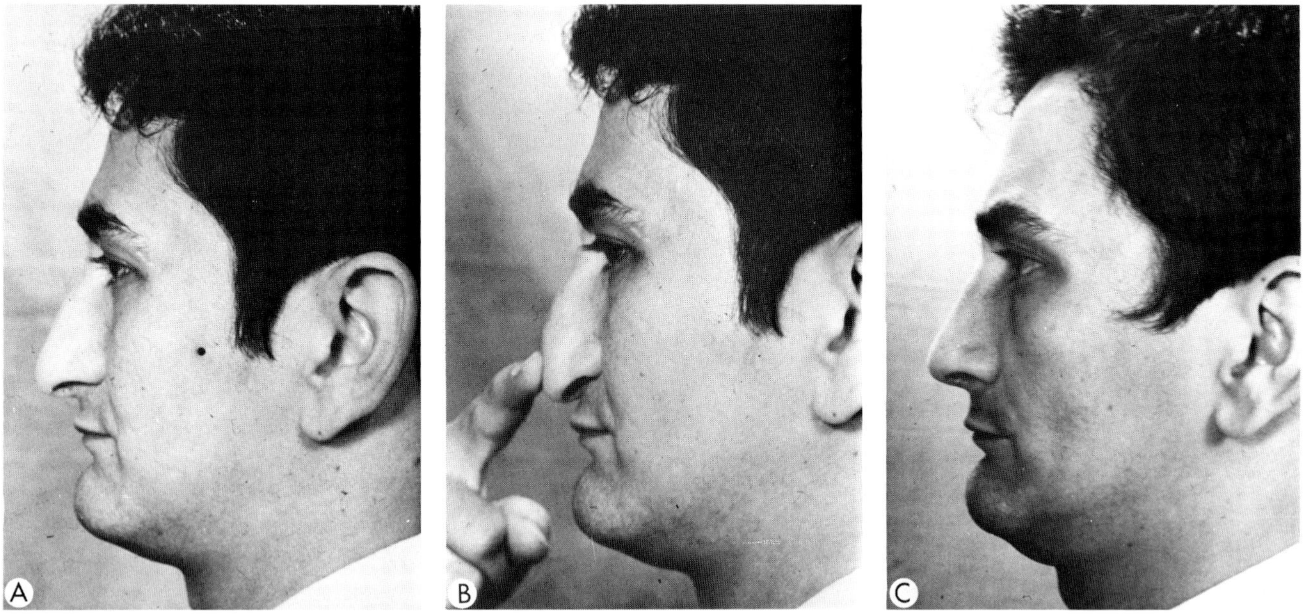

Fig. 11. (A) Preoperative view shows large lobule with a retracted columella. (B) With aging one would expect additional downward rotation. (C) Postoperative view showing a nose with increased stability.

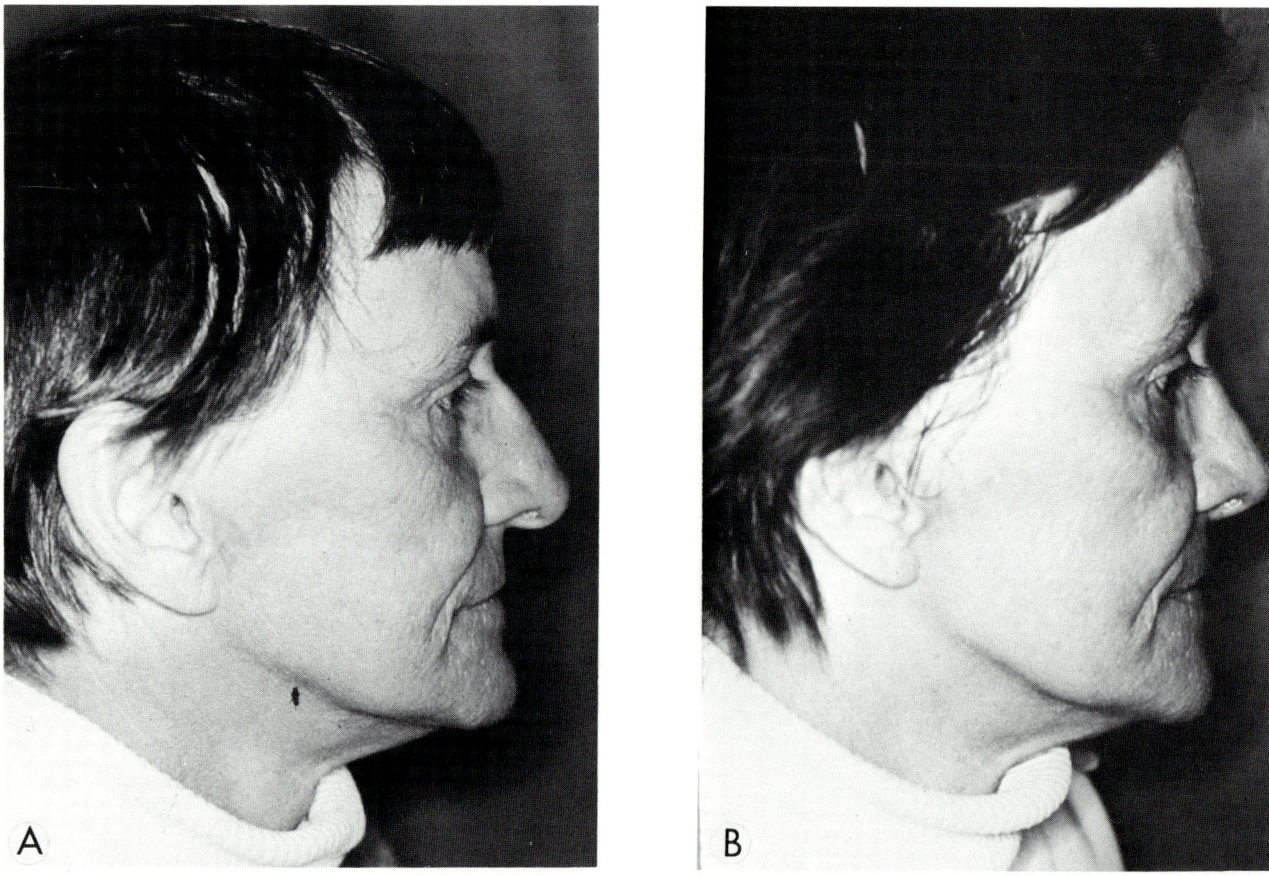

Fig. 12. (A) Preoperative view shows downward rotation of the lobule with columellar retraction. (B) Postoperative view shows youthfulness of the face by nasal shortening.

five years. He had a moderate septal deformity plus a large lobule which was already rotated inferiorly. A retracted columella further produced a weak cartilaginous nose which had already increased and would further increase with aging. The patient did not want any change in his external nose and temporarily deferred surgery until he clearly understood that his nasal physiology could not be adequately corrected without correction of his external cartilaginous deformities.

Case III

This is a 50-year-old white female (Fig. 12A–D) who had septal surgery elsewhere without relief of her nasal obstruction several years ago. She has continued to complain of difficulty in breathing. She also had cosmetic upper and lower lid blepharoplasties and a rhytidectomy elsewhere. With a physiologic septorhinoplasty she has relief of her nasal airway obstruction. Note also a younger appearance to the face achieved by the nasal reconstruction. This points to the need in some patients for nasal reconstruction as an important (and in this case) the most important part of facial rejuvenation.

Summary

The effects of aging are particularly manifested in the face. The vertical dimension of the lower third of the face decreases while this same dimension increases in the nose. The chin moves up, the nose droops down. In order to restore nasal physiology in these persons who present with this type of nose, a correction of the cartilaginous external nose is necessary.

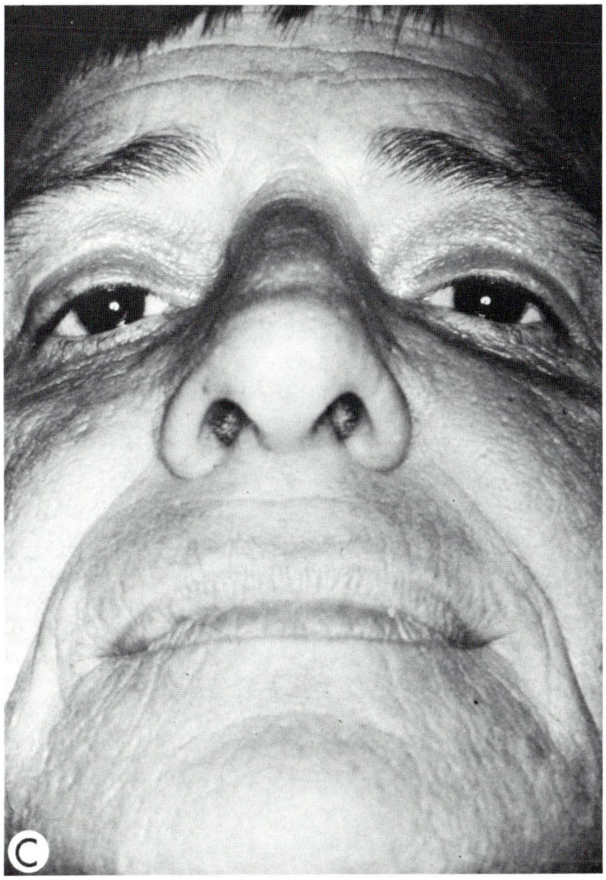

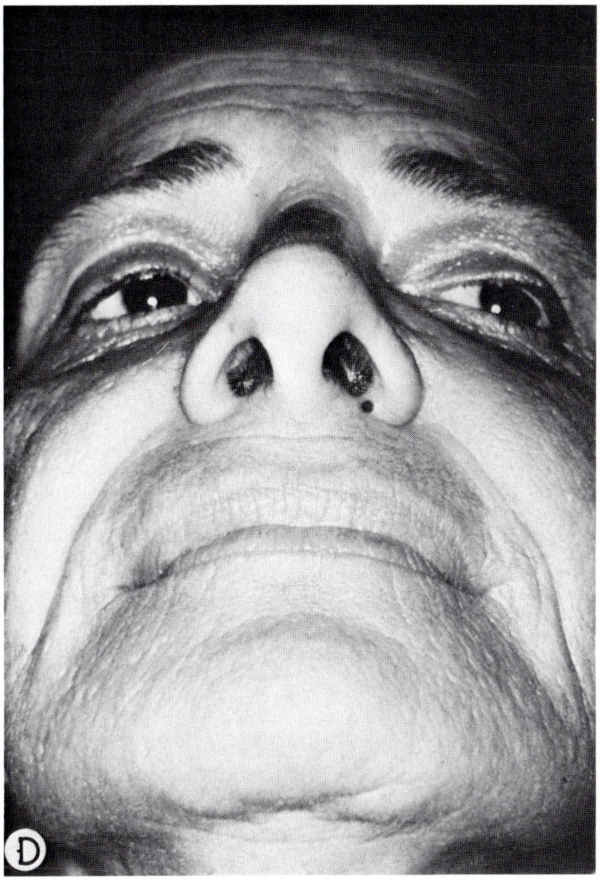

Fig. 12 continued (C) Basal view preoperative shows the effect on nasal airway by direction of naris opening. (D) Improved airway by changing the direction of the naris openings.

120 Cases of Revision Rhinoplasty

Fred J. Stucker, Philadelphia, Pa.

Introduction

Revision rhinoplasty is an enigma which tests the ingenuity and surgical dexterity of the best of plastic surgeons. Actual statistics on the percentage of revision rhinoplasties to initial procedures are difficult to find. The range has been reported to be less than five percent to in excess of twenty percent, and undoubtedly reflects the skill and experience of the surgeon.[1] More significantly, patient selection greatly influences the number of secondary rhinoplasties because a plastic surgeon deliberately avoiding the difficult rhinoplasty will have an artificially low incidence of revisions.

Safian outlined three rules to prevent postoperative complications in esthetic rhinoplasty.[2] His first rule warns against changing the normal basic anatomy or anatomical relationships of the eight component parts of the nose. While it is possible to reduce the size or modify the shape, he cautions that total removal of any of the eight components should never be done. Rule two advises one never to allow skin and lining membrane to meet or be left in contact without intervening tissue. The third rule states that nasal cartilage should never be destroyed. He denounced the morselizer as a means of destroying cartilage. Safian states that skin thickness is rarely responsible for failure in tip correction. He then mentions the uncontrollable factors involved in rhinoplastic surgery. These include excessive scar tissue contraction, hyperplasia of connective tissue and resorption of cut edges of nasal bones.

It is this author's opinion that skin thickness should be added to the list of uncontrollable factors. Thick skin has less elasticity and more connective tissue. It demands more extensive undermining for redraping. These factors contribute to dead spaces which fill with serum and blood. This may develop into fibrous tissue and scarring. Given the optimum rhinoplasty in which the evaluation and technical execution were flawless, a secondary procedure may at times be necessary on the basis of the uncontrollable factors alone.

Material, Methods, and Results

Preoperative photographs and intraoperative findings were recorded in 120 consecutive revision rhinoplasties. This analysis revealed 236 defects of a cosmetic nature. Airway problems were not included except where visible, i.e., alar collapse, pinched valve, and dislocated caudal septum. These 236 defects were arbitrarily placed in three anatomic areas: (1) upper one-third or bony dorsum, (2) middle third or cartilagenous vault, and (3) lower or caudal third. The latter included the tip, columella, and ala. There was a great deal of overlapping and at times some deformities defied classification.

Defects of the Upper Third

There were 66 abnormalities of the cephalic one-third in this series of 236 defects. These deformities included irregularities, asymmetry, open vault, wide dorsum, excessive and inadequate hump removal, abnormal nasofrontal angle and step deformities resulting from lateral osteotomies (Table 1). Defects of the bony dorsum presented the least difficult problem in diagnosis and correction at the secondary procedure. An exception to this is the management of nasofrontal angle problems which are among the most challenging. Of the three areas the least number of problems were encountered in this region.

Open vaults and broad bony dorsum were determined to result from one of two errors in the initial surgery. One was failure to achieve a complete fracture of the lateral bony process. Another was an unsuspected deflected perpendicular plate after the hump removal had been carried out. Postoperatively this structure tends to push laterally the nasal bone on the deflected side. Recognition and proper management is fundamental to obviate these conditions.

Managing the shallow nasofrontal angle is fraught with problems. It is not advisable to avulse the procerus muscle as this leads to an unsightly intracanthal swelling which may persist indefinitely. Removal of bone to deepen the angle can be carried out with chisels and bone-biter forceps. Occasionally, it may be necessary to obtain a more superior angle with the chisel. In this situation entry through a stab incision through the eyebrow is advised.

Defects of the Middle Third

Mid-third deformities were significantly more common. Supra tip prominence was present in 33 patients. This problem was generally due to a combination of soft tissue hypertrophy and inadequate removal of septal cartilage. Overriding of inadequately trimmed upper lateral cartilages was seen in five patients causing a polly beck. Excessive removal of the lower lateral cartilages in the region of the dome and hyperplasia of the mucosa have been mentioned as factors contributing to supratip prominence,[3] but were not seen in this series (Table 2).

A saddle deformity was noted in 20 patients and generally represented extensive removal of septal cartilage. Too generous a removal of the bony hump can also produce this complication. Saddle defects often manifest themselves as a rather late complication. Several cases were corrected by

Table 1. Defects of the Upper Third

Deformity	Numbers
Nasofrontal angle	4
Bony Saddle	6
Open or broad bony vault	16
Persistent Hump	11
Others (high osteotomies, spicules, unilateral collapse, deflection)	9
	46

Table 2. Defects of the Middle Third

Deformity		Numbers
Cartilagenous Saddle		20
Supra tip (a) soft tissue	(11)	
(b) upper lateral cartilage	(5)	
(c) septum	(17)	33
Valve collapse		6
Others (unilateral depression, asymmetry twisted)		12
		71

utilizing alar cartilage as well as other available nasal cartilage and bone. Other graft materials must be utilized in order to correct a saddle defect when there is an absence of adequate nasal structures. Other autogenous materials may be preferable but we have not hesitated to use alloplastic material on specific cases. Supramid mesh, (Dr. S. Jackson, Washington, D.C. 20014) because of its fibrous ingrowth, offers an alternative, especially over the mobile portion of the nose. In using this material in a total of 32 patients including both primary and secondary rhinoplasties it has had to be removed on three occasions. Time intervals have been 11 days, 31 days, and five months postoperative. Two of these patients had had multiple dorsal procedures which resulted in resorption of autogenous material and extrusion of alloplasts. The successful implantation in these cases is tenuous at best since one is dealing with a scarred avascular area over the dorsum. In any implantation it is critical to have the implants as far from the incision as is practical. Meticulous closure of the incisions and immobilization are also of paramount consideration. Dr. Richard Webster advocates the columellar splitting incision under certain circumstances.[5]

A saddle deformity may be made less apparent by decreasing the size of the tip. Minimal bony hump removal will at times make a cartilagenous saddle deformity less obvious.

Defects of the Lower Third

Deformities of the caudal one-third were the most common of all the defects noted (Table 3). These included arbitrary descriptions such as bulbous, wide, square, asymmetric, pinched, drooped, and abnormally projected tips. There were fifty-three tip deformities in this series. Alar asymmetry and collapse were identified in 17 instances. Hanging and retracted columellas were found 17 times. Thirteen patients required alar adjustments to achieve good cosmesis. Nineteen various other defects were noted for the lower third for a total of 119 deformities.

Secondary tip surgery tasks the technical facility and judgment of the surgeon more so than in any other area. Diagnosis of the underlying abnormality creating the deformity is often very difficult. The previous operative report is frequently of no value. There were several tips in this series which had not been violated by the primary

Table 3. Defects of the Lower Third

Deformity		Number
Tip		53
Deformity of lateral crus (a) asymmetry	(9)	
(b) collapse or pinch	(8)	17
Columellar (a) Hanging	(10)	
(b) Retracted	(7)	17
Alar base (needing alar adjustments)		13
Others (disarticulate caudal septum, shallow premaxilla, nasal labial angle defect)		19
		119

surgeon. It is likely these tip defects existed prior to the initial procedure rather than resulting from it. The most formidable challenges are those tips which have had extensive surgery with subsequent scarring and contracture.

Regeneration of the alar cartilages is not infrequently seen and can account for tip imperfections. Asymmetry can result if unequal regrowth occurs or it may be manifest as a developing bulbous tip after initial improvement. Regeneration has occurred in this series when the perichondrial layers were left intact, as with cartilage splitting techniques. When reentering a tip for revision it is wise to overcompensate for fibrosis and scarring. This can be accomplished by appropriate cartilage and scar removal. However, extreme conservativism is still indicated in the very thin skinned revision.

Columella deformities were diagnosed in 17 patients. Hanging columellas were routinely managed by full-thickness cartilage and mucosa excisions. Retracted columella presented a much more difficult management problem. Millard's chondromucosal flap[4] was utilized in conjunction with a Y-V advancement from the floor in three patients with satisfactory results.

Alar collapse is a perplexing problem caused by scar contraction and injudicious tissue removal. These patients are annoyed because of an obvious cosmetic deformity and a decreased nasal airway. Collapse of the lateral nasal wall in inspiration represents a disarticulation of the structure in the region of the nasal valve. These structures include the upper lateral cartilages, the lower lateral cartilages and the intervening accessory cartilages and ligaments. The nasal and alar muscles are also critical structures in this area. It is ill-advised to do extensive surgery in these areas unless necessary to correct a deformity. Insertion of a cartilagenous batten in the collapsed area from the patient's thin lower lateral cartilages is an excellent method of correcting this abnormality. Upper lateral cartilage or scar tissue may be adapted to solve this condition.

Conclusion

From the division of the nose into thirds it is immediately apparent that revisions are done most often for problems of the lower third of the nose (Table 4). This is not surprising when one considers the size and structures involved at the cephalic third as opposed to the caudal third. It is perhaps ironic that the hump deformity is the most frequent primary concern of the patient requesting a rhinoplasty. This series indicates that the bony deformity is the least difficult area to correct in cosmetic nasal surgery. The cartilagenous defects are somewhat more difficult to manipulate while the soft tissues represent the ultimate challenge to our skills. It should be pointed out that in revision rhinoplasties the most common deformities require the management of soft tissues and cartilages. Perhaps the surgeon performing the initial procedure makes some existing defects more obvious. He modifies the bony dorsum in an appropriate manner and does little to the tip. This situation is far easier to correct than excessive surgical trauma to the dome

Table 4. Deformities noted in 120 Revision Rhinoplasties

Defects of upper third	46
Defects of middle third	71
Defects of lower third	119
	236

area by the inexperienced. A large bony hump will mask other defects of the nose and profile. Occasionally, the recessed chin requiring mentoplasty becomes apparent only after the rhinoplasty.

Comments

A systematic, reproducible technique which is adaptable to most common deformities may have merit for the initial rhinoplasty. A single technique cannot be utilized for revision because of the myriad of defects. It is essential to add as little unnecessary surgical trauma as possible. The secondary procedures may be more appropriately approached by correcting only the problem or problems and avoiding tissues not involved. Many of these revisions will need no hump removal or lateral osteotomies. Minimal modification of the tip or columella may be all that need be done. The surgeon needs only expose the supra tip area if a polly beak is all that is in need of correction. Some patients have had multiple previous rhinoplasty procedures resulting in excessive scarring especially of the intranasal lining. Such cases preclude the usual endonasal approach. A satisfactory alternative is the columella approach as advocated by Webster.[5] It is important to elevate the dorsum with sharp dissection. Using a scissors will frequently result in tearing and avulsing tissue because of the scar. This unnecessary trauma will further complicate the results. It is very imprudent to attempt a revision if less than 6 months has elapsed since the previous surgery. Subtle changes over the months may negate the need for a procedure. Mature scar can be an aid to the secondary rhinoplasty surgeon if handled correctly.

Summary

Secondary rhinoplasties demand accurate diagnoses and a skillful conservative approach. It is important that the patient understand the capricious nature of soft tissue and cartilagenous healing. Optimum results very often cannot be achieved and it is paramount that the patient understands that perfection may be unobtainable.

References

1. Smith TW: As Clay in the Potter's Hand. Ohio Med J 63:1055, 1967
2. Safian: A New Anatomical Concept of Postoperative Complications in Esthetic Rhinoplasty. Plast Reconst Surgery 51:162, 1973
3. Raes D, Wood-Smith: Cosmetic Facial Surgery. WB Saunders Co., Philadelphia, 1973, 489
4. Millard D: The Versatility of a Chondromucosal Flap in the Naval Vestibuli. Plast Reconst Surgery 50:580, 72
5. Webster C: Columellar Incision in Revision Rhinoplasty. Plastic and Reconstructive Surgery of the Face and Neck, Vol 1, Grune and Stratton, New York, 1972

Maintaining Nasal Tip Projection

Eugene Bortnick, Kansas City, Kan.

Introduction

The delayed drooping downward of the nasal tip has been the bane of many immediate, apparently pleasing, postrhinoplasty results. This "tip ptosis" may occur as early as two weeks and as late as one year postoperatively.[1]

Attempts to prevent this complication fall into three catagories: avoidance of the surgical destruction of those anatomic elements which are believed to support the nasal tip, by surgically attempting to maintain or increase tip projection, and by exaggerating the amount of nasal hump which is removed to compensate for the normal settling of the nasal tip during the postoperative period.

The following is a progress report of an ongoing clinical study on the evaluation of some of the more commonly used surgical methods which have been recommended for the maintenance or reestablishment of nasal tip projection.

Anatomic Factors Which Maintain Tip Support

A study by Janeke and Wright defined four anatomic elements which maintained nasal tip support.[2] The most important of these factors was the fibrous attachment and overlapping relationship of the upper and lower lateral cartilages. The next most significant element was the fibrous attachment of the mesial crural feet to the base of the septum. Of less importance was the fibrous intradomal sling and the lateral alar areas which consist of fibrous tissue and sesamoid cartilages. This study was performed on cadaver dissections and did not take into account the weight and pull of the overlying skin nor the factors of scar tissue formation which occur in the healing process.

A more recent study, using the live patient, during and after rhinoplasty, reemphasized the importance of the overlapping relationship between the upper and lower lateral cartilages and the intimate relationship of the mesial crural feet and the septum.[3] In addition, this study demonstrated that removal of a large nasal hump would further reduce tip projection. Another significant but less well controlled factor was the formation and dissolution of scar tissue in the premaxillary area and along the transfixion incision which may, over the long postoperative period, cause a loss of tip projection.

Method

The present study comprised 75 patients who presented a variety of conditions commonly encountered in cosmetic rhinoplasty. Skin and cartilage texture and thickness, size of hump, and height

RHINOSEPTOPLASTY OPERATION RECORD

NAME________ Age____ Sex____

Pre-Operative Diagnosis:________

Nature of skin:____ oily____ thickness____ scars____

Nature of cartilage:________

Nasal Skeleton: Hump____ Width____ Nasal Spine____

Septum: Caudal____ mid-septum____ post-septum____ spurs____

Turbinates:____ Polyps____ Allergy____

Comments:

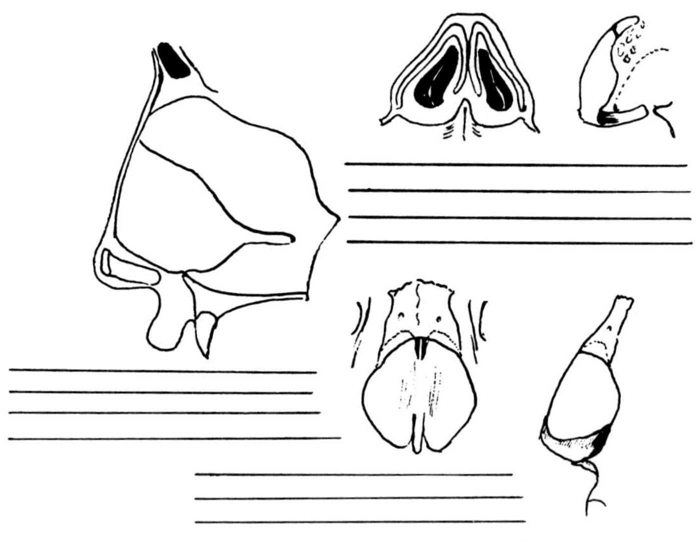

Post Operative Notes:

Fig. 1. The operation diagram presently being used.

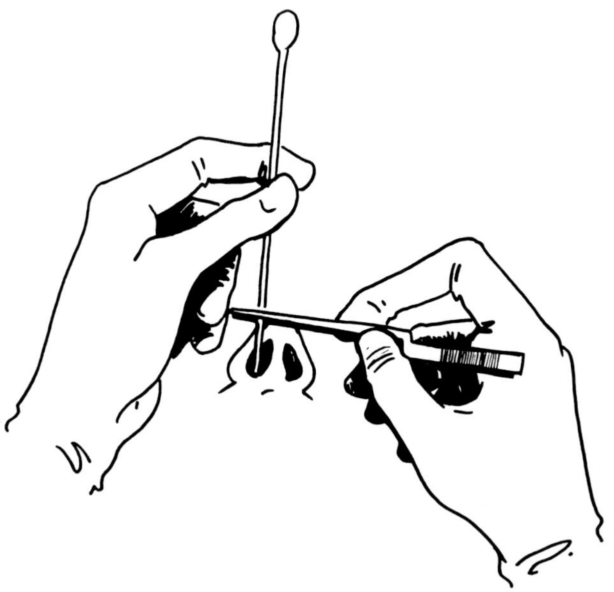

Fig. 2. A Q-tip applicator and a bayonet forceps are used to determine the nasal tip projection. Care must be taken not to apply pressure to the sill of the nostril during the recording.

of the nasal tip were recorded on an operation diagram (Fig. 1). The method of measuring the nasal tip is shown in Fig. 2. The measurements were recorded preoperatively and one year to 18 months postrhinoplasty. The surgical procedure was accurately recorded on the diagram immediately after surgery.

The pre and postoperative photographs and the operative diagrams were studied and the results recorded.

Results

Table 1 shows a record of the first 26 patients that comprise this group. Here is recorded the surgical procedure which destroyed nasal tip support, the technique employed in an attempt to maintain, reestablish, or increase tip projection, and the final results recorded in millimeters.

This study continued to confirm the conclusions of earlier studies that the single most devastating surgical maneuver to nasal tip support was the subtotal excision of the superior portion of the alar cartilages. Complete septal transfixion and removal of a moderately large nasal hump followed closely as surgical procedures which destroyed tip projection (Fig. 3).

Maneuvers which have been advocated to maintain or augment tip projection are: (1) avoidance of a complete septal transfixion, thus averting the supportive area of the mesial crural feet,[2,4,5] (2) "bunching" sutures placed at the base of the columella,[6] (3) "orthopedic" or "advancement", septocolumellar sutures, (4) insertion of implants or grafts placed inferior and between the mesial crura,[7] and (5) those methods which involve the borrowing of cartilage and occasionally vestibular skin from the dome and lateral crura and allowing this tissue to increase or maintain tip projection.[6] The maneuver of exaggerated cartilaginous hump and septal lowering, to allow the tip to project above the dorsum, was not considered in this study because it was felt that this method was not directly aimed at maintaining or augmenting tip support. This technique frequently necessitates the removal of tissue from the sill of the nostril because of the widening which occurs at the base of the nose. Measurements of tip projection would therefore be questionable.

The method which was most reliable in maintaining or increasing tip projection was that described by Goldman.[6] This method involves the delivery of the tip cartilages by way of a rim incision, division of the cartilages and vestibular skin at or lateral to the dome and the multiple suturing of this borrowed tissue in the midline into a cutaneous chondral "sandwich" (Fig. 4). Variations of this technique which utilize cartilage only, and not vestibular skin, are not as dependable in augmentation of the tip.

Subtotal excision of the alar cartilage, leaving an intact rim combined with a complete septal transfixion caused an immediate settling of the nasal tip of 2 to 3 mm. Attempts to reestablish tip support by placement of septal cartilage grafts were only partially successful.

An anterior septal transfixion or high septal transfixion, allowing the feet of the mesial crura to remain attached to the septum was successful in 70 percent of those cases in which these techniques were used (Fig. 5). Both of these methods were used in conjunction with a rim intact and subtotal excision of the lateral crura.

It was noted that the use of bunching or basilar sutures, combined with excision of tissue between the mesial crural feet, were of little value in maintaining tip projection. Similarly, "advancement

Table 1. Evaluation of Surgical Techniques on Nasal Tip Projection

Anatomy surgically destroyed[a]					Method used to preserve or augment tip support[b]					Result in millimeters	
Case	Age	S.L.C.	C.T.	A.S.	B.S.	D.C.	C.S.	A.S.T.	H.S.T.	Increase	Decrease
1.	46	X	X		X	X					1
2.	26	X	X	X	X	X				1	
3.	32	X		X		X		X		Same	
4.	17	X	X		X	X				1	
5.	25	X	X		X	X	X			1	
6.	16	X	X	X		X				1	
7.	24	X	X	X	X	X				Same	
8.	26		X	X	X	X				Same	
9.	15	X	X	X			X			1	
10.	16		X	X		X	X			1	
11.	18	X	X	X		X	X			Same	
12.	21	X	X	X	X	X				Same	
13.	20	X	X	X	X	X	X			1	
14.	17	X	X	X	X	X				1	
15.	39	X	X	X			X				1
16.	50	X	X	X	X		X				1
17.	25	X	X	X			X				2
18.	17	X	X	X		Intentionally Lowered					3
19.	18	X	X	X	X	X				Same	
20.	16	X		X			X	X		Same	
21.	21	X	X	X		Intentionally Lowered					2
22.	32		X							Same	
23.	40	X					X	X		Same	
24.	25	X	X	X		Intentionally Lowered					4
25.	23	Isolated Hump Removal						X		Same	
26.	16	X		X	X		X	X			1

[a] S.L.C., subtotal excision of lateral crus of alar cartilage carried out either through intercartilaginous incision or through a rim incision; C.T., complete transfixion incision with destruction of the attachment of the mesial crural feet to the septum; A.S., anterior septal lowering, usually with hump removal.

[b] B.S., basilar suture, always carried out with removal of tissue at base of columella; D.C., dome cartilage used to augment tip elevation and usually sutured together in the midline; C.S., cartilage strut placed inferior to the mesial crura; A.S.T., anterior septal transfixion, preserving the crural feet attachments; H.S.T., high septal transfixion, preserving the entire membranous septum.

sutures" and imbricating septal-columellar sutures were useful in approximating tissue edges but of no value in tip support.

Comments

Most of the surgical procedures performed on the nasal tip, during reduction rhinoplasty, can be divided into a rim intact and a rim divided technique. Both methods involve the sacrifice of varying amounts of the superior portion of the lateral crura.

The "rim-divided" technique usually involves the delivery of the alar cartilages by a marginal or rim incision together with an intercartilaginous incision. Under direct vision, various amounts of the superior part of lateral crura are trimmed, to reduce tip bulk. The cartilage and occasionally the underlying vestibular skin is divided at or lateral to the dome and the medial portions brought together in the midline and supported with mattress sutures. These surgical techniques do not rely on grafts for nasal tip projection. They must be used with caution in a thin-skinned individual because even minor surgical errors may become evident. The tip

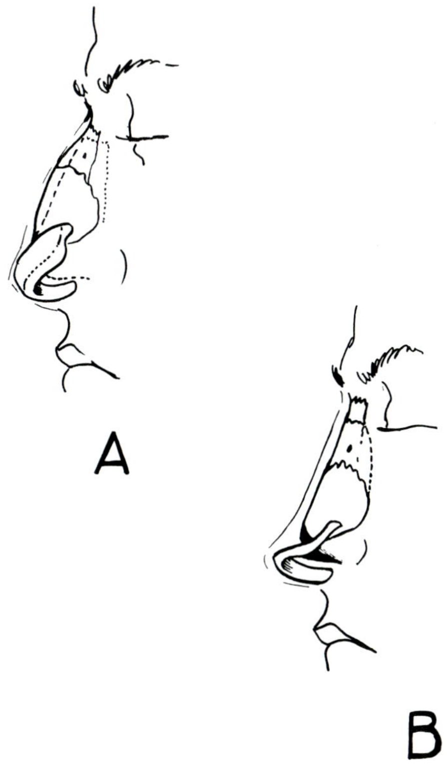

Fig. 3. (A) The proposed amount of bone and cartilage to be excised. (B) The tissue has been removed and a complete transfixion incision has been performed.

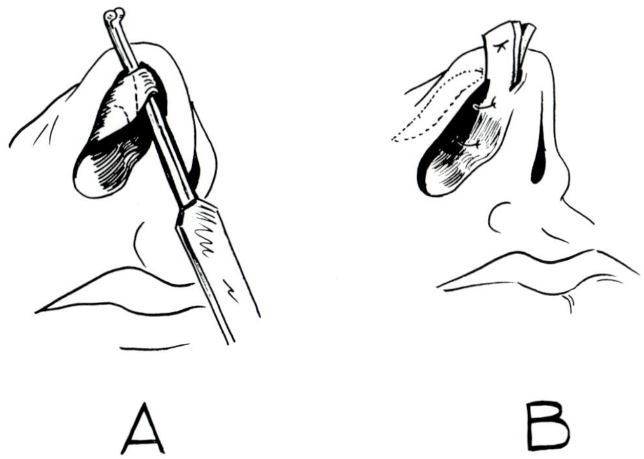

Fig. 4. (A) The alar cartilages are delivered through the nostril opening. (B) The cephalic portion of the lateral crus has been trimmed and this flap is returned to the vestibule. The dome and medial crura are sutured together in the midline.

of the nose may appear thin and pinched and occasionally the medial component may become warped or twisted. The cutaneous, chondral "sandwich" is best indicated when tip augmentation is desired in a thick-skinned patient.

Subtotal excision of the superior portion of the alar cartilage, leaving an intact inferior rim continuous with the mesial crus, has been advocated by many surgeons.[2,5,7] They feel that by leaving an intact rim of cartilage, the tip appears more natural. Because of the absence of the superior portion of the alar cartilage, the tip will rotate easily in a cephelad direction which may eventually cause flaring and widening of the nostril. Preservation of the membranous septum along its posterior one-third helps preserve tip support. Placement of grafts inferiorly and between the mesial crura has also been noted to preserve tip support.[2] The success of these supporting grafts depends upon their length and resilience. Short or easily fractured grafts are of little value. These grafts may also cause the appearance of a "hanging columella."

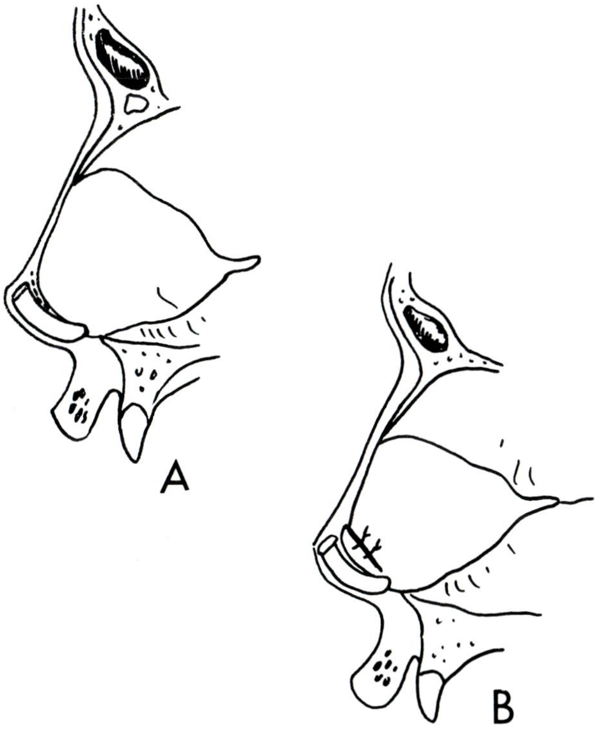

Fig. 5. When the attachments of the mesial crural feet are preserved, the tip projection is usually maintained. An anterior septal transfixion (A), or a partial high septal transfixion (B), preserves this critical area.

The utilization of "bunching" or "basilar" sutures, with or without the excision of tissue between the mesial crural feet, has only a transient effect on nasal tip projection. Advancement or orthopedic sutures and imbricating the mesial crura into a denuded septum does not appear to retard tip ptosis.

Summary

The drooping downward of the nasal tip following reduction rhinoplasty seems inevitable unless the surgeon understands the anatomic elements of tip support and takes measures either to preserve or reconstruct these supportive members. A clinical study was undertaken to evaluate the various rhinoplasty methods which were aimed at preserving and augmenting tip projection.

The older method of delivering the alar cartilages through a rim and intercartilaginous incision, dividing the cartilage and occasionally the vestibular skin, at or lateral to the dome, and approximating this "borrowed" tissue in the midline, has been demonstrated to give the most consistent results.

Subtotal excision of the alar cartilage and leaving the rim intact gives a more natural, nonsurgical appearance. If combined with a complete septal transfixion incision, the tip will settle 2 to 3 mm. Preserving the attachment of the mesial crural feet to the septum, and the use of anteriorly placed cartilage grafts helps maintain tip projection. Other surgical maneuvers are discussed but do not appear to be of lasting value in maintaining or augmenting nasal tip projection.

References

1. Tardy ME: Rhinoplasty tip ptosis: Etiology and prevention. Laryngoscope 83:923–929, 1973
2. Janeke JB, Wright WK: Studies on the support of the nasal tip. Arch Otolaryngol 93:458–464, 1971
3. Bortnick E: Evaluation of surgical techniques on nasal tip projection. Laryngoscope 84:1316–1324, 1974
4. Parkes ML, Berman HG: High septal transfixion to shorten the nose. Plast Reconstr Surg 45:487–492, 1970
5. Webster RC, White MF, Courtiss EH: Nasal tip correction in rhinoplasty. Plast Reconstr Surg 51:384–396, 1973
6. Goldman IB: Rhinoplasty Manual, Department of Otolaryngology, Mount Sinai Hospital, New York, NY
7. Anderson JR: A new approach to rhinoplasty. Trans Am Acad Opth Otol 70:183–192, 1966

Evaluation of the Goldman Tip in Rhinoplasty

Robert L. Simons, N. Miami Beach, Fla. and Irving J. Fine, Perth Amboy, N.J.

There is something spurious and misleading in the fusion of a man's name with an operative procedure, especially in the field of rhinoplasty. Few ideas are so simple or pure, few techniques so revolutionary or novel that a thorough search of the literature will not reveal the germinating seeds of the latest innovation to be scattered among the observations of earlier workers.

In 1954, Dr. Irvin B. Goldman while performing a revision rhinoplasty discovered that by freeing the earlier cut medial crura from their inadvertent lateral attachment to the septum, the nasal tip previously dependent and asymmetric suddenly assumed a more projected pleasing appearance. Enthusiastically, Dr. Goldman pursued this idea of dividing the alar cartilage to model the nasal tip.

Again, not a new idea. Others had separated the medial and lateral crura. Previously, however, the emphasis had been placed upon the lateral crura. Dr. Goldman centered attention on the medial crura adjusting tip projection by augmenting or reducing the size of the medial crus. In 1957 in the

Archives Of Otolaryngology, he published his paper, "The Importance of The Medial Crura in Nasal Tip Reconstruction".[1]

For almost 20 years, Irving Goldman taught thousands of students his method of rhinoplasty. With time and exposure the Goldman Tip became synonymous with the vertical transection of the alar cartilages.

Today there are few rhinoplastic procedures that generate as many controversial "Ayes" or "Nayes" as "The Goldman Technique." It is possible that misunderstanding and misapplication of the Goldman rhinoplasty has generated much of this criticism.

Utilizing over 30 years combined experience and observation with the Goldman technique, the authors of this presentation—and I don't believe that Dr. Fine would mind being singled out as the man closest to Dr. Goldman during his professional career or the major contributor to the total years of experience—we wish to make a few clarifying statements about the validity of this approach to rhinoplasty.

We will discuss "cons" as well as "pros." There will be no effort to suggest that this method of rhinoplasty is the only sensible one. Hopefully, we have all advanced beyond the days of the entrepreneur and the singular approach to all noses.

What is the Goldman nose? What are its advantages? Its limitations? Its drawbacks? When should it be employed and when not? These are the questions we will seek to answer.

What are the components of the Goldman technique? Simply stated: initial attention to creating a straight osseous and cartilaginous dorsum, followed by projection of the nasal tip above the profile line to produce the desired "double break" and triangular nasal base.

The supposition with the Goldman method is that tip projection can be created and maintained in proper relationship to the established profile line, rather than contouring bone and cartilage to fall in line with the initially modeled tip.

If it was Sam Foman who originally stated "He who masters the tip masters rhinoplasty," it was Irving Goldman who daily practiced that credo.

In the Goldman technique the entire tip pathology is delivered and examined through marginal incisions. The apex of the dome of the alar cartilage is identified, (Fig. 1). Then, depending upon the need for change in tip projection the alar cartilages are transected vertically either near or more generally lateral to the apecis of the lobular domes.

Separating the alar cartilage lateral to the dome adds height to the medial crura as they are sutured together to create a natural strut of support for the nasal lobule. As the joined medial crura are then positioned above the lateral crura and against the straight caudel end of the septum, the desired "double break" is attained (Fig. 2).

The "double break," a term first employed by James Barret Brown commonly refers to the break in the rounded columellar plane and the straight dorsal plane created by the properly tilted nasal tip (Fig. 3). Special attention is directed to the retrousse slant of the lobule away from the columella, and what is popularly termed a "double break" in reality represents a "single break."

This break is created naturally by the curved planes of the medial crura as they swing upward and backward to join the lateral crura in the dome region. Given strong medial crura with relatively thin skin one need not worry about tip projection or the absence of a "double break."

However, with a short columella evidencing inadequate medial crura, the Goldman method is often the answer to tip projection and lobular rotation. It is important to remember to stabilize the freed medial crura against a stong, straight caudel septum. One should not bastardize this procedure by combining it with another method that calls for loping off large segments of the septal angle. Unless the crura are adequately buttressed by the septum they will "droop" and the tip "poly" (Fig. 4).

How much can one "steal" from the lateral crura to increase tip projection? Two to three millimeters from the apex of the dome is a safe boundary line for borrowing (Fig. 5).

Through marginal incisions the exact apex of the dome is identified with a right angled hook and the crura lateral to the angled marker stabilized. The cartilage transection is symmetrically distanced and made in an oblique manner over grooved directors specifically made for this purpose. The 2 to 3 mm borrowing boundary is measured at the caudel border of the alar cartilage. The obliquity of the cut helps to narrow the supra lobular area. When the medial crura are sutured together their

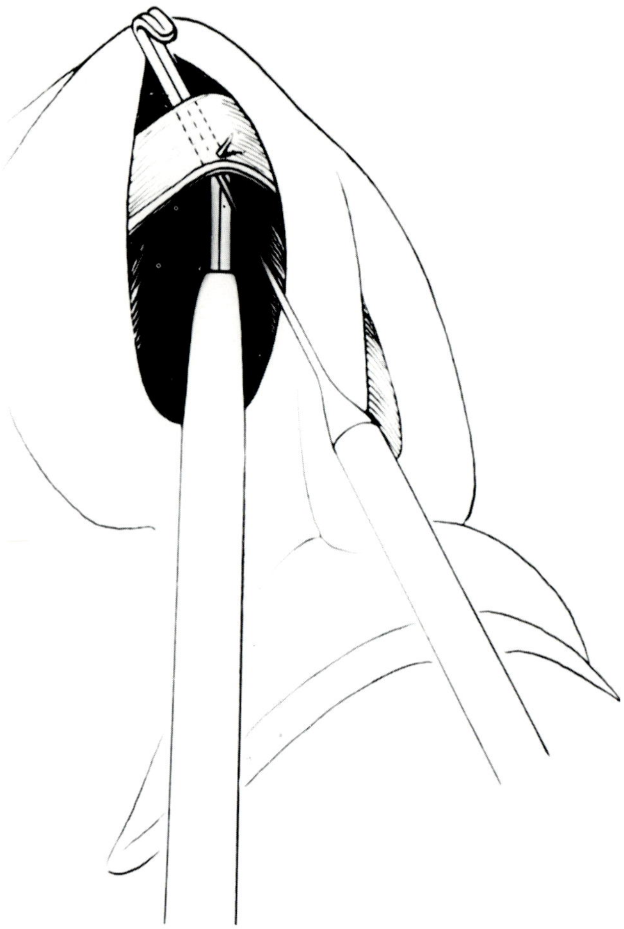

Fig. 1. Right-angled hook marks apex of lobular dome.

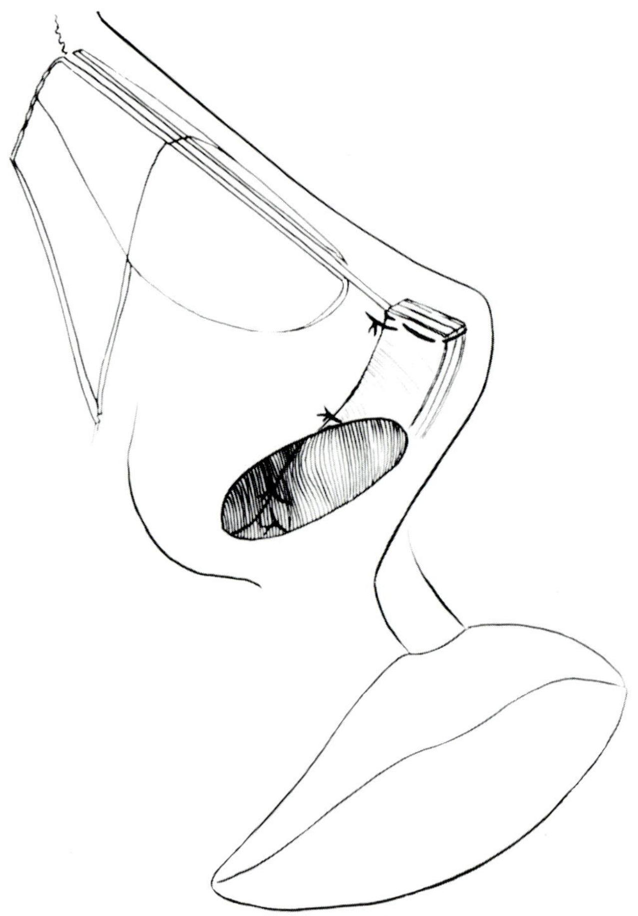

Fig. 2. Properly positioned medial crura against straight septum.

tops are trimmed so that the anterior portion is slightly elevated.

The alar cartilages are not delivered or repositioned prior to placement of the two lower septo-columellar sutures. Without this support the medial crural strut is too floppy and accurate judgment of its repositioned height most difficult.

If the tip appears overly projected the medial crura can be redelivered and trimmed. However, the reverse situation of inadequate projection is tough to correct. Therefore, one must take care to "steal enough," rather than later be caught "shorthanded" and find projection insufficient (Fig. 6).

Bringing the medial crura together not only increases projection and changes direction of the lobule, it also effects a narrowing of the tip and creation of a more triangular base (Fig. 7 A, B). Only small portions of the cephalic border of the lower lateral cartilage are trimmed—ideally only that amount denuded of vestibular skin and thus overlapping the upper lateral cartilages.

Again, one should not try and mix methods—combining a large resection of lateral crura with transection of the alar cartilages may lead to undesirable narrowing and pinching (Fig. 8). With the Goldman technique one depends less upon the variability of fibrosis for tip rotation and narrowing.

To talk about advantages of the Goldman technique, one begins with the stability of the nasal tip. The tip stays where positioned.

Indeed, for the rhinoplastic surgeon accustomed to overprojecting tips to compensate for postoperative drop, a warning must be issued not to overproject unless the skin of the nose is extremely thick (Fig. 9).

By controlling tip projection one can avoid excessive lowering of the nasal dorsum. Making noses smaller to meet low tips increases the need

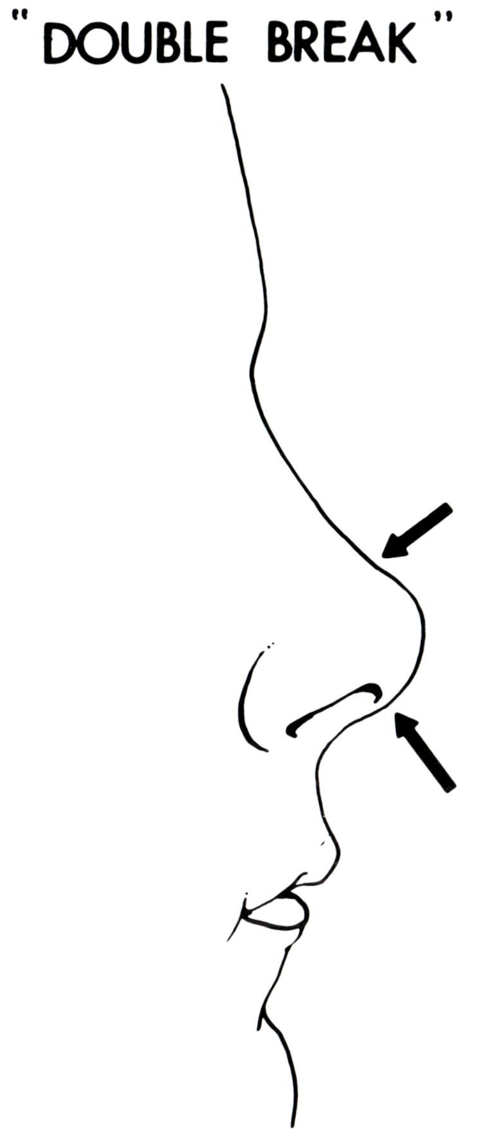

Fig. 3. Emphasis on tilt of lobule away from columella (lower arrow).

for alar resections. The Goldman technique elevates and narrows the nasal base by its tent pole action. The downward tilt of nostrils are redirected and the use of Weir resections, battens, and struts frequently obviated.

Delivery of the alar cartilages, furthermore allows examination of the lobular pathology with direct and symmetrical correction.

Provided these arguments are genuine, then what is the basis for the opposition to the Goldman procedure?

There is little question that the Goldman tip is more exacting and time-consuming than many other techniques. Marginal incisions have been criticized for causing loss of tip support, unequal nostrils, destruction of soft tissue facets, notching of alar rims and prolapse of alar cartilages. These are all real considerations but infrequent occurrences when the marginal incisions are executed with care.

Because the Goldman tip requires extensive dissection as well as division of the alar cartilages, both the chance to correct as well as commit tip asymmetry exists. One must divide, suture, and reposition in a symmetrical manner. Nasal packing is necessary for 3 to 4 days postoperatively to help secure the newly positioned medial crura.

Additional minutes of operative time, nasal packing and potential problems with marginal incisions, however, are relatively minor arguments. The disclaimer most often voiced against the Goldman nose is its postoperative unnatural surgical appearance, with a tendency for long term rounding of the tip.

It is certainly accurate that with this technique one trades a preoperative deformity for a dependable, albeit at times surgical, appearance. This is especially true in very thin skinned noses where the medial crural strut is less easily camouflaged.

However, a better understanding of this technique may avoid noses that slope to pinched, pointed, or rounded tips.

Since bone work proceeds tip surgery one must guard against extensive hump removal. Significant bone excision leads to aggressive cartilage removal and loss of support in the septal angle area. Along with drappage of skin, these factors lead to postop "ski-slopes and polys."

As indicated earlier, accurate borrowing of cartilage from the lateral crus, along with stabilization of the medial crura with a high septo-columellar suture is necessary to avoid rounding of the tip.

In certain thin skinned noses, the transected alar cartilage can be freed medially and the underlying vestibular skin kept intact. This modification, however, does not work well when the skin is thick and the tip drooping. Cutting through vestibular skin when observing the borrowing boundary of 2 to 3 mm does not lead to external pinching or internal scarring or blunting of the vestibular dome.

Considering the aforementioned limitations and the demanding, disciplined approach necessary for success for the Goldman procedure we do not

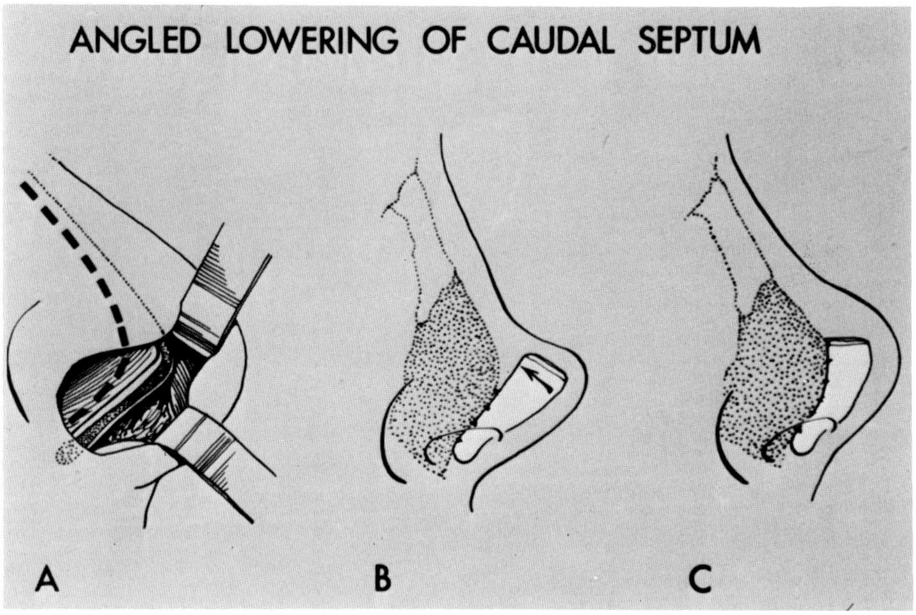

Fig. 4. "Polly" created by lowering septal angle.

recommend its use in all cases, no more than another rhinoplastic technique is the preferred method for all situations.

For which nasal deformity is the Goldman method most applicable?

There is little question the primary indication for the Goldman procedure is poor projection secondary to a short columella and/or the marked downward axis of the drooping tip.

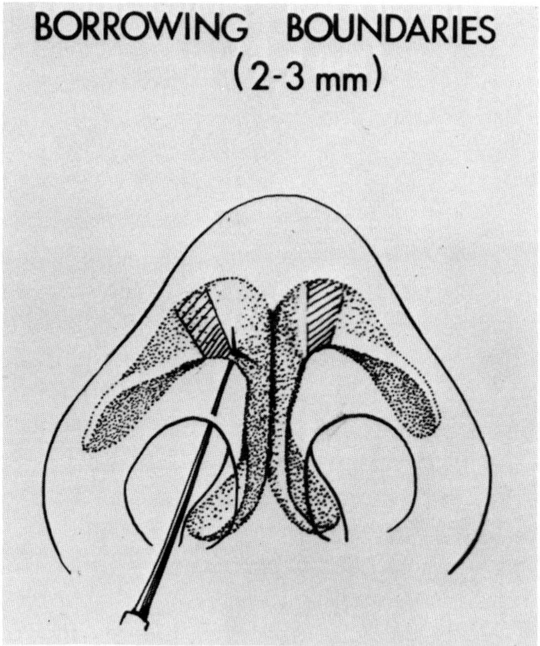

Fig. 5. Transection of alar cartilage measured from dome apex along caudel border.

With black noses it's important to remember that the alar cartilage is often frail and tip support further compromised by deficiency of the anterior nasal spine. In these situations additional support in the form of battens or crushed cartilage placed beneath the feet of the medial crura, is often necessary (Fig. 10 A, B).

For broad nasal tips at times presenting with an unattractive cleft between the lobular domes, the most direct solution is the Goldman tip (Fig. 11 A, B). Clefts can further be hidden by the placement of crushed cartilage beneath the lobular skin, a modification also employed to avert exaggerated flattening and angulation of the lobule caused by tension of elevated mesial crura in hypoplastic lobules.

Direct examination of the entire tip pathology is a significant aid in correcting asymmetries. Controlling the height of the medial crura can decrease as well as increase tip projection.

In secondary noses the ability to find the medial crura and remaining alar cartilages through a frequently unscarred marginal approach, can be of great benefit in helping to correct a problem of asymmetry or relatively poor tip position created by the previous surgery.

In summary, the Goldman rhinoplasty should not be considered basic either in terms of universal

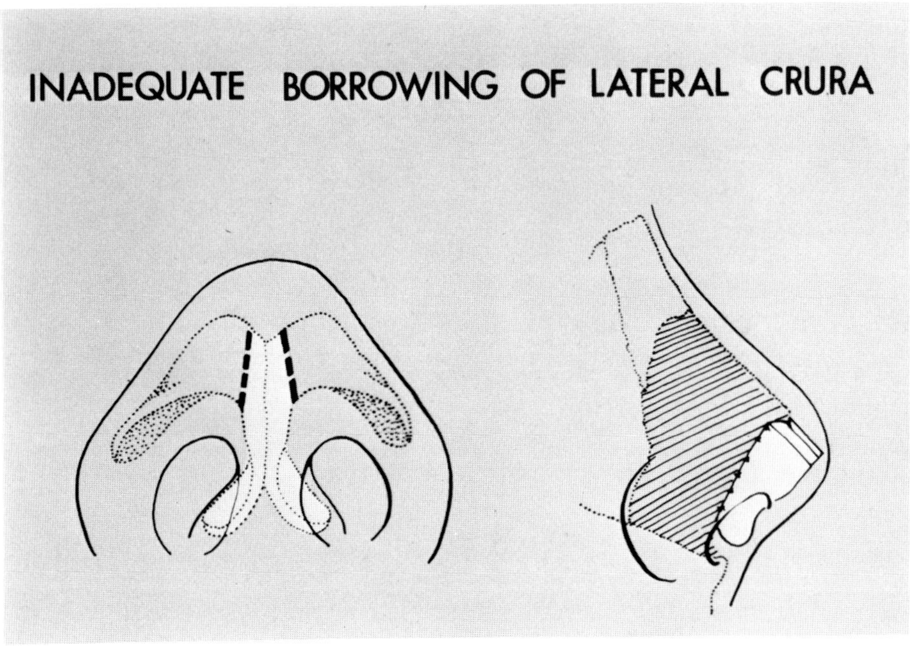

Fig. 6. Tip rounding caused by insufficient projection of medial crura.

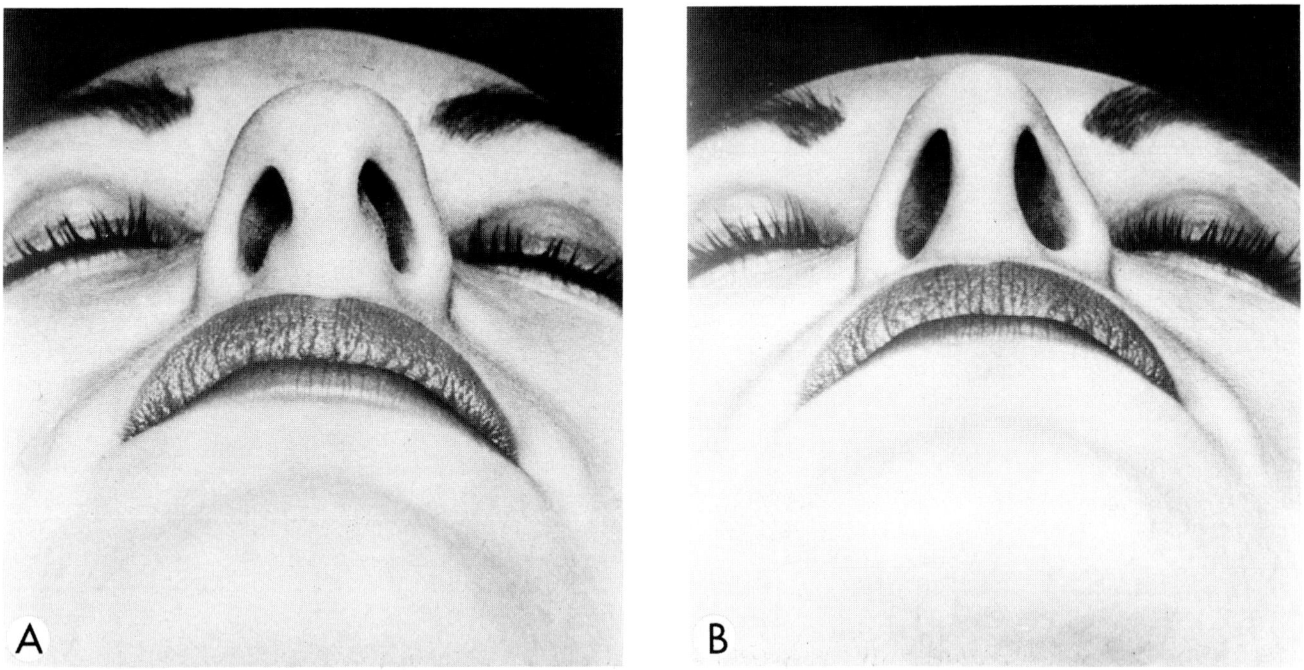

Fig. 7. (A) Preoperative base view. (B) Postoperative base view.

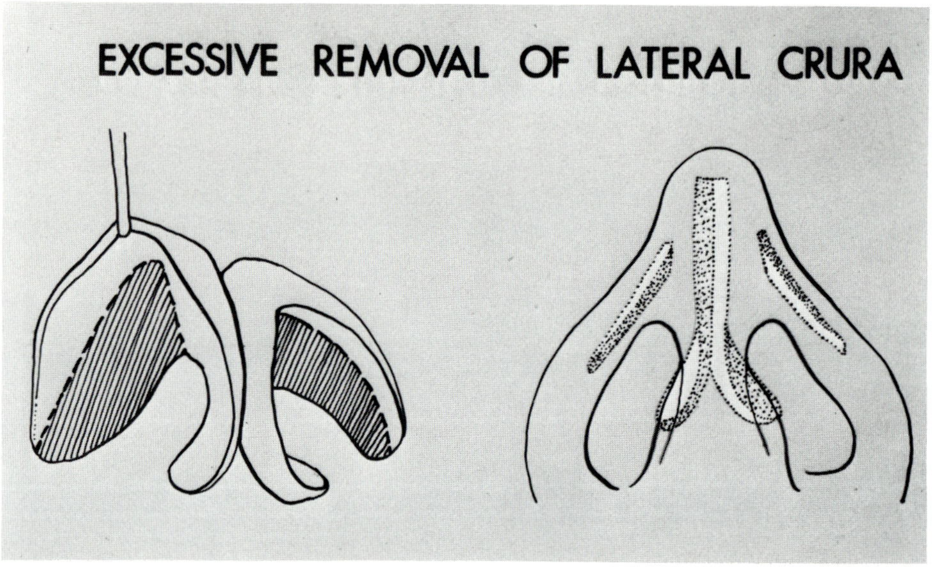

Fig. 8. *Removing large segments of lateral crura with Goldman tip may cause post-operative "pinching".*

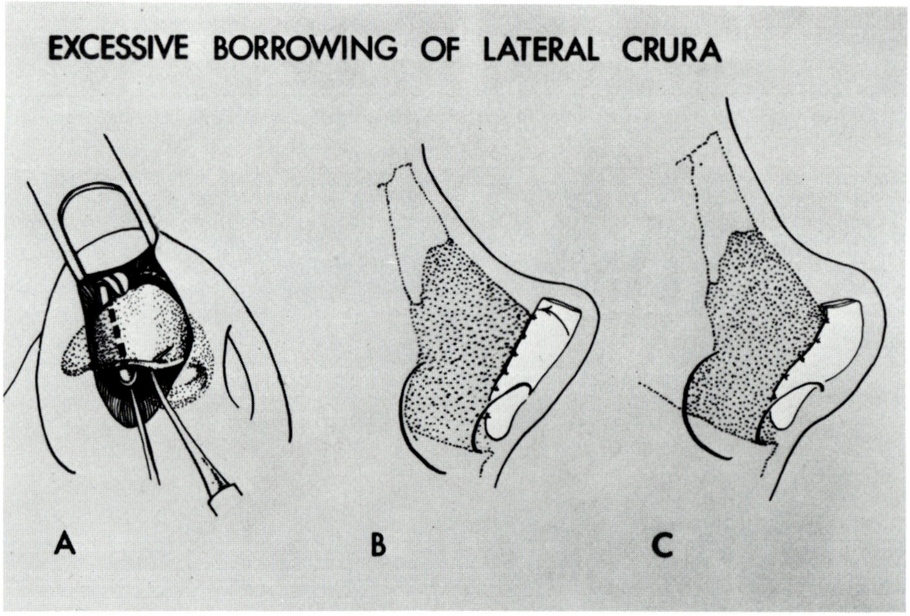

Fig. 9. *Rounding of crural strut overly extended above septal angle.*

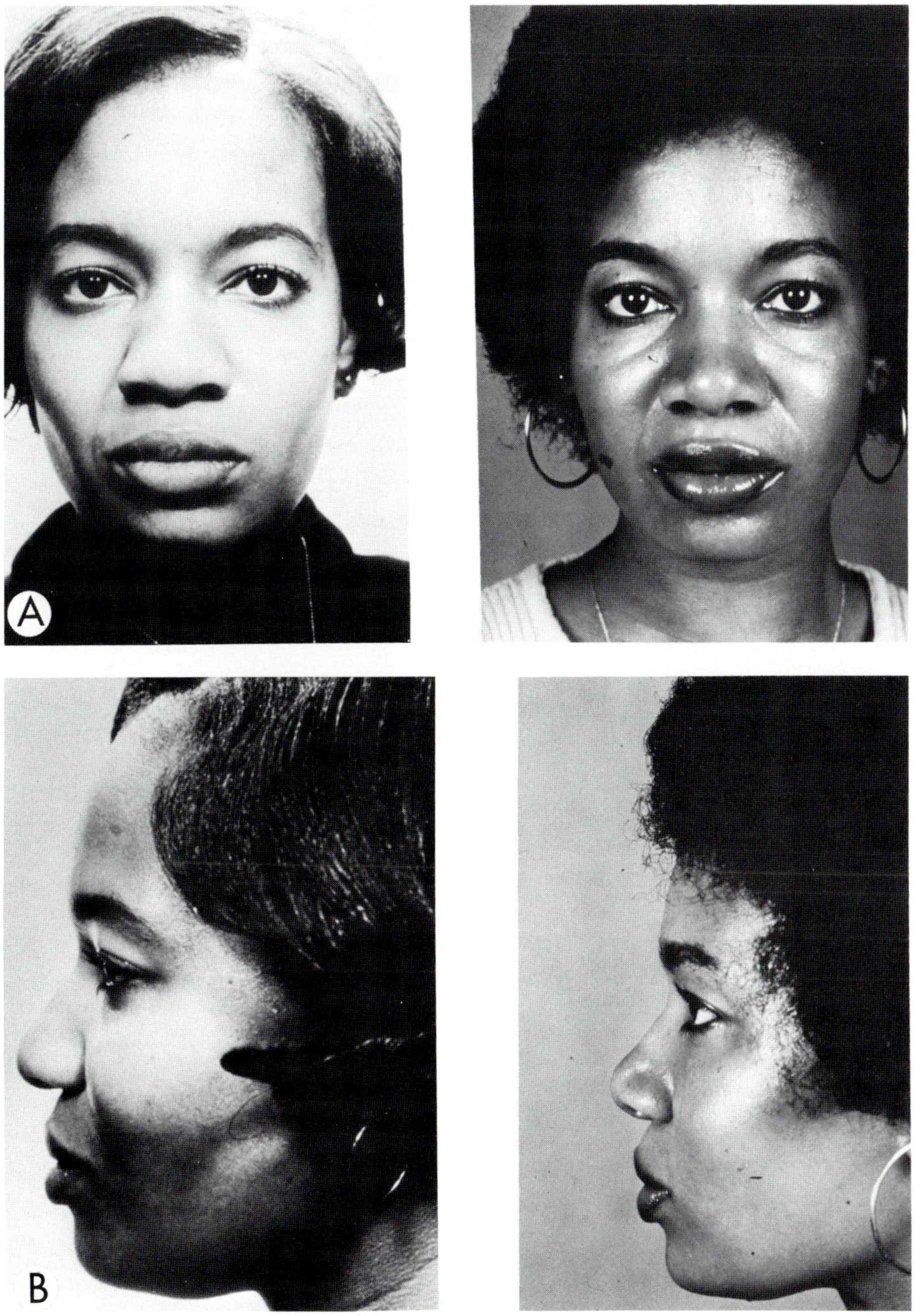

Fig. 10. (A) Pre and postoperative frontal views. (B) Pre and postoperative lateral views.

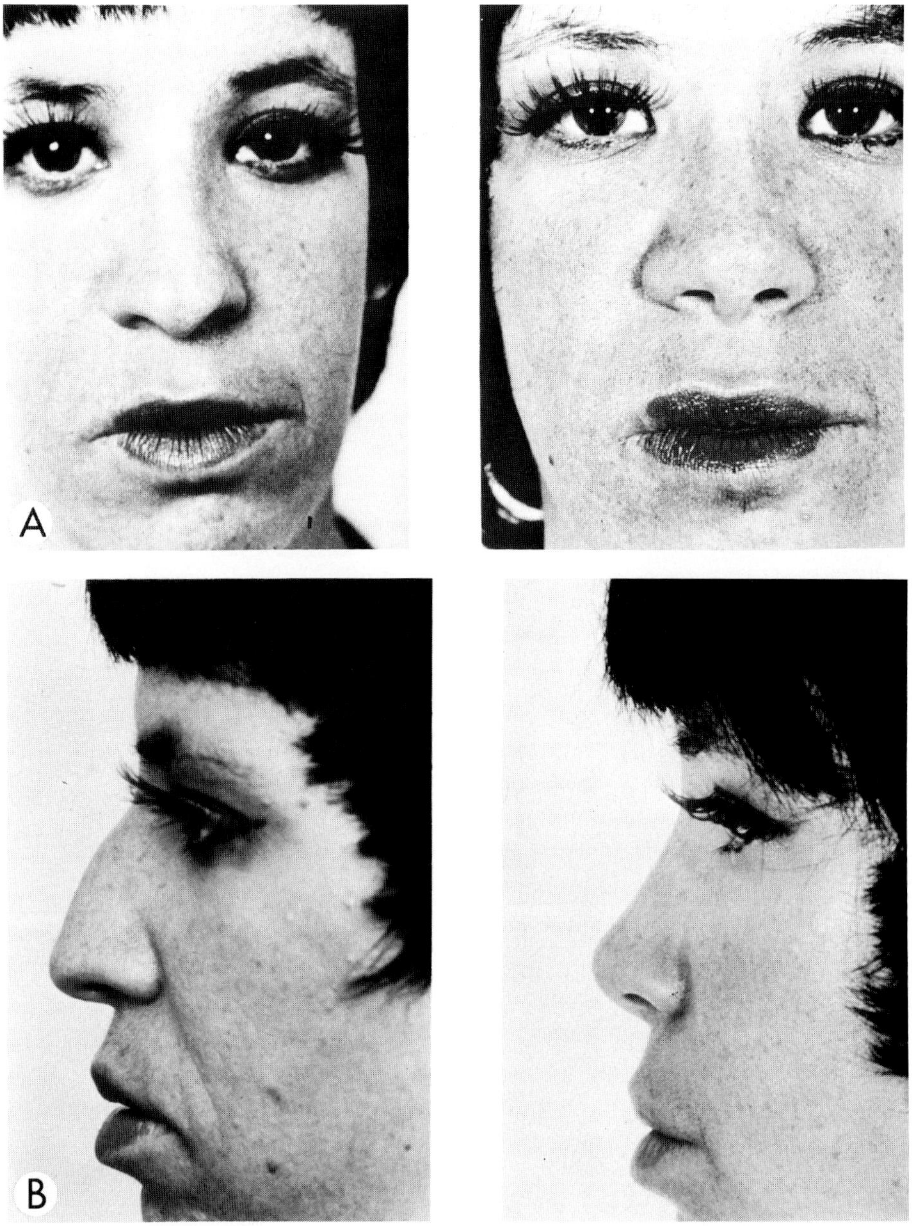

Fig. 11. (A) Pre and postoperative frontal views. (B) Pre and postoperative lateral views.

use or ease of performance. When, however, applied properly, generally in cases of significant tip pathology, the results are dramatically satisfying. This is not a method for all noses, but an extremely valuable asset in the armamentarium of the complete rhinoplastic surgeon.

References

1. Goldman IB: The importance of the medial crura in nasal tip reconstruction, Arch Otolaryngol 65:143–47, 1957
2. Goldman IB: The rim incision. Plastic and reconstructive surgery of the face and neck, Proceedings Of The First International Symposium, 1920, Grune and Stratton, New York, pp 130–134
3. Goldman IB: The Goldman nose. Plastic and reconstructive surgery of the face and neck, Proceedings Of The First International Symposium, 1920, Grune and Stratton, New York, pp 139–143

Evaluation of Nasal Tip Surgery: The Intracartilaginous and Rim Approaches

William H. Friedman, New York, N.Y.

Following rhinoplasty the surgeon anticipates a result which is satisfactory to the patient and outstanding by his own modest estimate. Unfortunately, an otherwise outstanding result may be marred by an imperfection of the nasal dorsum, lateral walls, alar base, or nasal tip. The latter represents a common problem, and is a site where even miniscule errors in operative technique are annoyingly visible. The most excellent techniques of hump removal, lateral osteotomy, septal resection, and upper lateral remodeling will be forgotten if the lower lateral rhinoplasty technique and result is not equally excellent.

The purpose of this study is to assess two technical approaches to the lower lateral nasal tip which are frequently performed and still controversial. Both are utilized in the excisional type of lower lateral rhinoplasty in which resection of the cephalic borders of the lateral crura of the lower lateral cartilages is accomplished. The excisional concept was introduced by Joseph[1] and is employed in most rhinoplastic surgery by utilizing either a rim (marginal) incision,[2] or an intracartilaginous (cartilage splitting) incision.[3] These incisions are also useful in a variety of other techniques such as the performance of the entire rhinoplasty through an intracartilaginous incision,[4] augmentation of the nasal tip by implantation of autogenous materials through a rim incision, or fashioning a bulky strut of sutured mesial crura (Goldman tip), also employing a rim incision. For this study, only those marginal and intracartilaginous incisions which were employed for simple excision of bulk of the cephalic border of the lower lateral cartilage are compared.

The Rim or Marginal Incision (Fig. 1)

This incision at the caudal margin of the lower lateral cartilage provides complete access to the lateral and mesial crura and the surgical dome. Delivery of the lower lateral cartilages allows the surgeon to inspect both major alar cartilages simultaneously and enables him to accurately assess the sesamoid lower lateral cartilage connections[5] under direct vision. A "V"-shaped wedge may be resected from the dome, or may be incorporated into the initial excision in hockey stick fashion. In this series excision through a rim incision was performed when: (1) the lower lateral cartilages were asymmetrical; (2) the lower lateral-sesamoid complex was to be preserved under direct vision; (3) if previous tip surgery had been performed through a cartilage splitting approach. Cases in which transsection of the surgical dome was performed with or without suturing of the mesial crura are not included since complications related to this technique are not necessarily the result of the rim approach.

The Intracartilaginous (Cartilage Splitting) Incision (Fig. 2)

The lateral crura of the lower lateral cartilages are approached directly in this incision. Vestibular skin and cartilage are transsected in an anterior-posterior direction parallel to the cartilage rim or nostril, depending on the type of excision desired.

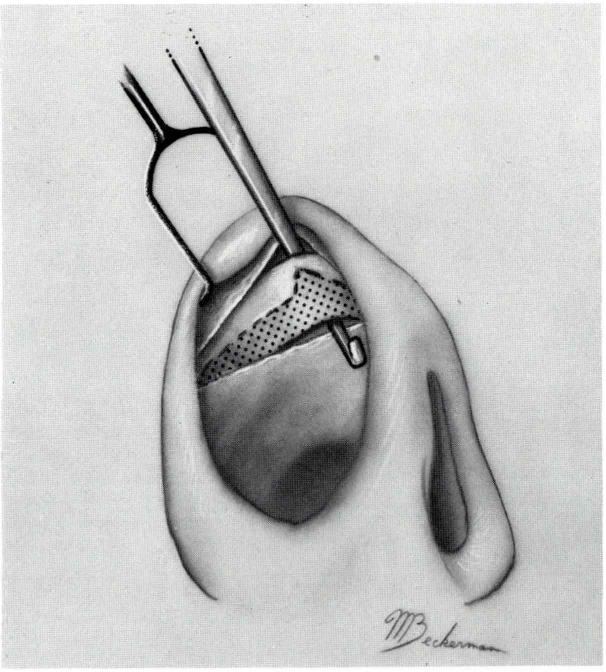

Fig. 1. The rim incision.

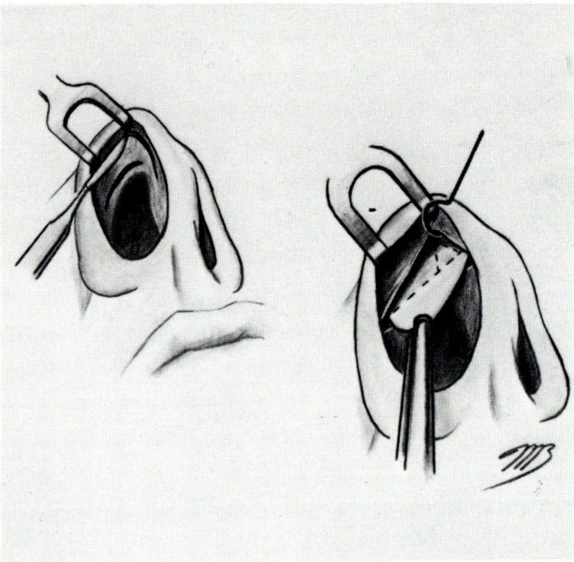

Fig. 2. The intracartilaginous incision (the rim is not exposed).

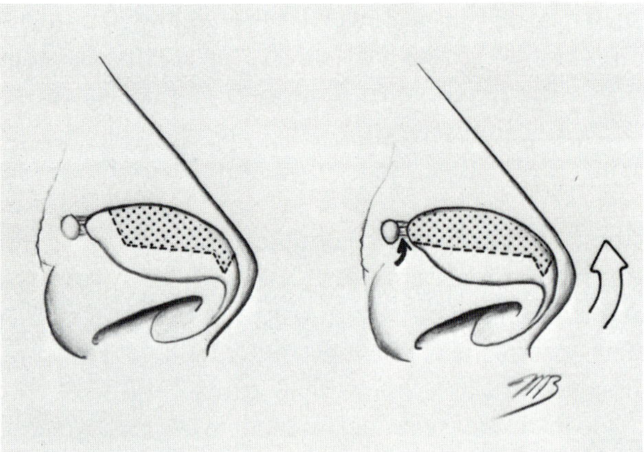

Fig. 3. "Rotation" of the nasal tip (the sesamoid lower lateral connection is either preserved or severed).

The incision lies approximately one centimeter cephalad to the nostril margin in most patients and either extends directly posteriorly, transsecting the posterior border of the lateral crus and lower lateral-sesamoid complex, or follows the curve of the caudal cartilage rim, sparing the connections between sesamoid and lower lateral cartilage. Up to ninety percent of the lateral crus can be resected in this fashion, and rotation of the tip is synergized by resection of the supporting structures posterior to the posterior crus margin. A "rotation point" can be selected without exposure of the rim margin and without delivery of the entire cartilage (Fig. 3). A "V"-shaped excision in the surgical dome area is accomplished as a second step by dissecting vestibular skin from the caudal remnant and removing a wedge of cartilage measuring 3 mm per side. This is a common approach and is suitable for most tip-excision type rhinoplasties. In this series the intracartilaginous approach was performed when: (1) simple debulking was required with facet installation; (2) when cephalic rotation of the tip was necessary with bilaterally symmetrical cartilages; and (3) when a previous procedure had been performed through a rim incision.

Materials and Methods

Private patients of the author and service patients at the City Hospital Center at Elmhurst were utilized. Two hundred patients who had undergone rhinoplasty in which an excisional approach to the lower lateral cartilages was utilized were selected. One hundred of these patients had rim or marginal incisions performed and one hundred had intracartilaginous or cartilage splitting incisions. A minimum of twelve months follow-up was secured. In evaluating the results, pre- and postoperative 35 mm slides were projected and the observations of the scrub nurse and surgeon independently noted. Five problem areas were characterized and catalogued, including: (1) tip ptosis; (2) pinching of the nasal tip; (3) alar retraction; (4) alar irregularities; and (5) bulk considerations. A sixth category was overall esthetic result.

Results

Viewing esthetic surgery in an uncompromising light, any deviation from the intended goal is a complication, whether or not the patient is satisfied with the result, or the surgeon feels he has done a good job "under the circumstances." Therefore, in evaluating the results of this surgery no consideration was given to the overall esthetic result until individual flaws had either been ascertained or excluded by the investigators. This principle was particularly applicable in comparing two different approaches to the nasal tip, since the patient was frequently unaware of the complication or was pleased with the result in spite of a photographically detectable complication.

There were twenty-nine nasal tip complications (14.5 percent) observed in the two hundred cases selected (Fig. 4). Sixteen occurred following rim incisions and thirteen following intracartilaginous incisions.

Tip Ptosis (Fig. 5)

Tip ptosis occurred in nineteen or 9.5 percent of patients in this series, and was the most frequent complication of the excisional technique either by a rim or intracartilaginous approach. Parrot beak formation, viewed as a species of tip ptosis, is included only as a distributional feature since the etiology of this deformity lies outside an exclusive discussion of lower lateral rhinoplasty. Eleven of two hundred patients (5.5 percent) developed a form of parrot beak. Six occurred following the rim incision approach and five following an intracartilaginous approach. Tip ptosis without parrot beak formation, consisting only of rounding or settling of the nasal tip was considered more relevant to excision of the cephalic border of the lateral crura of the lower lateral cartilages. This complication occurred in eight patients (4 percent), five following a rim incision and three following an intracartilaginous approach.

Pinching of the Nasal Tip (Fig. 6)

"Pinching" occurred in six patients (3 percent) with approximately equal distribution in both intracartilaginous and rim approaches. Although subjectively one might consider pinching at the postero-lateral compartment to be more likely if the vestibular incision is placed cephalad or closer to other incisions during the performance of rhinoplasty, this did not prove to be the case. Two patients developed postero-lateral pinching following a rim approach and only one patient developed this complication following an intracartilaginous incision. Pinching at the dome occurred in two patients following an intracartilaginous incision and in one patient following a rim approach.

Alar Retraction and Irregularity (Fig. 7)

Alar retraction or "flaring" of the alae following rhinoplasty occured in one patient in this series. "Notching" of the alar rim also occurred in one patient. Both occurred following rim incisions. This complication did not occur following an intracartilaginous incision.

Bulk Considerations (Fig. 8)

Inadequate debulking of the nasal tip occurred in two patients, both following intracartilaginous incisions. This complication did not occur following a rim incision. Removal of excess bulk from the cephalic borders of the lower lateral cartilages did not occur.

Corrective Rhinoplasty (Fig. 9)

Three patients underwent corrective rhinoplasty following excisional approaches to the nasal

RIM INCISION	(N=100)	16 (16%)
INTRACARTILAGINOUS INCISION	(N=100)	13 (13%)
TOTAL	(N=200)	29 (14.5%)

Fig. 4. Nasal tip complications.

		WITH PARROT BEAK	WITHOUT PARROT BEAK
RIM INCISION	(N=100)	6 (6%)	5 (5%)
INTRACARTILAGINOUS INCISION	(N=100)	5 (5%)	3 (3%)
TOTAL	(200)	11 (5.5%)	8 (4%)

Fig. 5. Tip ptosis.

		AT DOME	AT POSTEROLATERAL COMPARTMENT	TOTAL
RIM INCISION	(N=100)	1 (1%)	2 (2%)	3 (3%)
INTRACARTILAGINOUS INCISION	(N=100)	2 (2%)	1 (1%)	3 (3%)
TOTAL	200	3 (1.5%)	3 (1.5%)	6 (3%)

Fig. 6. Pinching of the nasal tip.

		ALAR RETRACTION	ALAR IRREGULARITIES	TOTAL
RIM INCISION	(N=100)	1 (1%)	1 (1%)	2 (2%)
INTRACARTILAGINOUS INCISION	(N=100)	0	0	0
TOTAL	200	1 (0.5%)	1 (0.5%)	2 (1%)

Fig. 7. Alar problems.

		INADEQUATE DEBULKING	EXCESS BULK REMOVED
RIM INCISION	(N=100)	0	0
INTRACARTILAGINOUS INCISION	(N=100)	2 (2%)	0
TOTAL	200	2 (1%)	0

Fig. 8. Bulk considerations.

		UNACCEPTABLE COMPLICATIONS	ACCEPTABLE COMPLICATIONS
RIM INCISION	(N=100)	1 (1%)	15 (15%)
INTRACARTILAGINOUS INCISION	(N=100)	2 (2%)	11 (11%)
TOTAL	200	3 (1.5%)	26 (13%)

Fig. 9. Corrective rhinoplasty.

tip. This represented a 1.5 percent unacceptable complication rate. Two patients underwent corrective procedures following the intracartilaginous approach, and one following a rim incision. Twenty-six of the total of twenty-nine complications were deemed acceptable and not requiring corrective rhinoplasty because of a complication of excision.

Conclusion

Only two of a variety of techniques for approaching nasal tip deformities are compared in this series. Many surgeons practice a single technique only, and they are likely to be confronted with nasal tip problems which are not amenable to a single technique. Since excision of the cephalic borders of the lower lateral cartilages is the most common technique for debulking the nasal tip, the surgeon is well advised to have at least two approaches at his disposal to accomplish this relatively simple task. In assessing two technical approaches, the strictest and most objective criteria were used and very little difference was discerned between the number of esthetic complications which occurred following rim or marginal incisions and those which occurred following intracartilaginous or cartilage splitting incisions. However, it may be stated that alar retraction and irregularity did not occur following the cartilage splitting approach and did occur, though rarely, following the rim approach (2 percent). Inadequate debulking of the nasal tip did not occur following a rim incision and did occur following the intracartilaginous approach, though rarely (2 percent). The relative locations of these incisions might predict these complications. Tip ptosis did not occur with significantly greater frequency in either of the two approaches. Pinching occurred with surprising frequency but at different sites than anticipated. Both incisions are extremely useful and in a much larger series[6] the author has utilized the intracartilaginous incision approximately twice as frequently as the rim incision for simple excisional approaches to the nasal tip. The rim incision, however, has proven to be a more utilitarian approach to the nasal tip for purposes of augmentation, dome transections, and mesial crural suturing. If these more sophisticated nasal tip problems are considered, the rim incision and intracartilaginous incision find in the author's experience approximately equivalent usage.

References

1. Joseph J: Nasenplastik und sonstige Gesichtsplastik (nebst einem Anhang über Mammaplastik und einige weitere Operationen aus dem Gebiete der äusseren Körperplastik; ein Atlas und Lehrbuch). Kabitzsch, Leipzig, 1931, pp 498–842
2. Converse JM: Reconstructive plastic surgery. WB Saunders and Company, Philadelphia and London, 1964, pp 718–721
3. Diamond HP: Rhinoplasty technique. Surg Clin Amer 51:312–331, 1971
4. Anderson JP: A new approach to rhinoplasty. A five year appraisal. Arch Otol 93:284–291, 1971
5. Janeke JB, Wright WK: Studies on the support of the nasal tip. Arch Otol 93:458–467, 1973
6. Friedman WH, Oliver M, Biller HF: Evaluation of nasal tip surgery. The Laryngoscope, Vol 8, No 9:1539–1549, Sept 1975

The Sandwich Tip

Donald J. Huttner, Denver, Colorado

We are all "Fiddler's on the Roof" of the nose. If one had to choose a central theme for the story of the fiddler, it may be the destruction of traditional thoughts and teachings. This presentation is a breakdown of traditional surgical approaches to the nasal tip. As we all know one of the most difficult nasal tips to improve is the one that is bulbous, projecting, and broad. This tip, post-surgically, may be a disappointment both to you and your patient. When the tip cartilages are large and bowed, the tip usually appears ugly. This type of tip is the one most suitable for the "sandwich" approach. In the past two years I have used this type of tip with satisfactory to excellent results.

This discussion will not involve at which point in the rhinoplasty the tip procedure should be done. However, support can be given to approaching the nasal tip initially.

The "sandwich tip" is a variation of the Lipsett tip. The easiest way to understand and teach this tip to residents is through the "sandwich" analogy.

A standard Joseph intercartilaginous incision and transfixion is used with this nasal tip. The first actual incision, after local anesthetic injection, is 0.5 cm from the margin of the alar rim (Figs. 1, 2). This is the "modified rim" technique as compared to the rim incision proposed by Lipsett.[1] It cuts directly through the vestibular lining and cartilage on the initial incision. Through this incision a small curved scissors is inserted and the overlying skin of the nasal tip is separated cephalically from the cartilage (Fig. 3). The incision starts laterally one-third of the way above the alar base and extends just beyond the soft triangle. The 0.5 cm strip of cartilage can be varied as to its width depending upon the particular nose. This strip of cartilage is known as the bottom piece of bread in our "sandwich." This lower lateral cartilage is then rotated laterally out of the nose. The movement allows direct visualization of the lower lateral cartilage.

The next incision is an anterior posterior cut through both the cartilage and vestibular skin at the angle (Fig. 4). The actual point of the incision can be varied. If one is attempting to gain projection, this incision should be made lateral to the angle in order for the medial crura to come together in a tent pole fashion. If the projection needs to be reduced, an incision is made medial to the angle. After the incision is made the lateral cartilage can be thought of as a unipedicle flap. The laterally pedicled flap can be carved and resected.

The next step in the procedure is the one that deserts traditional teaching. The upper half of the

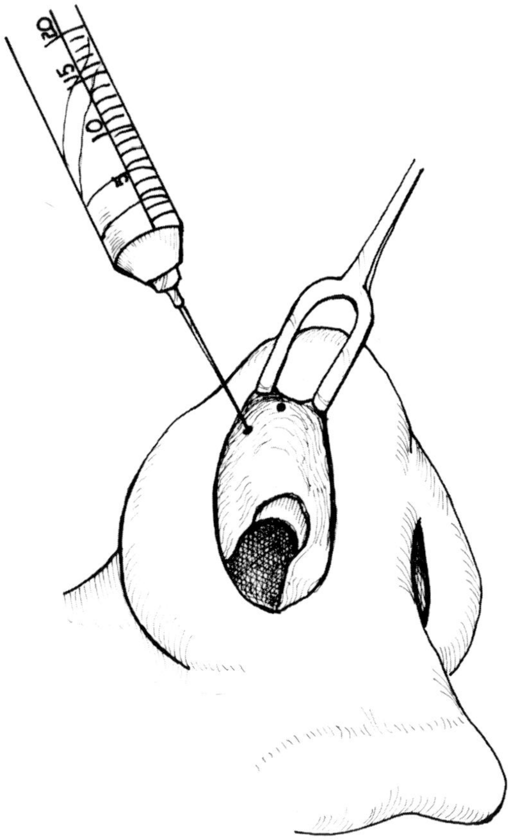

Figure 1.

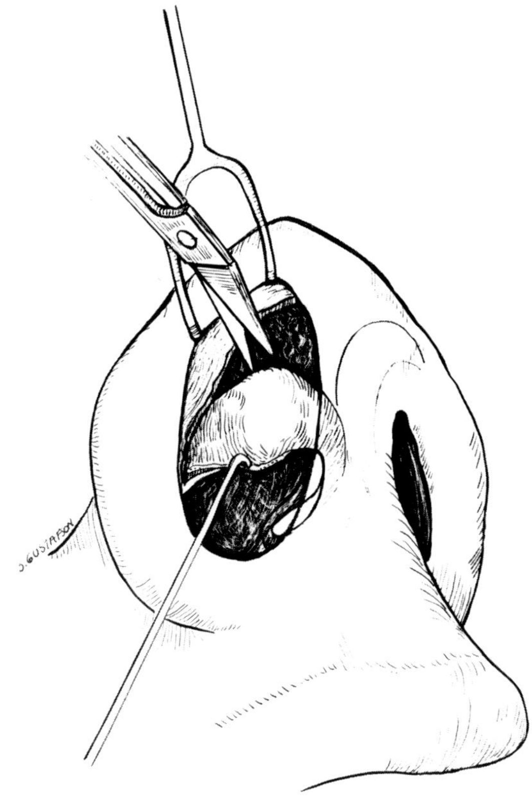

Figure 3.

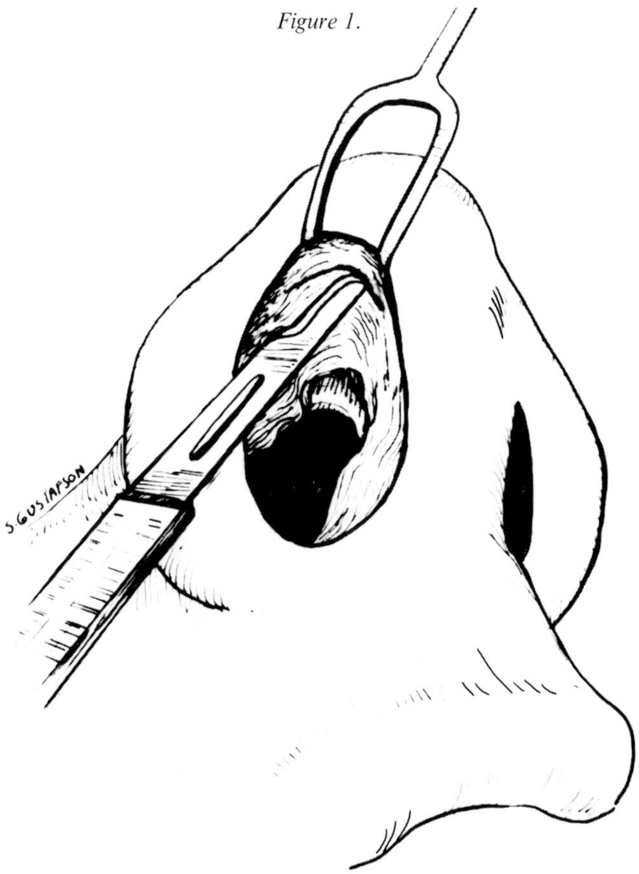

Figure 2.

flap is excised and discarded including both vestibular mucosa and cartilage (Fig. 5). In the "sandwich" analogy it could be said that the upper slice of bread is removed.

After this step, the remaining flap is furrowed as suggested by Lipsett in order to reduce its projection (Fig. 6). These cuts are made through the cartilage, but not through the vestibular mucosa. The furrowed flap is the meat portion of our sandwich. An attempt is then made to return the flap to its normal position in the nose. Many times excision of a small amount of cartilage and mucosa at the medial end of the flap must be performed in order for the flap to fit smoothly into the vestibule (Fig. 7).

The next step is suturing the furrowed flap to the 0.5 cm alar rim. These two areas must be well aligned and sutured together (Fig. 8).

This procedure provides a well defined nasal tip which appears as a separate entity from the dorsum of the nose. A double break appearance

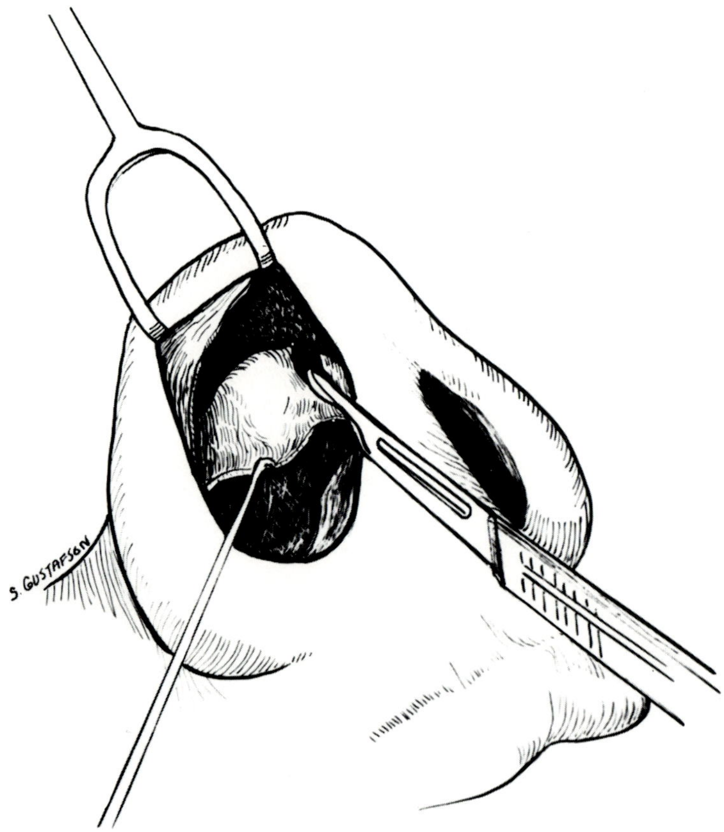

Figure 4.

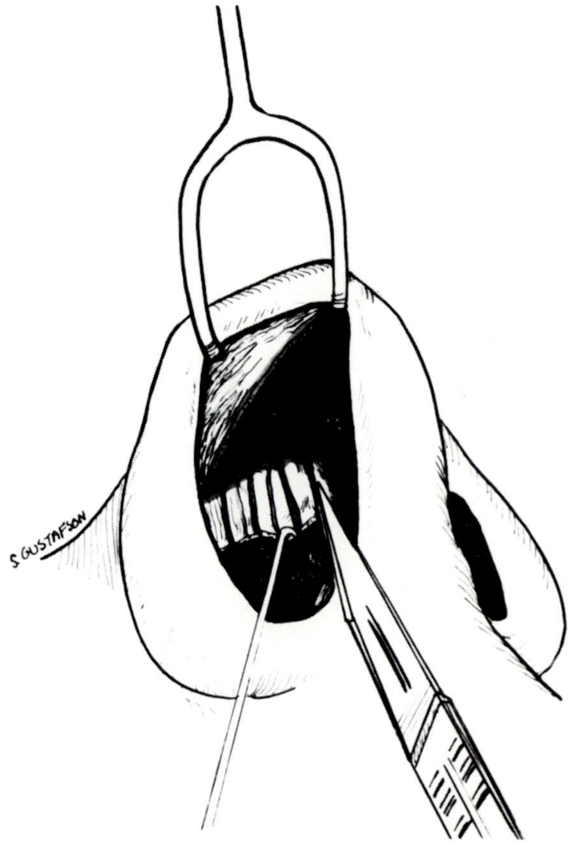

Figure 6.

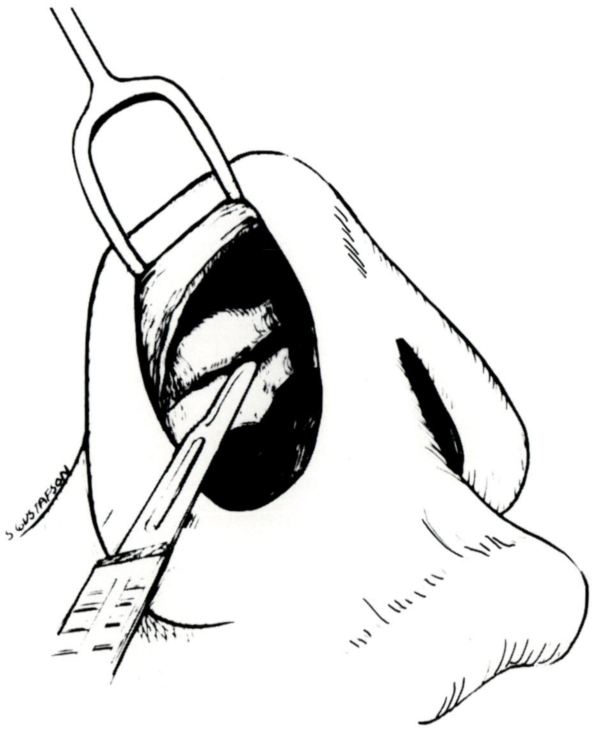

Figure 5.

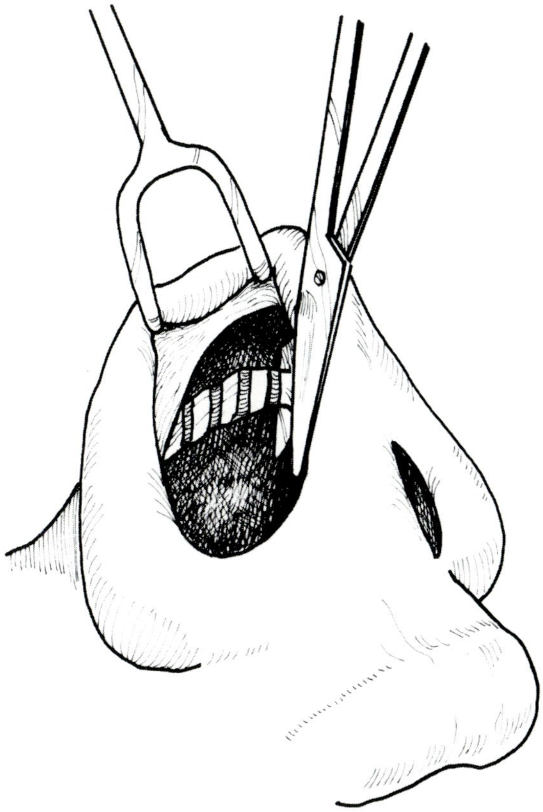

Figure 7.

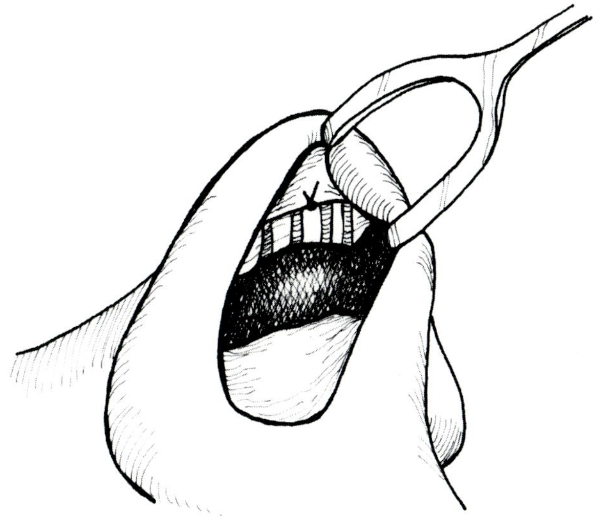

Figure 8.

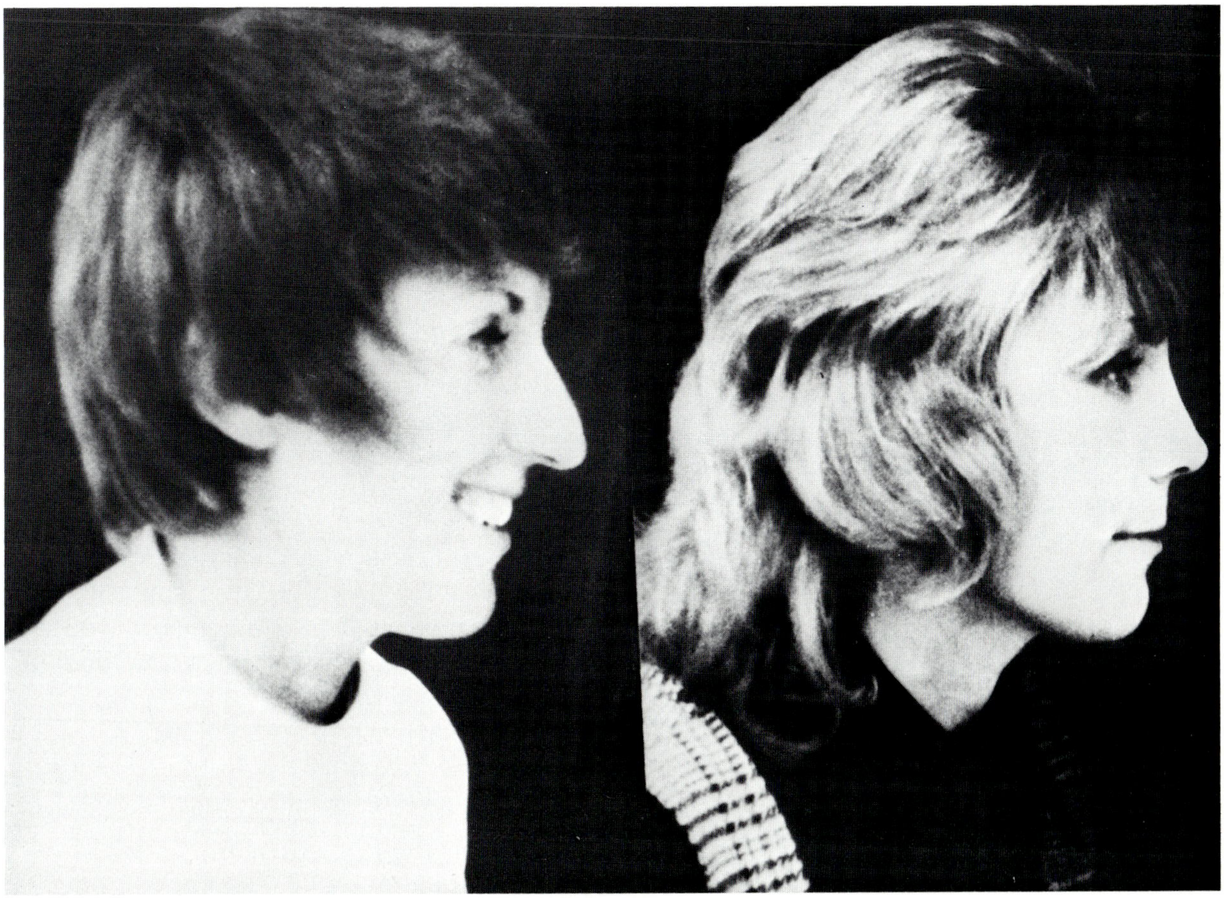

Figure 9.

occurs since the gap of the vestibular mucosa allows for excellent contraction and draping. Three weeks after surgery there is no evidence of any bare or denuded space inside the nose. Scarring, stenosis or valve obstruction has not occurred with this procedure. The noses do not have a pinched appearance. The tip appears to be quite natural with no evidence of surgical intervention.

The "modified rim" technique, as pointed out by Dr. Parkes,[2] prevents alar notching and maintains the subtle sensuous facets of the nasal tip. There appears to be an asymmetry of irregularities. "Modified rim" incision combines all the advantages of the rim incision and cartilage-splitting technique without their inherent disadvantages.

There has not been any problem as to breathing. The nasal valve has not become impaired. A problem did develop when the suture broke and the furrowed flap fell into the vestibule area.

This tip procedure goes against traditional teaching of plastic surgery of the nose. It has always been thought that removing the vestibular mucosa would meet with disaster. I do not believe that this is the case. As in the Fiddler, maybe one can find happiness for both himself and the patient when he defies tradition by using this procedure on the bulbous tip (Fig. 9).

References

1. Lipsett EM: A new approach to surgery of the lower cartilaginous vault, Arch Otolaryngol 70:42, 1959
2. Parkes ML: Current concepts of rhinoplasty, Plastic And Reconstructive Surgery of the Face and Neck, Vol 1, Grune and Stratton, New York, 1972

Epistaxis After Rhinoplasty—Its Prevention

Ralph L. Dicker and Victor R. Syracuse, New York, N.Y.

Introduction

The rhinoplastic surgeon who performs many rhinoplasties will eventually encounter postoperative nasal hemorrhage. The scope of this presentation is to consider the prevention or avoidance of this annoying and, at times, dangerous complication.

Prevention of postoperative bleeding may be divided chronologically into five phases:

1. preventive preoperative preparation—history, physical examination, and laboratory screening tests;
2. preventive surgical techniques;
3. preventive outer nasal dressings;
4. preventive inner nasal dressings;
5. preventive postoperative management.

Preventive Preoperative Preparation

Screening History

A personal history to evaluate hemostasis in adult patients should answer these questions: (1) Have you had any blood diseases, anemias, leukemias? (2) Any bleeding from mucous membranes? (3) How often do you notice a new bruise on your body? What is the largest bruise that you have developed, following such minor injury, that you did not recall the injury until after you saw the bruise? Do you develop bruises at sites of immunization or injection of drugs? (4) Any abnormal bleeding from minor or major injuries or operations, e.g., late bleeding after the 3rd postoperative day? Has bleeding after dental extraction lasted longer than 24 hr or recurred after 3 or 4 days? (5) Have you had any transfusions? (6) Do you have excessive or prolonged menstrual bleeding? (7) What drugs are you taking? Aspirin, heparin and coumarin interfere with blood clotting. (8) Is there a family history of hemophilia? The hemophilias are the most common hereditary bleeding disorders in the United States. Therefore, a history of abnormal bleeding in a male member on the maternal side of the family deserves particular attention.

Physical Examination

1. Blood pressure.
2. Look for petechiae[2] and ecchymosis particularly on the lower legs and ankles. Petechiae offer evidence of increased vascular fragility secondary to thrombocytopenia.
3. After ascertaining the blood pressure, the same instrument performs the "Hess Test," widely used to measure capillary resistance or fragility of the walls of small vessels under pressure. The cuff pressure is maintained between systolic and diastolic, at no more than 100 cm of mercury for 5 min. If a circle drawn 2.5 cm in diameter on the flexor surface of the forearm, below the bend of the elbow, contains more than 5 petechiae, 5 min after releasing pressure, the result is recorded as positive. This test is suggestive of capillary fragility.
4. Capillary fragility test using a petechiometer (Fig. 1) may be substituted for the Hess Test.
5. Small body scars are discussed as to how the lacerations occurred and how long they bled.
6. Abnormal elasticity of the skin and hyperextensibility of the joints are evidence of hereditary connective tissue disorders associated with vascular bleeding.
7. Look for evidences of hereditary telangiectasia and stigmata of chronic liver disease: spider angiomas, liver palms, dilated abdominal veins, enlarged liver, and spleen.
8. The nose is examined to exclude extranasal or intranasal processes which predispose to bleeding, such as angiomas, ulcers, or polyps.

Laboratory Screening Tests[3]: Platelets (Fig. 2)

The role of platelets[4] or thrombocytes in hemostasis or blood coagulation is of *vital* importance. They are needed numerically to form hemostatic plugs and qualitatively to provide factor No. 3 (thromboplastin) for intrinsic clotting. If the history and physical examination are completely negative, after the routine complete blood and differential cell count, only one additional laboratory test is really needed, namely, a review of a well-made and well-stained peripheral blood film to assure that adequate numbers of platelets are present. Oil immersion fields in which RBC are just touching should contain 3 to 10 platelets and small clumps of platelets (a result of beginning aggregation that should be seen in many fields).

Variations in platelet morphology must be noted and evaluated: larger platelets suggest increased or abnormal production. The most common platelet abnormality is thrombocytopenia. An excess of platelets (thrombocytosis) can also result in bleeding though less often. Patients with the highest platelet counts, e.g., 1,000,000 per cubic millimeter usually bleed the most. When platelets appear reduced on the film, if the technician does not have the experience to make a rapid estimate, the electronic platelet counter should be used if available. Platelet counting should undoubtedly be used routinely.

There are various drugs that alter the platelet count and morphology of the platelets:

Drugs Which Cause Decreased Production of Platelets[5] (Thrombocytopenia)

1. Sulfonamides
2. Tolbutamide (Orinase)
3. Chlorthiazide (Diuril)
4. Acetazolamide (Diamox)
5. Chloramphenicol (Chlormycetin)
6. Phenylbutazone (Butazolidin)
7. Mephenytoin (Mesantoin)
8. Gold

Drugs Which Are Associated With Immune Destruction of Platelets (Thrombocytopenia)

1. Sulfisoxazole (Gantrisin)
2. Tolbutamide (Orinase)
3. Chlorthiazide (Diuril)
4. Meprobamate (Miltown)

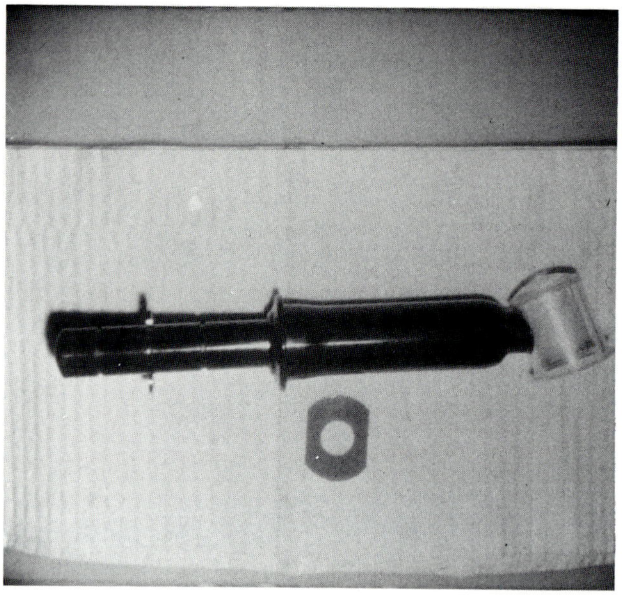

Fig. 1. Capillary resistometer or petechiometer of E.E. Brown, Ashland, Oregon.

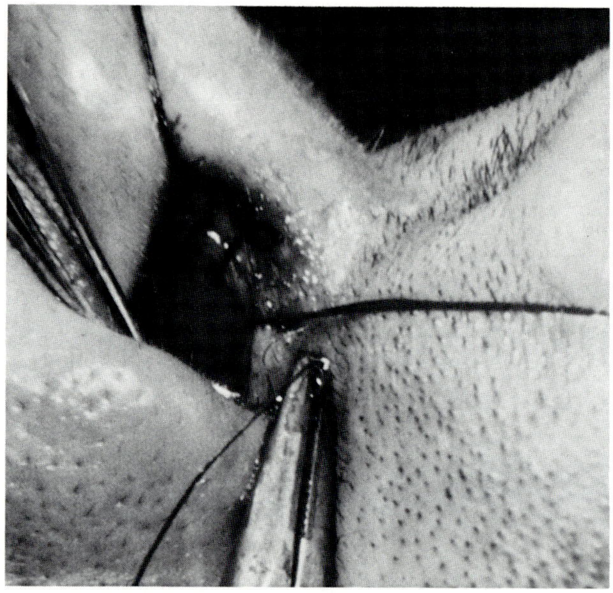

Fig. 3. Approximation of columella to septum with numerous sutures to prevent postoperative bleeding.

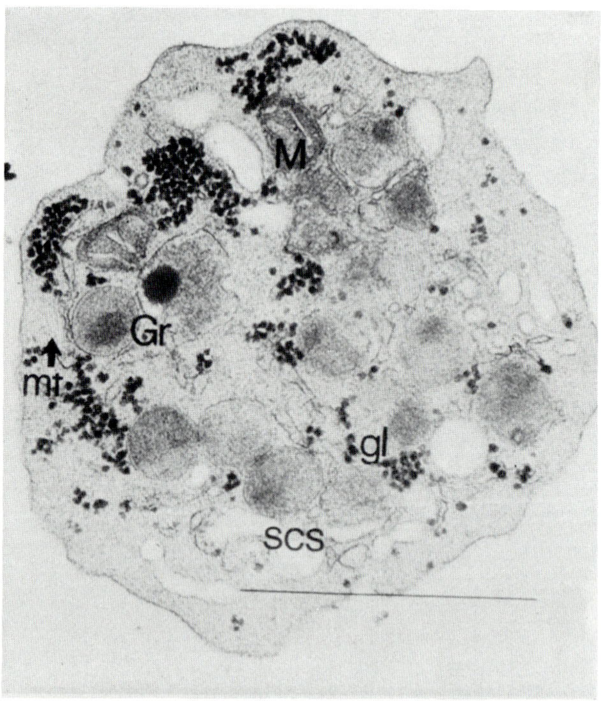

Fig. 2. Electromicrograph of a platelet.

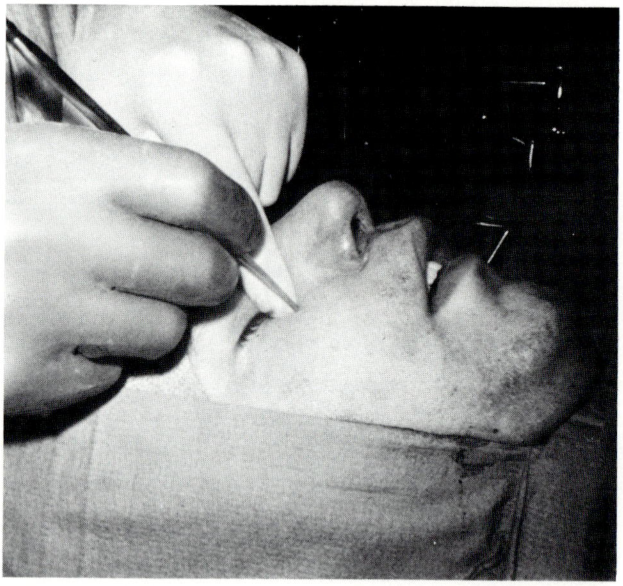

Fig. 4. Site of entrance for external osteotomy with a 3 mm chisel. External osteotomy or infracture with chisel is less traumatic than infracture with use of saw.

5. Digitoxin (Linozin)
6. Quinidine
7. Phenacetin
8. Phenylbutazone (Butazolidin)
9. Gold

Drugs Which Alter Platelet Function

1. Acetylsalicylic Acid (Aspirin)
2. Sulfonpyrazone (Antrin)
3. Diazepram (Valium)
4. Chlordiazepoxide (Librium)
5. Benadryl
6. Dextran
7. Tricyclic Antidepressants
8. Phenothiazines (Thorazine)
9. Dypyridamole (Persantin)

When the platelet count falls from the normal range of 150,000 to 350,000 to about 50,000 per cubic millimeter (thrombocytopenia) a potential bleeding tendency is present; at 20,000 there is a serious bleeding tendency; between 15,000 and 5,000 there is a risk of serious bleeding. When platelets fall below 5,000 per cubic millimeter the patient is in imminent peril of fatal nervous system bleeding and of massive gastrointestinal hemorrhage. Therefore, accurate platelet counts become more important in managing a severely thrombocytopenic patient.

The order of laboratory screening testing is:

1. Complete blood count and blood-film differential count.

2. Platelet count on blood film as previously described.

3. Quick's Prothrombin Time. The normal prothrombin time is 11 to 15 sec. Common causes of a prolonged prothrombin time are vitamin K deficiency, certain liver diseases, specific coagulation deficiencies and coumarin drug therapy.

4. Partial thromboplastin time (PTT). This should replace the popular but inadequate whole blood "clotting time," a test not relegated to medical history. The PTT test measures the *whole* clotting process and is abnormal when any one factor is 30 percent below its normal value. It detects previously undiagnosed hemophilia. The normal values for this tests are 35 to 45 sec. Values of 45 to 50 sec are considered borderline, while results over 50 sec are considered abnormal. It is important to assert that values 2 to 3 sec beyond a laboratory's upper limit of normal cannot be disregarded and requires further study of the case.

5. Fibrinogen level[3]: The Dade Thrombin Method decrees a norm of 200–400 mg percent.

For more substantial confirmation of these screening tests, they should be repeated on a fresh specimen of blood to avoid the risk of false results.

Ideally surgeons and hematology consultants should form a more permanent and continuous working team. Every surgeon, whether he knows it or not, is part hematologist, for he deals with abnormalities of the blood potential or preexisting in every one of his patients.

Preventive Surgical Technique

There should be a 5–10 min waiting period after the local anesthesia (Carbocaine or Xylocaine with adrenalin) is infiltrated into the nasal tissues. The waiting period is helpful in reducing the amount of bleeding when the operative incisions are made. Since bleeding in the first 48 hr is usually from any of the nasal incisions or osteotomies, each operative step is calculated to minimize hemorrhage. Of primary importance after the initial nasal incisions is the elevation of the tissues of the dorsum of the nose very close to the skeleton to avoid the vascular and muscle layer.

Vestibular Sutures (Fig. 3)

Contrary to the usual timing of suturing the columella to the septum *following* the infracture, the authors perform the procedure *before* the external osteotomy and infracture. This step is helpful for early hemostasis to control bleeding up to this stage of the operation. As usual this apposition is accomplished by several interrupted sutures through the thickness of both. However, the authors do not stop here. We find it very valuable to secure still closer coaptation of the right and left vestibular incisions by an adequate number of 5-0 interrupted silk sutures.

Lateral Osteotomy (Fig. 4)

The lateral external osteotomy is performed with mallet and a chisel that has a sharp 3-mm cutting edge, gently penetrating the skin, just lateral to the mid-nasomaxillary groove. The chisel is angled and guided subcutaneously to this groove, penetrating through bone at various points along its course, thus severing the lateral nasal wall along its base, from the remaining process of the maxilla. At this point the infracture of the nasal bones is performed. The small initial wound is closed with one 6-0 silk suture. The authors believe that this method is the least disturbing to the continuity of the tissues involved, least traumatic and, therefore, least likely to give rise to profuse bleeding. There is less bleeding with the infracture after an external osteotmy because the soft tissues are not severed totally as with the use of the Silver chisels or saws.

Sources of Postoperative Rhinoplastic Hemorrhage[6] (Fig. 5)

1. Bleeding from the septum, usually anterior and inferior, or Kisselbach's area is due to severance of the branches of the nasopalatine artery, inferior labial artery, and descending palatine artery.
2. Bleeding arising from between the upper and lower lateral cartilages is due to severance of the branches of the infraorbital artery, the orbital branches of the internal maxillary artery, and the lateral nasal branches of the external maxillary artery (facial).
3. Oozing of blood around the pyriform opening is due to severance of the alar branches of the external maxillary artery.

Preventive Outer Nasal Dressings[7,8]

External Pressure Dressings—Suspension Dressings

When the combined surgical procedures of a reduction rhinoplasty have been accomplished and all free or excised tissue fragments at the dorsal space have been meticulously extracted with the rasp (debridment), the operation is still unfinished without the ultimate proper dressings. These are imperative to prevent crowding of unattached structures, dead spaces, formation of bird-beak deformities and for hemostasis. These are an admixture of outer pressure and suspension dressings combined with vestibular packing that exerts gentle counter pressure from within.

Preliminary cleansing of the skin and application of tincture of benzoin compound will favor firmer adhesion of outer dressings for which we favor 0.5 in. micropore paper tape.

Preventive Inner Nasal Packings

Initial packing is removed from each fossa. Blood clots are removed by gentle suction. With a bayonet forceps, a folded and flattened "cigarette" packing of xeroform gauze 0.25 × 4 in. is placed in each anterior nasal fossa, in the anterior olfactory fissure, just beneath the dorsum. This must be done gently without separating the upper lateral cartilages from the septum—a mere apposition. These are intended to prevent hemorrhage and adhesions from this region. Then from a 14-gauge French rubber catheter a 6 in. section is removed. One such tube is inserted in each nasal fossa having a 0.75 in. protrusion from the nares (Fig. 6).

A 0.5 in. wide xeroform vaseline strip of gauze is packed fairly snugly around each tube to fill the anterior nasal fossa and vestibule. Lastly, the operator squeezes the lobule between the thumb and index finger of each hand to rotate the lobules upward and to mold the packing more firmly in the vestibule.

The floor nurse is instructed to keep these tubes clear by injecting through them several cubic centimeters of sterile physiologic saline. This makes swallowing more comfortable. A moustache of rolled dry gauze is then fixed over the nostrils, below and above the projecting tubes to absorb seepage.

Preventive Postoperative Management

The written postoperative orders are as follows:

1. Head elevated 14 in.
2. Continuous iced compresses to the eyes.
3. Light diet today, regular diet tomorrow.
4. Analgesic p.o. (without aspirin)—Darvon Plain 65
5. Synkavite 2 cc (75 mg) b.i.d. I.M. for 2 days

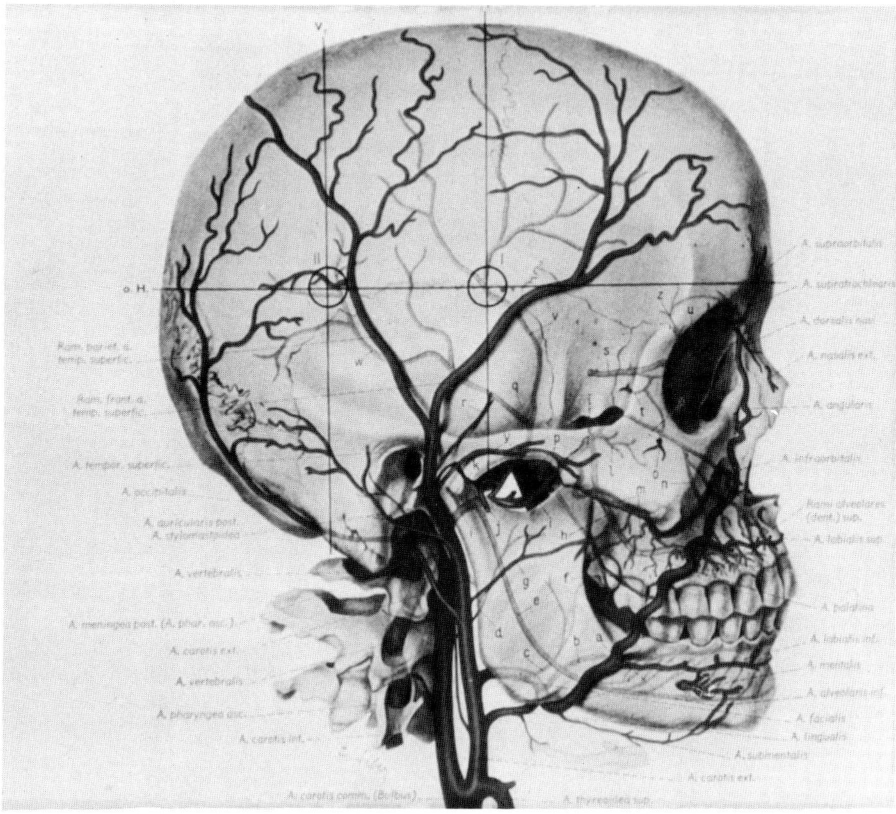

Fig. 5. Semischematic representation of the large arteries of the head: Sources of postoperative rhinoplasty hemorrhage.

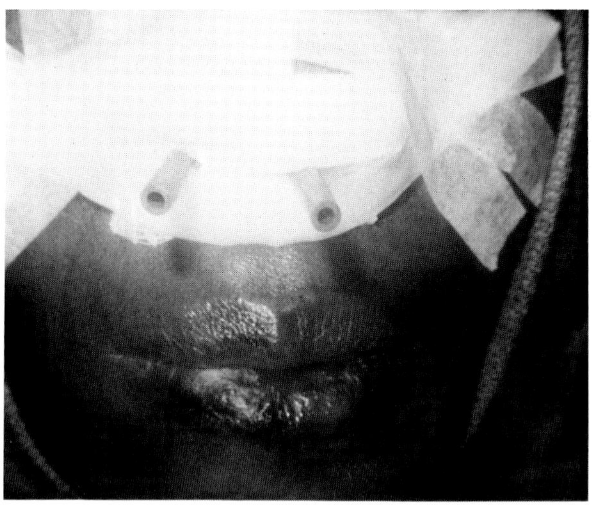

Fig. 6. French no. 14 Catheters, 6 in. Section inserted into nasal passages for easier swallowing and more effective intranasal packing. This aids in prevention of postoperative bleeding.

6. Penicillin -C I.M. or oxy-tetracycline p.o. in adequate dosage for 10 days.
7. Chymoral (100,000 units) İİ tab., q.i.d., p.o. for 3 days.
8. BRP tomorrow.
9. Two cc of sterile physiologic saline injected through nasal catheters q.i.d. to keep them open.
10. Thera-combex with ascorbic acid 500 mg, b.i.d., p.o. during convalescence.
11. Benadryl 50 mg, b.i.d., for 3 days
12. Fluid Extract Cascara Sagrada Aromatica, 2 drams by mouth the following evening.

Patient remains in the hospital on an average of three whole days and continues his hospital medications at home for three to four days. On the second postoperative day packings and tubes are gently teased out and removed from the nasal fossae. On the 4th or 5th day, look for xeroform cigarette packing in the roof of the nasal fossae under the dorsum. These can be removed gently or allowed to fall away naturally. If the cigarette packings are not removed or have not become sufficiently loosened to extrude themselves after 5 days, loosen them gently to remove them.

Summary

Ordinary prudence suggests avoidance of postoperative hemorrhage after rhinoplastic surgery. It will alarm even a confident patient and the family who sense the obvious concern of the surgeon. It may also jeopardize the final cosmetic result. Therefore, in the first place, the best insurance against an unexpected bleeder going to surgery is adequate preoperative screening.

To summarize:

1. Adequate history and physical examination.
2. Adequate hematological screening.
3. Approximating with numerous 4-0 black silk sutures columella to caudal septum.
4. External lateral osteotomy for infracture.
5. "Cigarette" packing in the olfactory airway under the dorsum.
6. Adequate external dressing.
7. Firm vestibular packing.
8. Suitable medications to promote coagulation.

All contribute to better hemostasis in the prevention of postoperative bleeding.

References

1. Rapaport SI: Introduction to hematology (Harper & Row), New York, NY, 1971, p 315, Feb. 25, "Electron Micrograph of a Platelet" (Courtesy of Joseph Goodman, Veterans Administration Hospital, San Francisco, California.)
2. Brown EE: Evaluation of a new capillary resistometer: The petechiometer. J Lab Clin Med, St. Louis, 34:12, pp 1714–1717, 1949
3. Laufman H, Erichson RB: Hematological problems in surgery, Philadelphia, W.B. Saunders Co., 1970, pp 53–62
4. Nour-Eldin F: Blood coagulation simplified, 2n ed, London, Butterworth & Co., 1971, pp 82–85
5. Sharkey I, Brughera-Jones A: Evaluation of potential bleeding problems in dermatologic surgery, J Dermatologic Surgery, 1:41–44, 1975
6. Pernkoph E: Atlas of topographical and applied human anatomy, Volume I, Head and Neck, p 22, Feb. 22, "Semi-schematic Representation of the Large Arteries of the Head." Philadelphia, W.B. Saunders, 1963
7. Parkes M et al: Rhinoplastic Dressings. EENT Monthly 52:5, 1973, pp 166–170
8. Smith, TW: A Rhinoplastic Dressing Pad, EENT Monthly 46:635–648, 1962

When to Stop in Rhinoplasty

Jacob S. Aronoff, New York, N.Y.

In my early years of rhinoplasty, errors in technique were not unusual, e.g., too great a reduction in profile, comminution of nasal bones, or a niche in the nares from a poorly executed rim incision. However, many of the bad results of those years stemmed only from poor judgment in attempting to do too much to achieve perfection. I still see the same judgment errors being made by residents and younger surgeons. Sam Fomon stated it well—"the operation starts the night before in your office."

Before proceeding to the factors that should make one stop during the operation, I shall briefly discuss those that should make one cancel or, at least, delay the surgery.

Psychiatric Status of the Patient

This is a most basic factor in evaluation. It has been discussed frequently.[1–3] Suffice it to say, we are not only aiming for a beautiful nose, but for a happy patient—and the latter does not necessarily result from the successful anatomic result.

Psychosomatic or Vasomotor Nose

The stabilization of the vasomotor process prior to surgery will diminish both the operative bleeding and the amount and duration of the post-operative reaction. My chief reliance is on a rotation trial of the various antihistamines to determine which is the optimum one for the particular patient. Results in over 12,000 patients have shown that no single antihistamine works in more than 28 percent of patients. However, by means of a rotation, almost 80 percent of patients can be stabilized.[4–6]

Physical Immaturity of the Nose

This is obviously a reason for delaying the rhinoplasty. The question can be determined by the relationship of bony and cartilaginous components of the nose. The usual percentage would be 35 to 40 percent bony profile and 60 to 65 percent cartilaginous profile. Any significant diminution of the bony portion would be good reason for delay of the operation.

Revision of Rhinoplasty

This is an important part of the specialty. One must remember to delay the surgery until the healing process is complete. The lobule should be soft and supple, and it should be easy to roll the skin over the underlying cartilaginous and bony framework (Figs. 1 and 2). One can expect the patient to be impatient, but not the surgeon. Gillies and Millard stated it well—"never do today what can honorably be put off till tomorrow".[7,8]

Poor Rapport with the Patient

No comment is required on this point in elective sugery such as rhinoplasty or other aesthetic surgery. We shall now consider the reasons for limiting the amount of surgery.

Poor Tissues

Poor tissues, i.e., thick skin and thin, soft cartilage. These findings might militate against any surgery on the lower alar cartilage, but not against changes in the bony pyramid (Fig. 3).

Normal or Excessive Naso-Labial Angle

Here the transfixion should be partial, i.e., carried down only 40 to 50 percent of the usual distance in order to minimize the amount of scarring and retraction that would further increase the angle (Fig. 4).

Relationship of Upper Alar Cartilages to Septum

If profile correction need not be too great, then upper alar cartilages do not have to be separated from the septum. This prevents the need for the traditional amputation of these cartilages and preserves the major nasal valve and respiratory efficiency. However, if the profile correction is considerable, the preservation of the attachments to the septum becomes impossible.

Combination of Short Columella and Dependent Tip

The coexistence of these two findings results in a higher than normal frequency of a "polly beak" deformity. I would advise limiting the degree of change in the nasolabial angle and discussion of this limitation with the patient before surgery (Fig. 5).

Projecting Tip

It is imperative that this pathology be corrected before any profile changes are made. After the projection has been reduced by appropriate resection of the lower lateral cartilages, inferior spine, etc. only then can profile reduction be done. The latter reduction may very frequently be limited because the tip projection cannot be fully corrected (Fig. 6).

Asymmetry of Alae

Many noses reveal differences between right and left alae as regards their level and angle of insertion into the face.[9] This is usually not noticed before surgery by the patient—only after the operation. The surgical correction is a classic example of "search for perfection" which cannot be obtained. It is preferable to point out this asymmetry before the operation and then avoid it (Fig. 7).

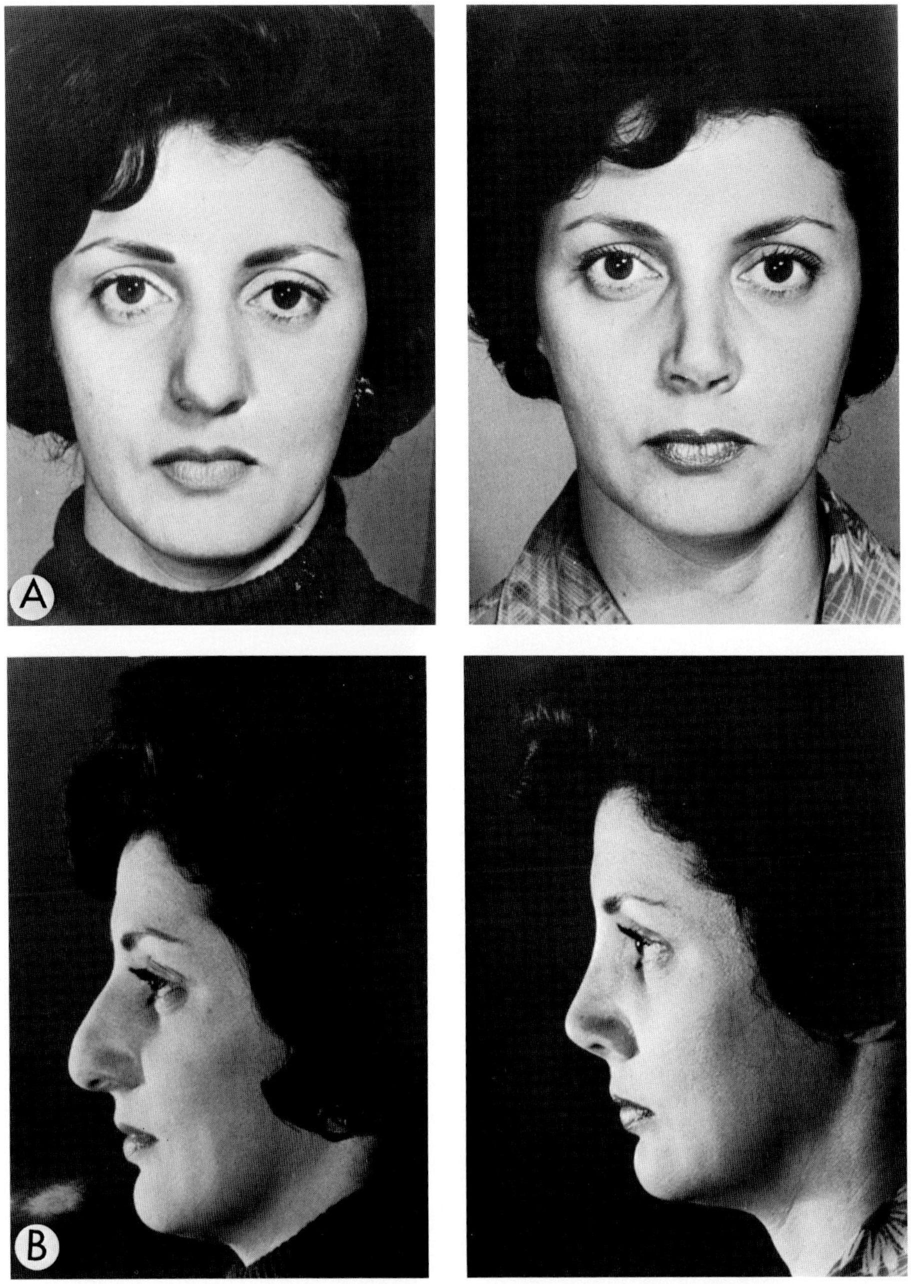

Fig. 1. *Rhinoplasty was followed by severe, persistent swelling despite intensive therapy with antihistamines and steroids. Revision one year later revealed much scarring in both lobule and profile areas. The result could possibly have been improved by further delay of the revision surgery.*

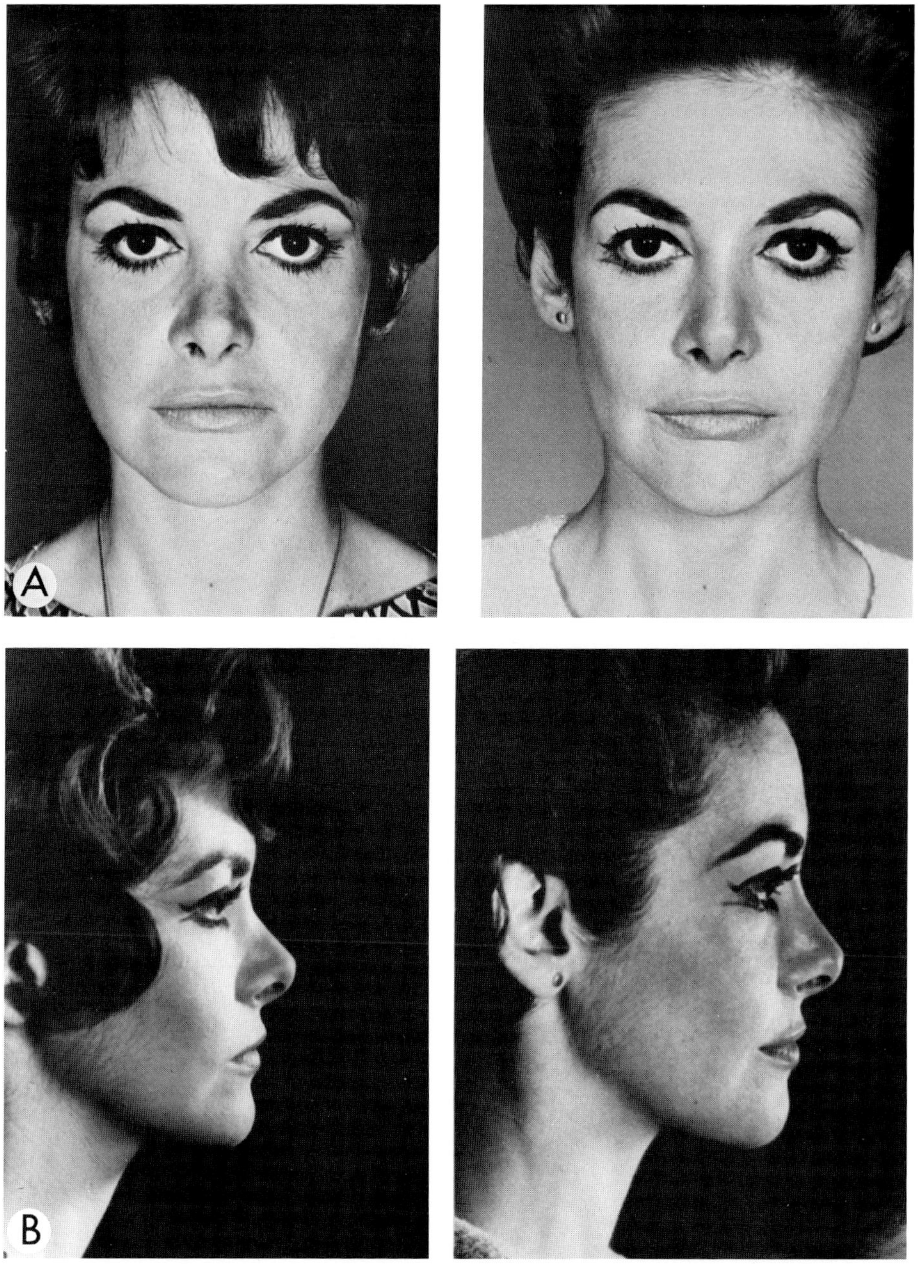

Fig. 2. Rhinoplasty 19 years previously had resulted in partial loss of the right nasal bone and localized saddling. Correction of the deformity was accomplished by three injections of 0.2 cc of silicone fluid 360 at two week intervals.

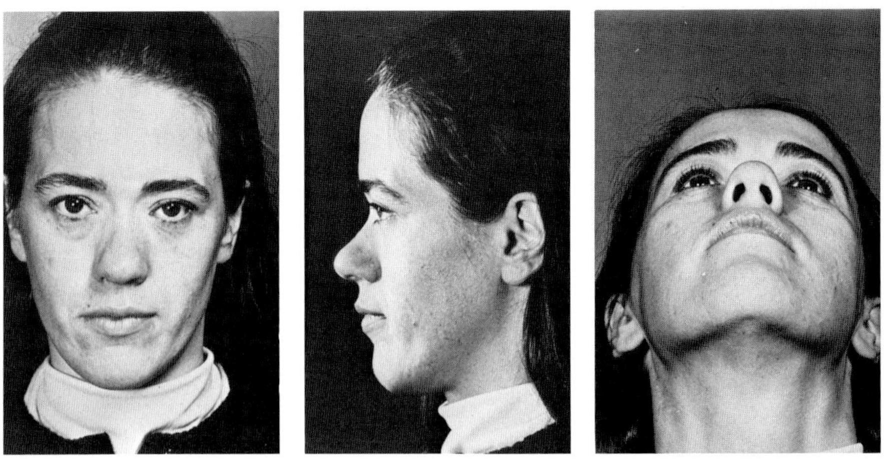

Fig. 3. The thick skin and atrophic cartilage of the lobule prevent the possibility of significant improvement.

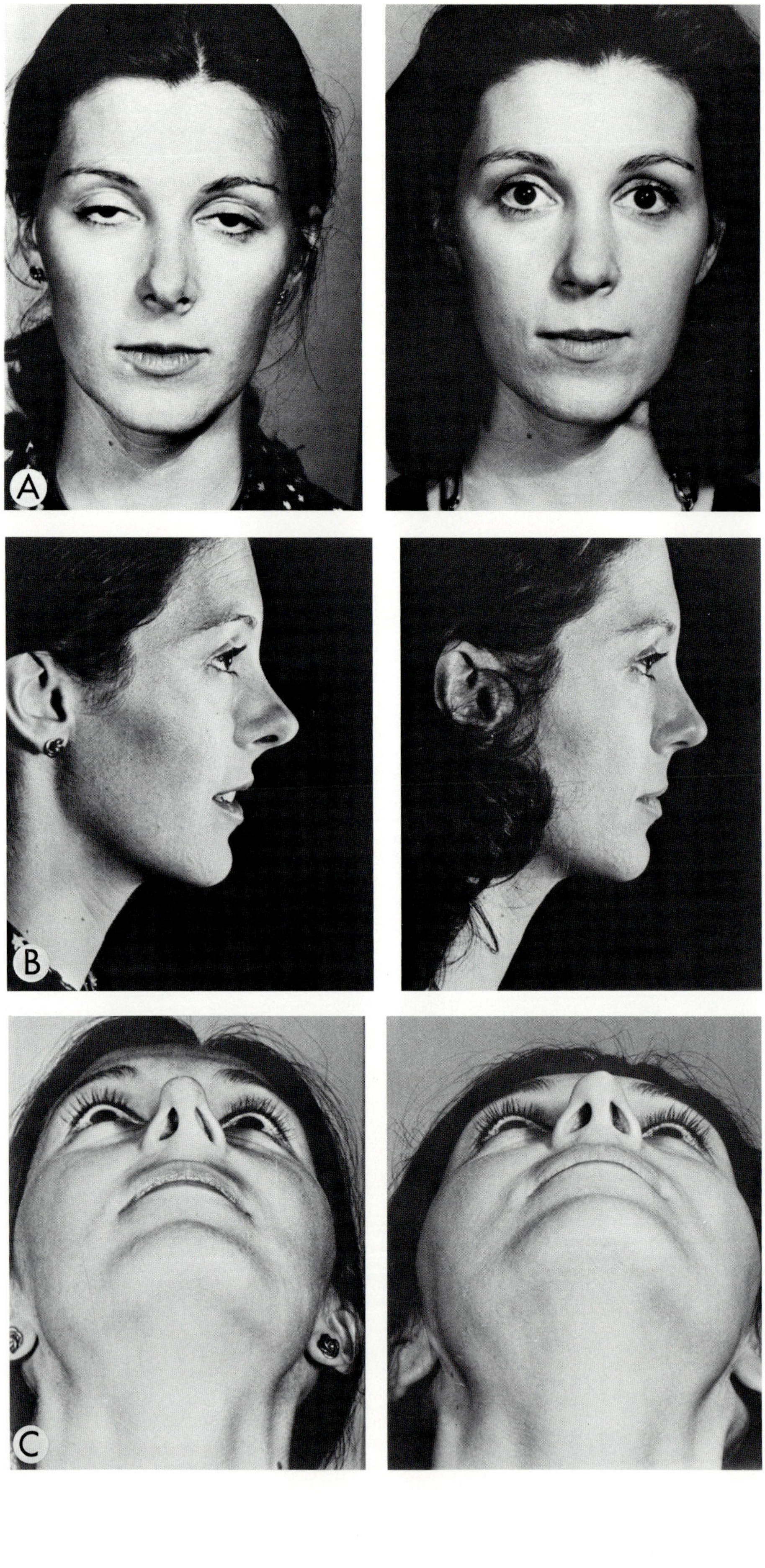

Fig. 4. The original rhinoplasty effected a good result. Nasal trauma eleven years later resulted in significant deformities of nose and septum. To prevent any change in the nasolabial angle, a partial transfixion incision was used for the revision procedure.

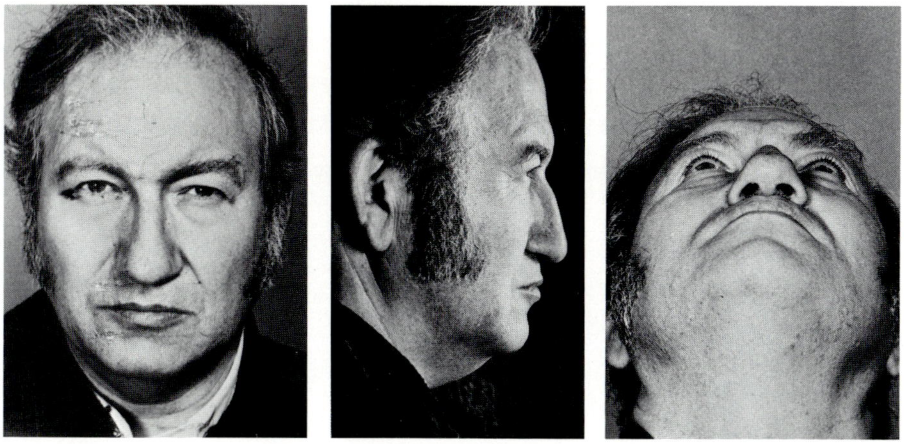

Fig. 5. This patient required septal surgery. However, the nasolabial angle was only partially corrected. A polyethylene strut was also inserted into the columella to diminish local "stress" and the possibility of a "polly beak" deformity. The surgery was therefore limited largely to improving respiratory function and minimally for cosmetic reasons.

Wide Alae

The Weir procedure or vestibule resections should be limited or avoided if the patient has wide, high cheekbones, i.e., increased transverse diameter of the face.

Deviated Septum

When the deflection is severe and, especially, if it involves septum close to the profile line or anterior to the insertion of the upper alar cartilages, I would advocate a two stage procedure. The first operation should be confined to correcting the septal pathology. The septal surgery is done with a minimal amount of resection. The use of the Rubin septal morselizer is helpful. With a six to eight week interval, any changes in the profile and columella should be apparent and therefore permit a better evaluation of the changes required for the second stage rhinoplasty. Another reason for two stage surgery is that the intranasal packing required in the septal surgery could interfere with optimum results in rhinoplasty. Intranasal packing in rhinoplasty is best confined to the vestibules and only for a 24 hr period.

Profile Implants

The extent of the intercartilaginous incision should be limited to the size of the implant. The area of soft tissue elevation in the profile area should also be similarly limited to prevent mobility of the implant, regardless of the type of material used.

Rhinoplasty in Older Patients

There are two nasal findings that contribute to the aged appearance, i.e., dependency of the tip and hypertrophy of the lobule. Therefore, the rhinoplasty in older patients can be frequently confined to these problems, if the bony pyramid pathology is not too prominent. This applies especially where the rhinoplasty is being performed as an adjunct to eyelid and face lift surgery.[10]

With all the points mentioned in this paper, I would take the liberty of paraphrasing Fomon's dictum to "the operation begins when the patient first enters your office." Parkes stated it succinctly: "perfection is the enemy of good" (Figs. 8 and 9).

Summary

Five reasons for cancelling or delaying rhinoplasty are discussed.

Ten physical findings that should make the surgeon limit the extent of his rhinoplasty are also discussed.

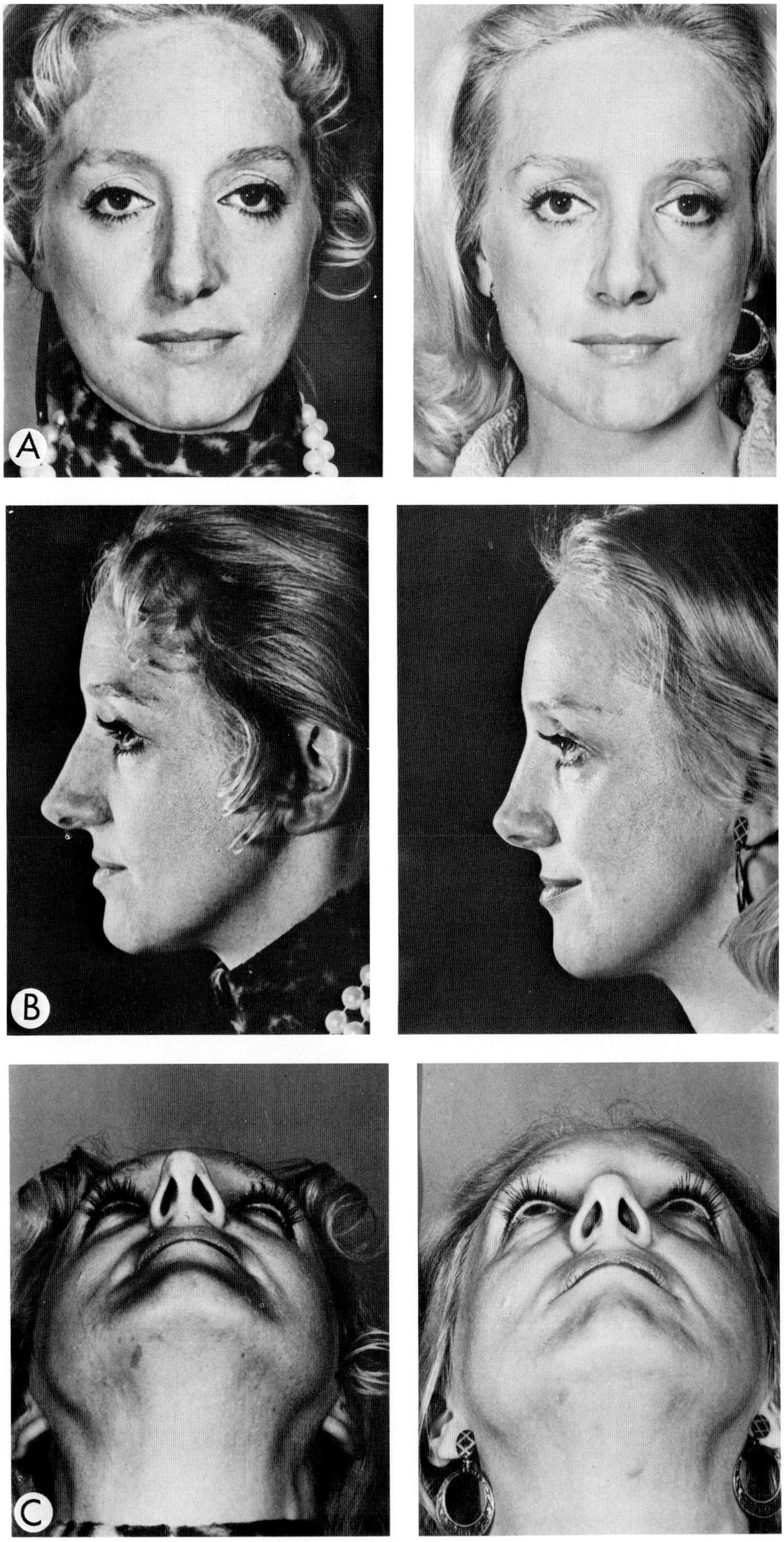

Fig. 6. Correction of the projecting tip in this case was facilitated by the excellent quality of the lower alar cartilages. This allowed for significant reduction of the tip projection and, therefore, also for the profile projection.

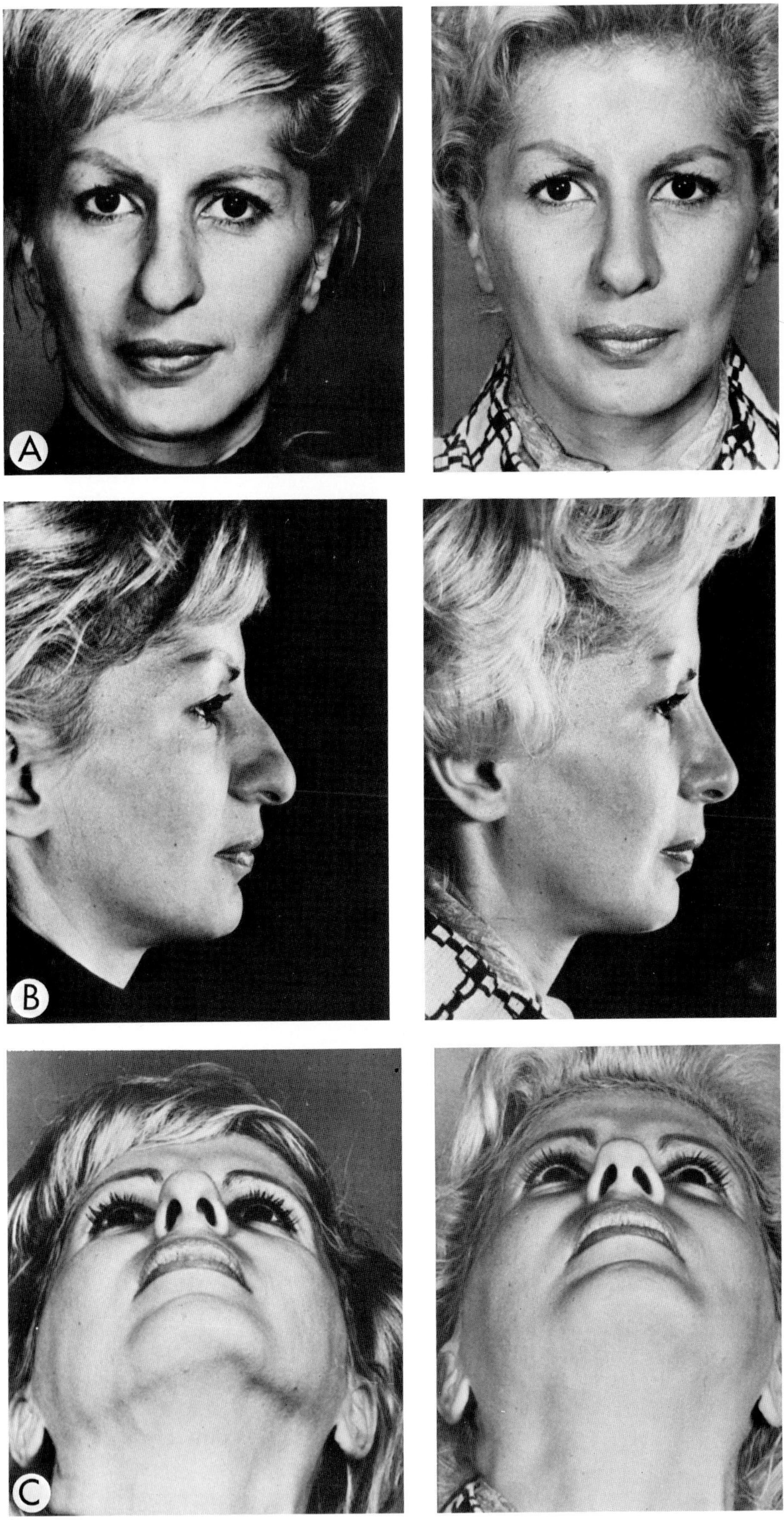

Fig. 7. Alar asymmetry in this patient was increased by an unresolved Bell's palsy. Rhinoplasty was confined to correcting the other considerable nasal deformities.

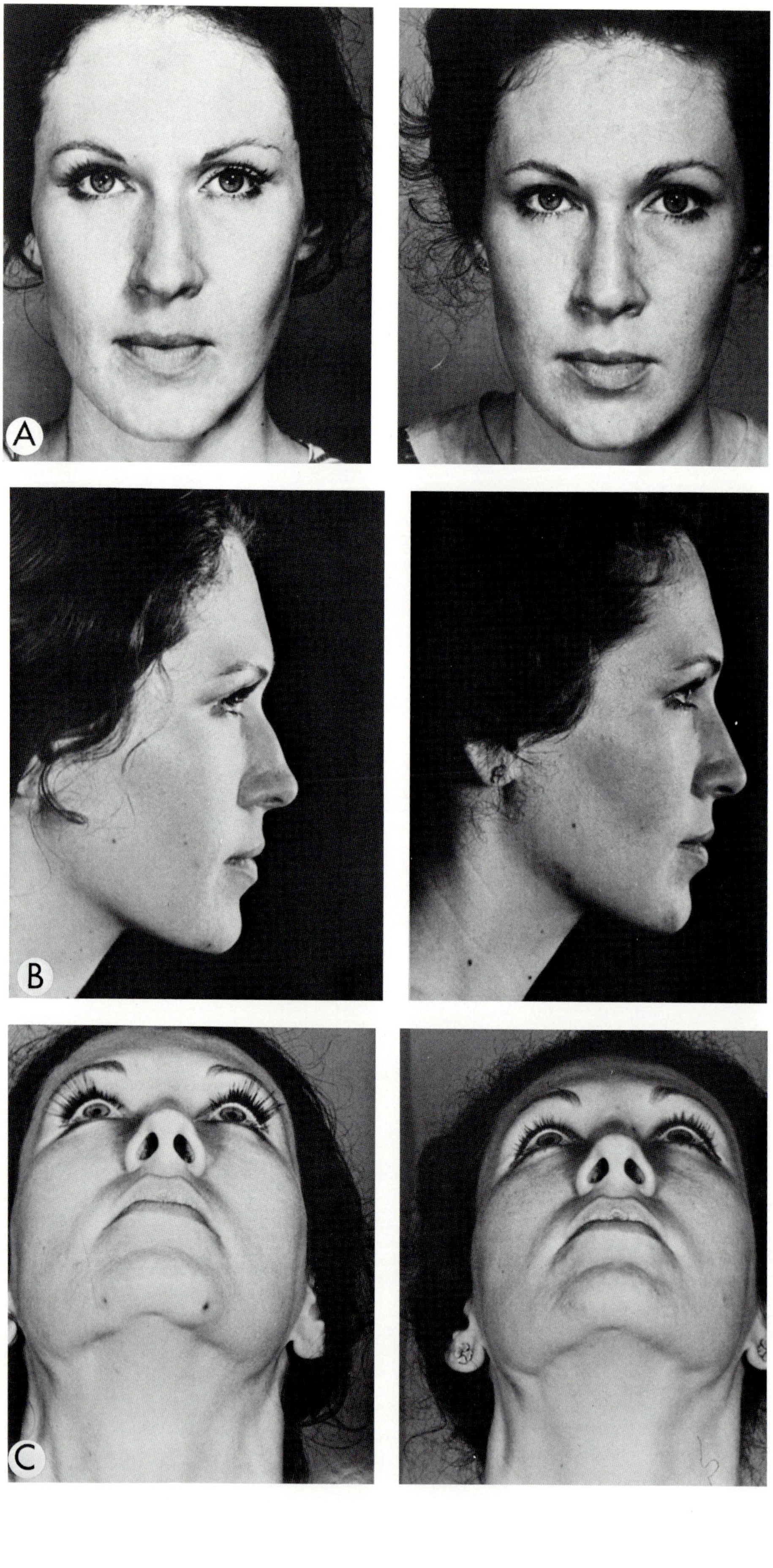

Fig. 8. This patient is very tall and no shortening was done. The upper alar cartilages were not cut. The minimal change in the profile was performed with rasps.

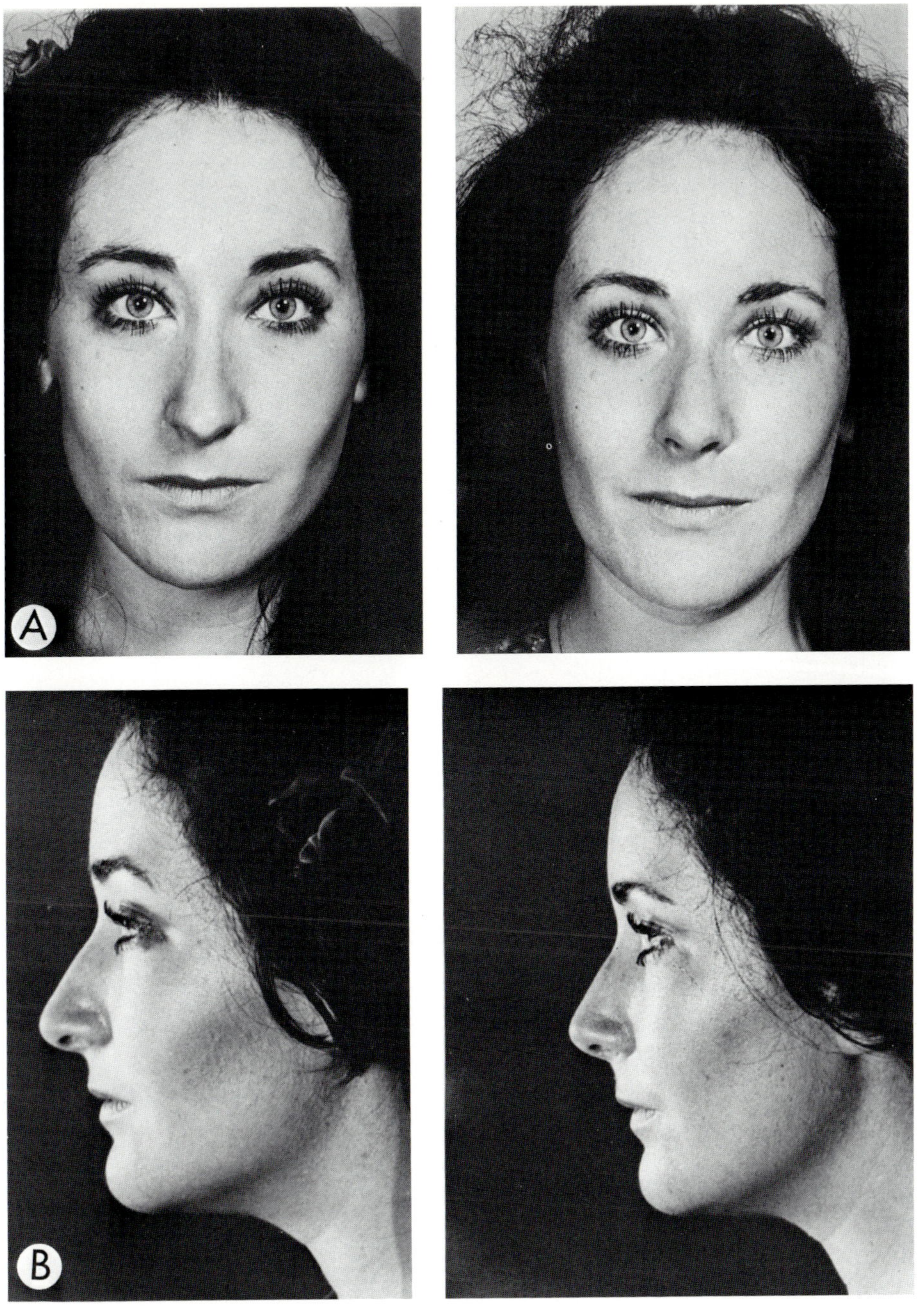

Fig. 9. Rhinoplasty in this case was conservative and limited largely to the lobule. The upper alar cartilages were not separated from the septum nor were any osteotomies performed.

References

1. Linn L: Psychiatric aspects of plastic surgery, Chap 6, Psychology of physical illness, New York, Grune and Stratton, 1952
2. Schilder P: The image and appearance of the human body. Psyche Monographs #4. London, Kegan, Paul, French, Trubner and Co., 1935
3. Aronoff JS: Psychological aspects of facial plastic surgery, Transactions of the 1st International Conference of Facial Plastic Surgery, NY, Aug 1970
4. Aronoff JS: Psychosomatic aspects of otolaryngology, Trans Int Congr Otolaryngol, Aug 1961, Paris
5. Aronoff JS: The nervous nose in rhinoplasty, Arch Otolaryngol 81:26
6. Aronoff JS: Psychosomatic aspects of rhinoplasty and blepharoplasty, International Society of Aesthetic Plastic Surgery 2nd Conference Jerusalem, June 1973
7. Gillies HD, Millard DR, Jr: The principles and art of plastic surgery, Boston, Little Brown 1957
8. Rogers BO: Chap 20, Rhinoplasty, in Unfavorable results in plastic surgery, edited by Goldwyn RM, Boston, Little, Brown and Co. 1972
9. Gorney M, Harries T: The preoperative and postoperative consideration of natural facial asymmetry, Plast Reconstr Surg 54:187
10. Parkes M: personal communication

Rhinoplasty for the Nasal Deformities

V.P. Sood, New Delhi, India

Otorhinolaryngologists are frequently consulted by patients who have a nasal deformity with or without nasal obstruction. It is not uncommon to see that the mechanical obstruction for the nasal blockage is relieved by surgical intervention and associated external nasal deformity is generally ignored.

An understanding of the anatomical features and structural support of the nose is important in knowing how to manage nasal deformities. Avoidance of injury to the nasal musculature and the preservation of dynamics of the nasal cartilages is an important consideration in nasal surgery.

Nasal deformities may be associated with psychological upsets. At times surgery may not be needed, but instead, the patient requires psychiatric help.

Materials and Methods

Fifty cases have been operated upon in the department of Otorhinolaryngology, All India Institute of Medical Sciences for various types of nasal deformities in the last two and one-half years. The cases were operated under local anesthesia, except those who required removal of the piece of bone from the ilium for the reconstruction of dorsal bridge line.

The correction was done by standard Joseph rhinoplastic approach along with septoplasty as follows.

1. Bilateral intercartilaginous and transfixation incisions.
2. Deskeletalization of the nasal dorsum.
3. Medial and lateral osteotomies.
4. Septoplasty was done in those cases who had deviation of the nasal septum with or without crooked nose. In septoplasty the mucopericondrium was separated from one side only through the transfixation incision. The cartilagenous septum was detached from the bony septum so as to make the cartilagenous septum free in its posterior and inferior attachments. The deviated bony septum was either fractured or partially nibbled. This was followed by swinging door technique as described by Converse.

The upper lateral cartilage was detached from the septal cartilage on each side and trimmed suitably.

The tip was corrected by exposing and trimming the alar cartilage through the alar marginal incision.

In ten cases, crooked nose was corrected (Fig. 1). In eight cases, hump was reduced (Figs. 2, 3).

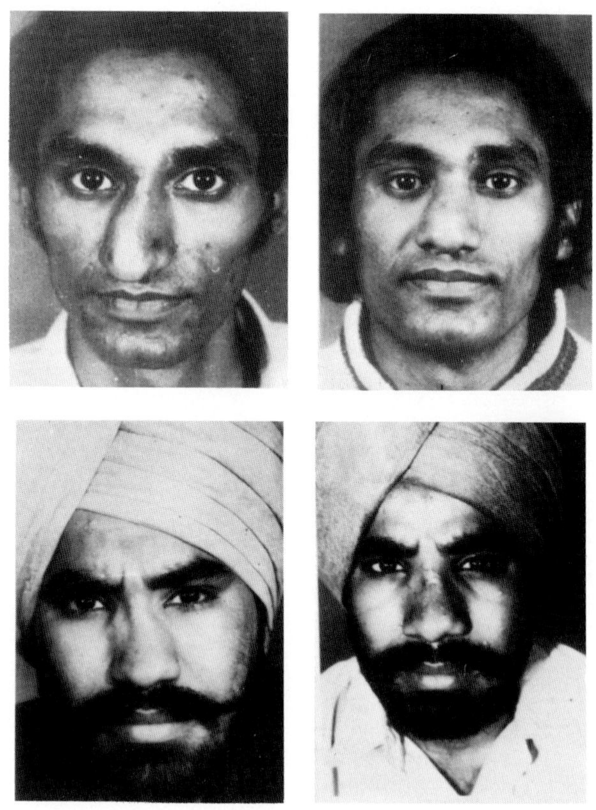

Figure 1.

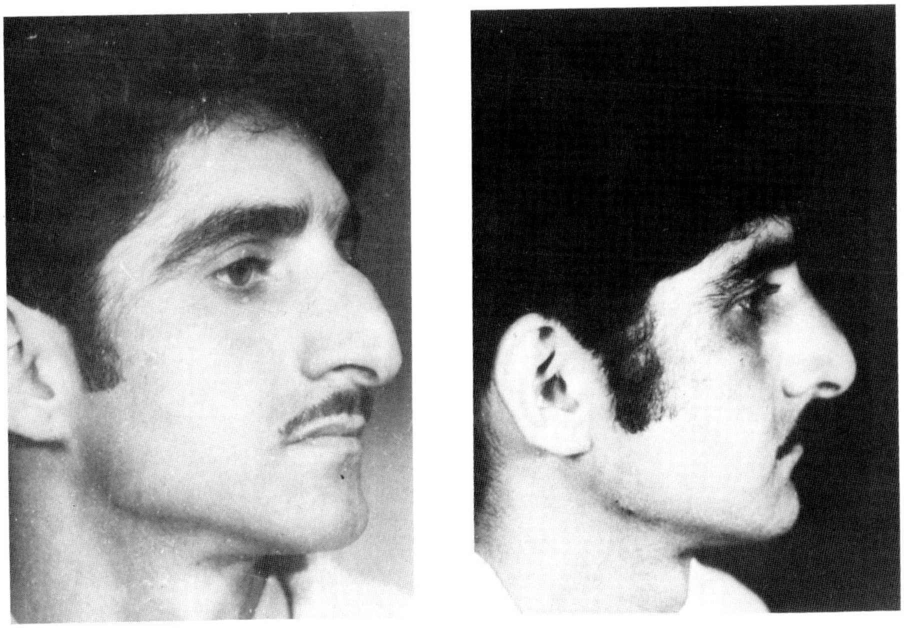

Figure 2.

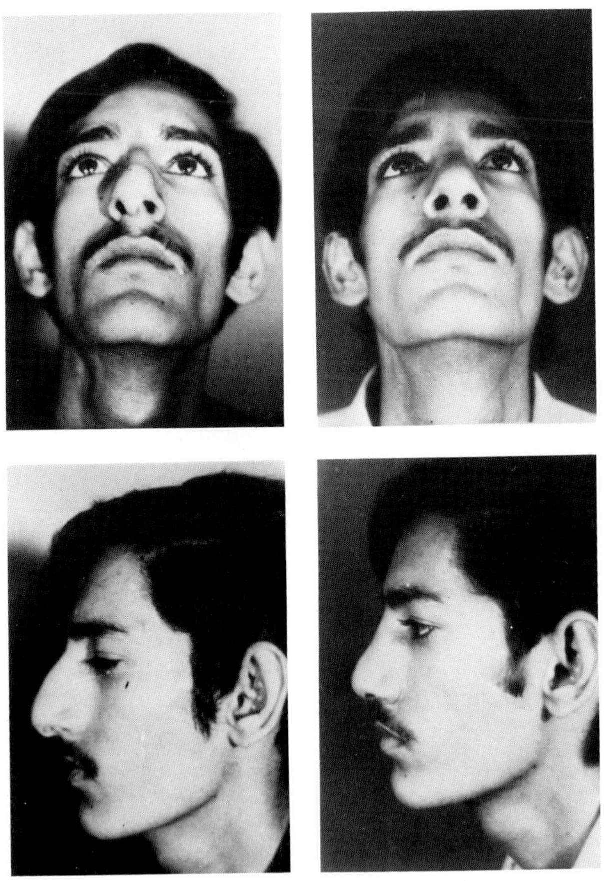

Figure 3.

In twelve cases there was depression of nasal bridge line. One case, in this group, had severe fronto nasal injury with collapse of the nose. The open reduction of the fractures and glabellar reconstruction along with the reconstruction of dorsal bridge line was done in this case.

The grafts were inserted in the dorsal bridge line through the alar marginal incision. In three cases columellar grafts had to be inserted to raise the tip (Fig. 4). In eight cases there was only supratip depression which was corrected by inserting homologous pieces of septal cartilage (Fig. 5). The septal tissues in our operation theatre during septal surgery are not discarded but preserved in 70 percent alcohol for subsequent use in ossiculoplasty and rhinoplasty.

I have found the alar marginal incision better than other types of incisions. The mid-columellar and intercartilaginous incisions were tried earlier and abandoned. These cases could not be followed up hence these are not included in the present series of cases. In mid-columellar incision sometimes scar is apparent. The intracartilaginous approach is good for inserting the graft if the depression is only in the bony part and the nasal tip does not require any lifting. In four cases a tilted nasal tip was corrected by fashioning the alar cartilages by using alar marginal incisions, (Fig. 6). Two of these cases

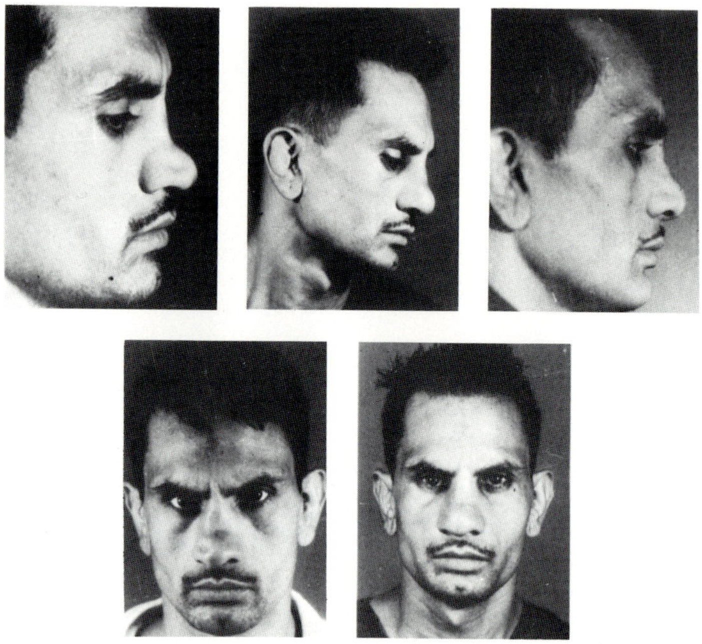

Figure 4.

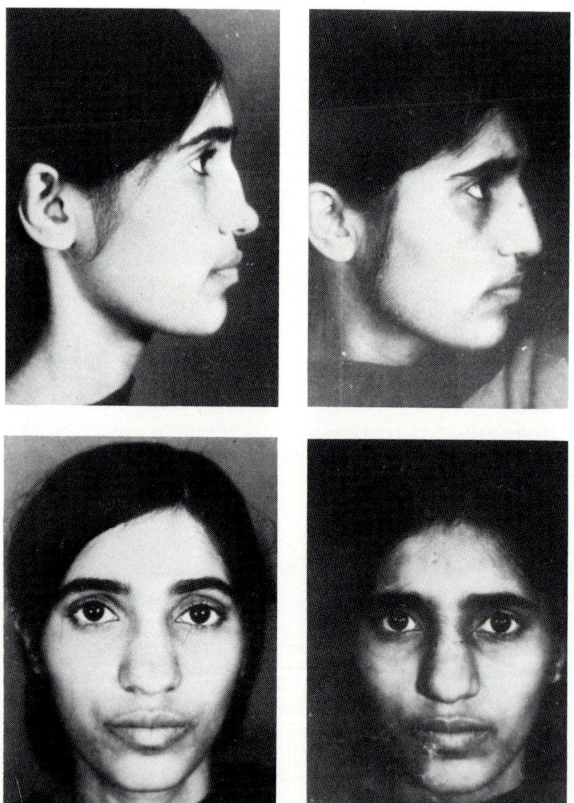

Figure 5.

were associated with anterior septal dislocation, which was corrected simultaneously. Three cases had bony thickening of the lateral wall which was rubbed off using a rasp.

In two cases an alar defect was reconstructed. The nasal defect was corrected by using a free composite graft removed from the pinna. The composite graft was preferred depending on the gratifying experience gained in the previous two cases done sometimes in the past for the partial alar defect. The margin of the helix gives beautiful contour mimicking the rounded contour of the alar margin.

Two cut noses were reconstructed using forehead flaps (Figs. 7, 8).

The youngest patient was 10 years old and had multiple fractures of the nasal bones and frontal processes of the maxilla with collapse of the nose. The correction in this patient has been planned in two stages. The first stage has been done. The second stage will be done later, after adolescence. The oldest patient was 38 years old.

I shall quote another case which of course did not require any corrective surgery. This was a young married female patient having good educational background. She presented with the complaint of having some nasal deformity following pregnancy two years back. I could not detect any

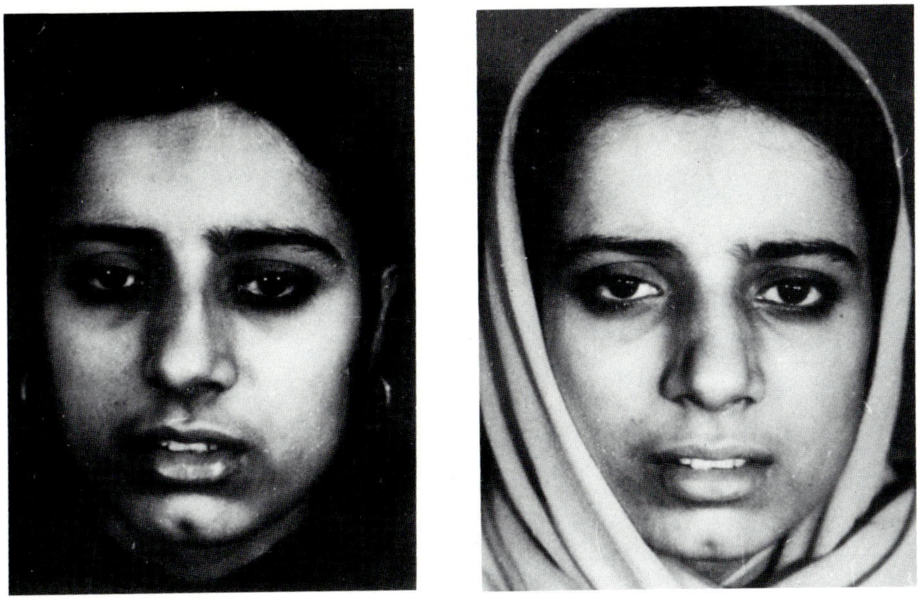

Figure 6.

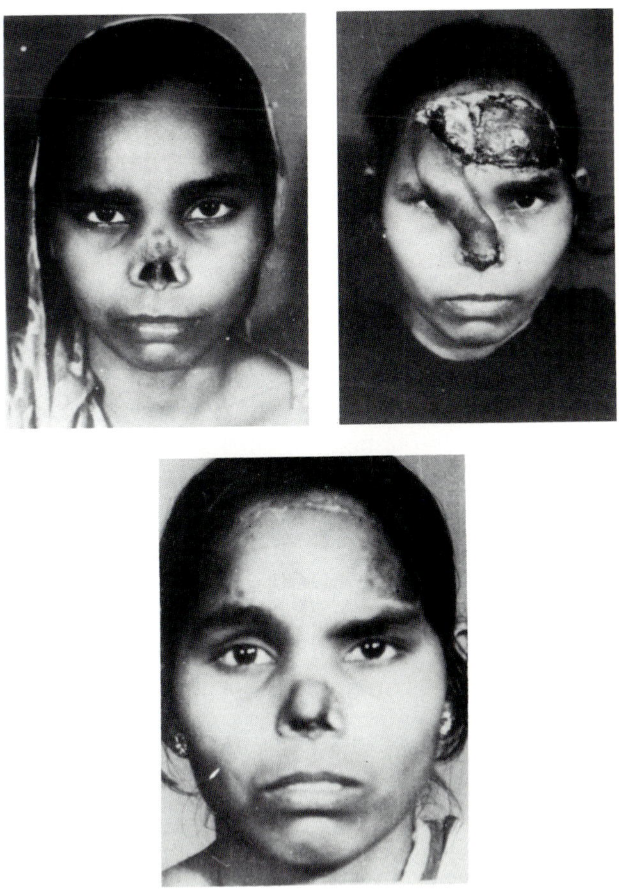

Figure 7.

Table 1. Showing Types of Nasal Deformities Corrected

Type of deformity	No. of cases
Depressed nose	12
Hump nose	8
Lateral deviation	10
Tilted nasal tip	4
Hump with lateral deviation	5
Hump with drooping nasal tip	2
Bony thickening lateral wall	3
Alar defect	2
Cut nose	2
Square tip	2
TOTAL	50

Table 2. Showing Age and Sex Distribution

	Sex		
Age	Male	Female	Total
10–20	12	8	20
21–30	15	7	22
31–40	5	3	8
Total	32	18	50

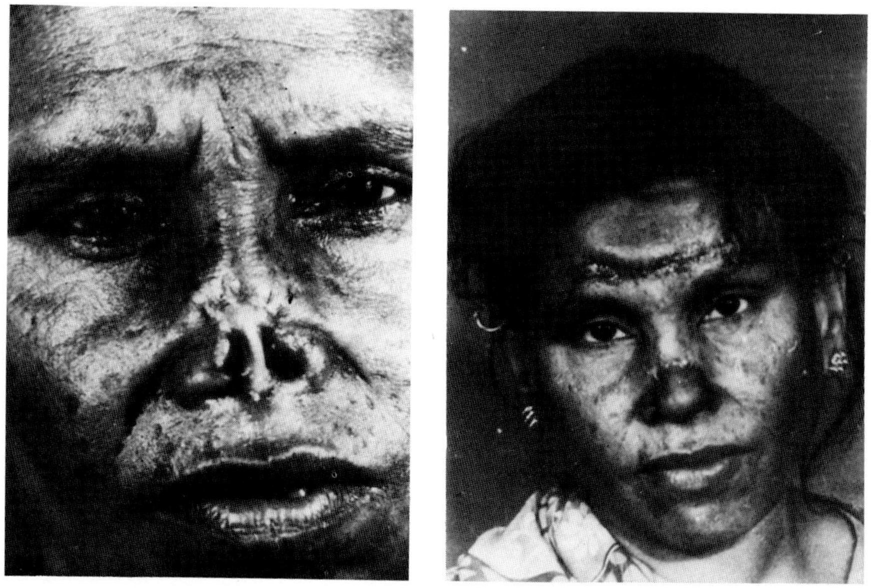

Figure 8.

physical deformity in the nose, rather her nose perfectly matched her face. The lady insisted that her nose was definitely deformed. Her husband had already failed to convince her. She was not prepared to seek psychiatric help in spite of our best efforts.

Discussion

The selection of the rhino-septoplastic technique must be carefully chosen in order to achieve the best results in correcting the deformity. Rigid rules cannot be made and each situation must be individualized for their respective deformities. There are many opinions whether rhinoseptoplasty is to be combined in the same sitting or to be staged. In the present series of cases septoplasty was combined in the same sitting whenever it was required. The current opinion appears to be in favor of correction at the same sitting in majority of cases, Clarke[2] and Parisier[3]. The one stage operation for combined septum and external nasal deformity is not suitable in those cases when surgical intervention is likely to interfere with nasal spine of frontal bone or cantilever of the nose.

The rhinoplasty should be delayed in adolescents until sufficient maturation has occured. Age, sex, heredity, and general body development are some of the factors to be kept in mind before taking decision for operation. All our operated cases except two in the present series were older than 18 years. Bloom[4] has recommended the age for boys 18 to 21 years old and girls 16 to 18 years old as optimum age for rhinoplasty. In eight cases in the present series homologous septal cartilage preserved in 70 percent alcohol has been used for the reconstruction of the supra tip depression. Six cases have been followed for more than a year without any untoward reaction. Some workers have recommended the use of Teflon in glycerin paste for the correction of saddle nose, Wilson[5] and Schell[6]. Clarke[2] has used processed heterogenous bone and cartilage transplants removed from embryo calf bone with good results. I do not have any experience of using plastic materials and do not like to use plastic implants because of their remote possibility of eliciting carcinogenic reaction, Wilson[5]. The use of plastic material can be considered as a temporary means to correct the depressed nasal deformity on the children before proper rhinoplasty after the age of maturation. The use of preserved homologous septal cartilage appears to have good promise according to my experience. The long-term follow up of the patients will show us the extent of shrinkage of graft. The results of the rhinoplastic surgery should be evaluated after six months because the postoperative thickening of the soft tissues subsides after a long interval, and the change in the final shape of the nose due to fibrosis will manifest by that time.

Many times occasions do arise when surgeons have to seek psychiatric opinion for the cases of rhinoplasty. Occasionally one encounters a case when the desire for operation may be indicative of psychological disturbance, as it happened in one of our cases.

It is well known that in certain personalities a disfigurement can produce abnormal psychogenic developments and there is frequently a need for early correction of disfigurement so as to prevent personality change.

The concept of the symptom being used as an excuse or scapegoat for deeper emotional difficulties have been stressed by Hay.[7] There is a tendency in some patients to blame their appearances for many happenings in everyday life. In one of the cases a patient blamed pregnancy and attributed that there has been some change in the appearance of her nose after the pregnancy.

Smith[8] has nicely dealt about the selection of the patients and psychological implications for rhinoplasty. Both rational and irrational forces prompt the request for rhinoplasty.

In two of our operated cases psychological problems were involved. One patient had been postponing marriage because of an ugly looking nose. In another case of a boy aged 14 years the depression of the dorsum of the nose followed septal abscess. This boy stopped going to the school and was upset because of his nasal deformity. Though this is not an ideal age for correction but reasons for operation were so compelling that with minimal possible surgical interference I inserted the graft to shape the depressed dorsal bridge line. This boy resumed his studies happily after the correction.

Summary

Experience with a group of 50 patients for various types of nasal deformities operated upon is highlighted. There are many psychological implications involved to the patients for rhinoplasty. In my experience septoplasty should be combined with rhinoplasty at the same time as far as possible. The preserved homologous septal tissues for the correction of supratip depression was found quite satisfactory. The results of the rhinoplastic surgery are gratifying and should be evaluated after the lapse of at least six months.

References

1. Converse JM: Reconstructive plastic surgery, Vol. II. Philadelphia & London, W. B. Saunders, 1968
2. Clarke GM: Specially processed heterogenous bone and cartilage transplants in nasal surgery; J Laryny 83:275, 1969
3. Parisier SC: Correction of deviated nose. Arch Otolaryngol 92:60, 1970
4. Bloom SM: Rhinoplasty in adolescence. Arch Otolaryngol 92:66, 1970
5. Wilson TG: Teflon in glycerine paste in Rhinology. J Laryng 78:953, 1964
6. Schell JJ: Polytef injection for nasal deformity. Arch Otolaryngol 92:554, 1970
7. Hay GG: Psychiatric aspects of cosmetic nasal operations. Brit J Psychiatr 116:85, 1970
8. Smith TW: The selection of patients for rhinoplasty. Arch Otolaryngol 94:56, 1971

Aesthetic Problems in Surgical Technique of the Nasal Tip

Lionello Ponti, Rome, Italy

In recent years, functional and aesthetic nasal surgery has greatly progressed as a result of many courses of specialization and of abundant literature on this subject. Even though the fundamental operating techniques are commonly known, nevertheless some technical and aesthetic problems remain unsolved. It is still difficult to insert a new nose on a determinate face and above all it is difficult to foretell the kind of nose suitable to that face. Only experience, self-criticism and wisdom may lead us to satisfactory results even though imperfect. We must also consider that patients with ugly noses often present with some deformities of the osteo-cartilaginous septum and functional respiratory insufficiency, a defect we must eliminate, not only for physiological reasons, but also because it is very difficult to build a straight and regular nose on a distorted foundation.

Once the patient's constitution and facial anatomy are evaluated, we must take into consideration the nasal pyramid on the whole, its position on the face, its length, breadth and prominence and relation to the forehead, cheek-bones, upper-lower lip, jaw, eyes, etc. It must be considered, in fact, that very little disproportion between the new nose and the other segments of the face can cause an artificial appearance.

Without resorting to casts of the face, it is important to take a series of standard photographs of the patients face on a dark background including frontal, both lateral profiles in repose, and smiling and basal view. Thus, photographic analysis can be properly performed using geometric lines such as the Frankfort and frontomental lines which may be very useful to the beginner.

By transferring the lines of the whole face in photographic transpariences we can trace and predict the new nose and also perhaps realize the surgical limitations of a particular nose in advance.

At this point, besides analyzing all the abovementioned problems, the surgeons personal artistic and surgical tastes may be applied to the particular patient even though they do not correspond to the exact geometrical dictates.

In the preliminary discussion, one often encounters difficulties in persuading the patient to follow his aesthetic suggestions. The majority of patients, in fact, consider a nose beautiful only when it is very small. This is perhaps a psychological belief of those who undergo aesthetic nasal surgery. Nevertheless, the surgeon would not be acting in the best interest of the patient if he adhered to his patients desires.

In nasal analysis, the surgeon must consider the following factors:

1. The anatomical constitution of the nose itself.
2. The anatomical balance of the face.
3. The patient's age.
4. The patient's occupation.
5. The patient's personal concept of beauty and his psychological condition.

It is essential that one diminish the possibility of technical failures and disappointments as much as possible.

If one evaluates the aforementioned factors and carefully analyzes the following variations in nasal quality and contour, then, one may be in the position to plan the appropriate surgical procedure.

1. A very large nose with thick, flabby, or sebaceous skin may be reduced very little in proportion, so that it would be opportune to project a smaller nose with blunted angles and the patient must be informed thereof, so that he will be prepared (if he accepts) to a modest improvement. It is wise to know that a very deflected nose since infancy cannot become perfectly straight. The surfaces of the deviated bones, in fact, have grown, one convex, and the other, concave, and even after accurate osteotomy they will maintain their abnormal curvatures.

2. The lower third part of the face is perhaps one of the most important parts on which the surgeon must reconstruct the new nose. Thin lips, microgenia, small mouth and protruding teeth exclude construction of a small nose with an obtuse noselabial angle. If the defect only concerns the chin we must compensate for this with a graft at the chin articulation; mentoplasty may be performed through an intraoral or submental external approach, both with autoplastic material. After having come to a decision with the patient we must study the nose after having drawn the appropriate lines of the profile of nose and chin on the photographs. If the chin, on the other hand, is too developed, we must reduce the nose as much as possible.

3. The age of the patient must be considered both from a physiological and surgical risk as well as an aesthetic point of view. Rhinoplasty performed before age sixteen for females and eighteen, for males, are generally subject to postoperative deformities; it is clear that the growth centers may undergo osteogenesis because they have been stimulated or liberated from anatomical formations which restricted them. The extirpation of the convexity some months after the operation, may give

rise to a vertical crest by regrowth of the perpendicular lamina of the ethmoid, liberated from the roof of its bones and may fill the nasal-frontal angle with newly formed bony tissue.

4. Many people undergo an operation of rhinoplasty both for their own satisfaction and also for professional reasons; professional men, artists, shopmen, employees, the one for not being ugly, the other to be more photogenic, etc. It is clear that for each case a particular nose must be projected; to the artist's nose one must extirpate more convexity and, on the other hand, make more obtuse the naso-labial angle of a mother of a family.

5. Many people are not satisfied with their rhinoplasty even though it is the result of an operation correctly performed and is balanced to the face. So it happens that such patients undergo revisions in other places obtaining inferior results. The surgeon must evidently be firm in his decision and prefer to lose the patient rather than to perform an inferior operation.

6. It is not rare that apparently normal people in reality conceal a psychopathy and it is certainly not easy for the surgeon to discover it during a brief preoperative interview. To take precautions in this area the surgeon must appreciate such an eventuality for each patient. Slight symptoms may be observed; for example, a patient does not exactly know what he wants, he says he cannot live with that nose, etc. Once the suspicion is aroused, it is absolutely essential to have a psychiatric evaluation and permit prior to surgery.

Operating Techniques

While we are still adhering to the teachings of Joseph as regards the fundamental operative techniques, many authors have described personal techniques for the correction of the alar cartilages. Each one of these procedures can have its indication but cannot, in itself, solve every problem. It is essential, therefore, for the surgeon to make himself master of those techniques with which he can obtain the desired changes with the slightest aesthetic and functional risk.

Following these concepts, we have subdivided the patients into three fundamental groups:

1. Rhinoplasties requiring great modifications of the nasal tip.
2. Rhinoplasties requiring moderate modifications of the nasal tip.
3. Rhinoplasties requiring little modifications of the nasal tip.

The first group includes large noses, prominent noses, those with thick skin, long nostrils, or those with hypoplastic tips, short columella or presenting significant asymmetries and also results of imperfect operations.

The second group includes those cases in which the nasal tip requires a little more projection or a little rotation upwards in addition to reduction of nasal tip bulbosity.

The third group includes those nasal tips which are almost normal and require only a little reduction of the alar cartilaginous complex. In these cases the medial crura must already be in a satisfactory position and cannot be modified.

Considering the problem exclusively from a technical point of view, we must recognize that the greater the modifications the easier becomes the possibility to incur complications like asymmetries, irregularities, or exuberant scars. The aim of the surgeon is to obtain the best results by taking less risks.

It must be kept in mind that by corrective surgery of the nose one must be very careful in sacrificing bony and cartilaginous structures. These support tissues are necessary to the reconstruction of the new nasal pyramid and their reduction must be well calculated and performed only when absolutely necessary.

The empty space caused by the removal of such structures is not always covered by a measured draping of skin, but is often replaced and amply filled by fibrous tissue, which rounds the edges, and makes the skin, covering the nose, irregular.

We have, therefore, adopted a different technique for every group of the described cases. For the first group that includes very bulbous tips, short tips, and in revisions, we use the Goldman technique by which one can directly inspect the medial crus to extend or shorten and also to engraft them under direct vision. Such procedures present some problems because they require the marginal incision the whole mobilization of the lateral crura and their interruption at the level of the dome. Then, we run the risk of slight dislocations and consequently of asymmetries of nares contours but, on the other hand, this procedure permits us to easily correct the obvious asymmetries and, to restore, in case of revisions, a reasonable tip through true cartilaginous grafts.

The surgical steps are:

1. Marginal cut which runs along the inferior edge of the lateral crus and involves a portion of the inner margin of the medial crura.
2. Careful undermining of the lateral crura and of the dome from the nasal tip skin.
3. Extraction of the dome with a hook which is through all thicknesses including the vestibular skin, more or less laterally, according to that which is required to extend the medial crus.
4. Extraction of two medial crura through the right nostril and their approximation with a mattressed 4 or 5-0 cat-gut suture.
5. Moulding of the medial and lateral crura.
6. Suture of the vestibular skin at the level of the lateral crura.

For the second group, which includes noses that require moderate modifications in, more or less, of the projection of the tip, we use a personal technique coming from a combination of the Goldman with others. This technique differs from Goldman because in it we do not sever the vestibular skin but only the cartilaginous layer, and the medial crura are sutured between them without including the skin in the suture. Evidently, the medial crus, stripped of the skin, is weaker and unable to support and resist the contraction of a thickened, nonelastic cutaneous covering. This procedure is not advisable in seborreic skins and in revisions. Nevertheless, it is very useful in many cases and the vestibular skin serves as an "internal splint" and, therefore, it is more difficult to have distortions or asymmetries.

The surgical steps are:

1. Marginal cuts and uncovering of the alae as in Goldman's technique.
2. Extraction of dome and cutting of the cartilage without touching the cutaneous surface.
3. Partial cut more or less extended laterally according to the amount of projection that is required from the medial crura.
4. Moulding of the lateral crura.
5. Extraction of both medial crura from the right nostril and suture of these with cat gut.
6. Possible further support sutures of the medial crura posteriorly and moulding of these.
7. Suture of the vestibular skin at the level of the lateral crura.

For the third group which requires slight modifications, when the projection of the medial crura are exact and not wide, we use the "cartilage-splitting" approach. This is a very simple technique and gives superior results in the aforementioned group of cases and eliminates many of the possible complications of those cases performed through the marginal incision approach.

The surgical steps are:

1. Intracartilaginous cut, parallel to the lower edge of the lateral crus, more or less caudal, according to the necessity. The cut is extended from the dome for about 2 cm laterally through the vestibular skin and the cartilage. These incisions should be equally parallel and equidistant from the caudal margins of the lateral crura.
2. Careful division of vestibular skin from the lower cartilage in its superior of cephalic portion.
3. Freeing of the superior segment of cartilage from the skin of the nose.
4. Section of the cartilage at the level of the dome and laterally sideways, from the internal to the external side for a variable distance as required by the individual case.
5. Cut of remaining cartilage of the lateral crus from the skin of nose.
6. Suture of the bipedicled vestibular skin delivered from the cartilage to the skin and remaining alar cartilage.

Summary

An attempt is made to summarize the author's experience with several thousand cases of surgery of the nasal tip. Both socio-psychological and pragmatic evaluations of methods of management of varieties of nasal tips are presented. The point is stressed that each surgical technique utilized should be tailored to the specific deformity and not the deformity tailored to the technique.

Rhinoplasty and Orthognathic Surgery

Jack P. Gunter and William H. Bell, Dallas, Tex.

Cosmetic surgeons have long recognized the importance of facial symmetry and proportion. Of the factors which influence facial proportion, none is more important than the relationship between the middle and lower thirds of the face. It is essential that these two areas be in harmony with each other if the face is to have an aesthetically pleasing appearance.

A technically "successful" rhinoplasty may not achieve good facial balance if there is coexisting jaw deformity which remains uncorrected. In the past, the cosmetic surgeon has relied mainly on artificial implants to correct associated jaw deformity and his concern has been directed primarily toward the mandible. With the recent advances in corrective jaw surgery techniques, however, this is no longer acceptable. Orthognathic surgery has added a new dimension to the field of cosmetic facial surgery. With the use of such techniques, the jaws or segments of the jaws, consisting of the teeth encased in bone, can be repositioned in any direction to restore a normal function and facial harmony. The maxilla or mandible can be raised, lowered, advanced, retracted, widened, or narrowed. Dentofacial deformities corrected by a combination of rhinoplasty and orthognathic surgery may achieve dramatic results in respect to facial appearance, occlusal relationships, and patient personality.

When nasal and jaw deformities are present in the same patient, the problem is best approached by a multidisciplinary team of specialists. The patient is seen by the involved specialists, and a diagnosis is made from a coordinated analysis of the clinical, cephalometric, and occlusal studies. A long range corrective plan is then formulated with each involved specialist aware of the objectives of the other team members and all working toward a common goal: to obtain the best aesthetic and functional result for the patient.

When orthodontic treatment is indicated, it is usually the initial step in the corrective plan. Occasionally, orthodontic appliances may be needed postoperatively to stabilize the teeth and jaws after they have been repositioned surgically.

When nasal and jaw surgery are indicated in the same patient, it is desirable to perform both during the same operative procedure. In most cases, however, this is not feasible. It is possible only when the jaw surgery can be performed without compromising the oral airway, and if there is no repositioning of the anterior portion of the maxilla. An uncompromised oral airway is essential because rhinoplasty usually results in obstruction of the nasal airway for a few days after surgery. If the teeth have been wired together, or if there is a significant amount of edema in the upper airway area, adequate pulmonary ventilation may become a problem.

Rhinoplasty is not performed at the same time that maxillary surgery is performed. If the anterior part of the maxilla has been moved, there is usually some edema around the base of the nose which makes it difficult to evaluate the configuration and projection of the nasal tip during the rhinoplasty. In most of these cases, nasotracheal intubation is preferred, and although the tube can be changed at termination of the jaw surgery, it has frequently caused some distortion of the nose and septum. Additionally, when the vertical height of the anterior maxilla is decreased, there is usually an unpredictable amount of splaying of the nasal base that occurs. At the time of surgery, it is impossible to determine how much of the splaying is due to actual movement of the nasal base and how much is due to edema, thereby making it impossible to judge accurately the amount of narrowing needed. It is preferable to wait until the anterior maxillary segment stabilizes and the edema subsides before performing rhinoplasty in these cases (usually two to three months postoperatively).

The following are cases of associated nasal and jaw deformities which have been treated by combined rhinoplasty and orthognathic surgery.

Case 1

A 26-year-old woman desired rhinoplasty to improve her facial appearance. Her nasal deformity included a moderate sized dorsal hump, an excessively projecting nasal tip and lack of definition of the tip. She also had a slight recession of the chin (Fig. 1A and 1B). In addition to rhinoplasty, a chin augmentation using a 6 mm solid silastic implant was placed intraorally. (Fig. 1E)

Postoperatively, a good result was obtained from the rhinoplasty. The chin augmentation succeeded in projecting the chin and creating better definition between the lip and chin. This improved the balance between the middle and lower thirds of the face. (Fig. 1C and 1D)

Case 2

A 16-year-old girl had undergone several years of orthodontic treatment prior to cosmetic surgery consultation. Although her occlusion was good, she was dissatisfied with the overall appearance of her chin, lips and nose. The lower third of her face was slightly elongated in the vertical dimension as compared to the middle third. Most of the excess was beneath a line drawn through the oral commissures. She had a prominent nasal spine associated with an increased columellolabial angle and a straight dorsal profile with a high nasal dorsum (Fig. 2A and 2B). The lower anterior facial height was reduced 8 mm by reduction genioplasty,* (Fig. 2E) along with rhinoplasty.

Postoperatively, a shortened facial height was attained from the jaw surgery. The rhinoplasty reduced the nasal dorsum, decreased the tip projection and relieved some of the tension appearance of the upper lip (Fig. 2C and 2D).

Case 3

A 28-year-old female was initially seen for treatment of her malocclusion. All study parameters showed the typical dental-facial features of mandibular prognathism (Fig. 3A and 3B). Her prominent and asymmetric chin, malaligned teeth, and prominent "hooked" nose necessitated a treatment plan of orthodontics and surgery. Total time for the preoperative orthodontics** was three months.

Treatment was planned so that bilateral mandibular midbody osteotomies (55 mm left side; 8 mm right side) to retract the mandible were done concomitantly with rhinoplasty (Fig. 3E). Orthodontic arch wires were used to fix the mandibular bony segments in the desired position at the time of surgery and in the immediate postoperative period when the nasal airway was compromised. This treatment plan facilitated rhinoplasty by obviating the immediate need for intermaxillary fixation. Five days after surgery, when the nasal airway was patent, the mandible was immobilized in the desired position. The surgical-orthodontic treatment produced a balanced soft tissue profile, facial symmetry and occlusal balance (Fig. 3C and 3D).

Case 4

A 21-year-old female was seen with the typical dental-facial characteristics of mandibular prognathism associated with maxillary deficiency. A broad nose with a bulbous tip, a hypoplastic-appearing midfacial region, and prominent chin were the dominant facial features (Fig. 4A and 4B). Cephalometric studies corroborated the clinical findings. The lower anterior teeth were positioned approximately 12 mm anterior to the maxillary dentition.

The treatment plan was to first align the maxillary and mandibular teeth by orthodontics. The maxilla would be surgically advanced 6 mm by LeForte I osteotomy and the mandible simultaneously retracted 7 mm by bilateral mandibular body osteotomies (Fig. 4I). Eight months following the jaw surgery, the patient had a better

* Genioplasty was performed by Dr. Robert V. Walker, Dallas, Texas.

** Orthodontic treatment performed by Dr. Phelps J. Murphey, Dallas, Texas.

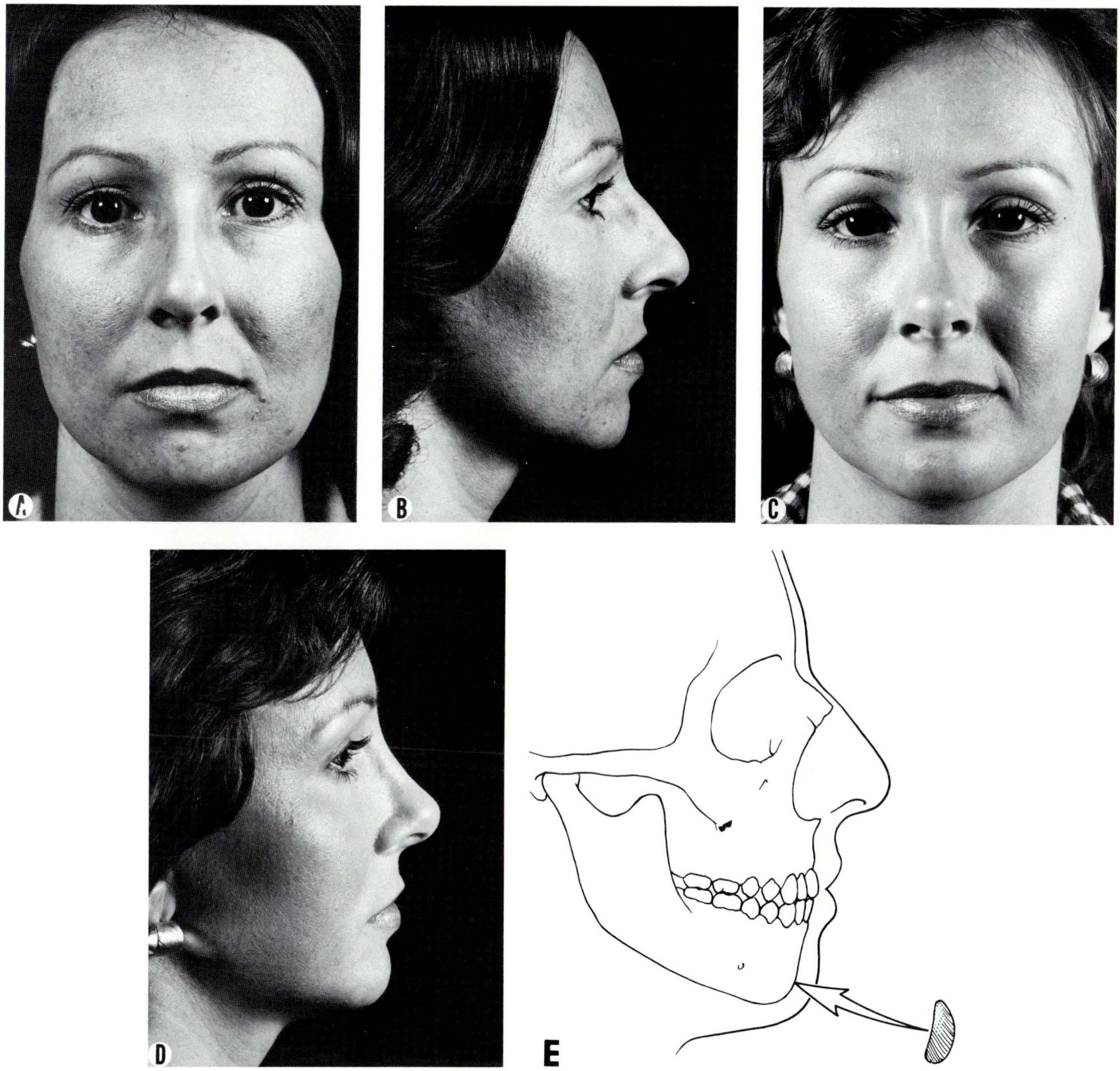

Fig. 1. (A, B) Preoperative appearance. (C, D) Postoperative appearance. (E) Diagrammatic plan for implant insertion.

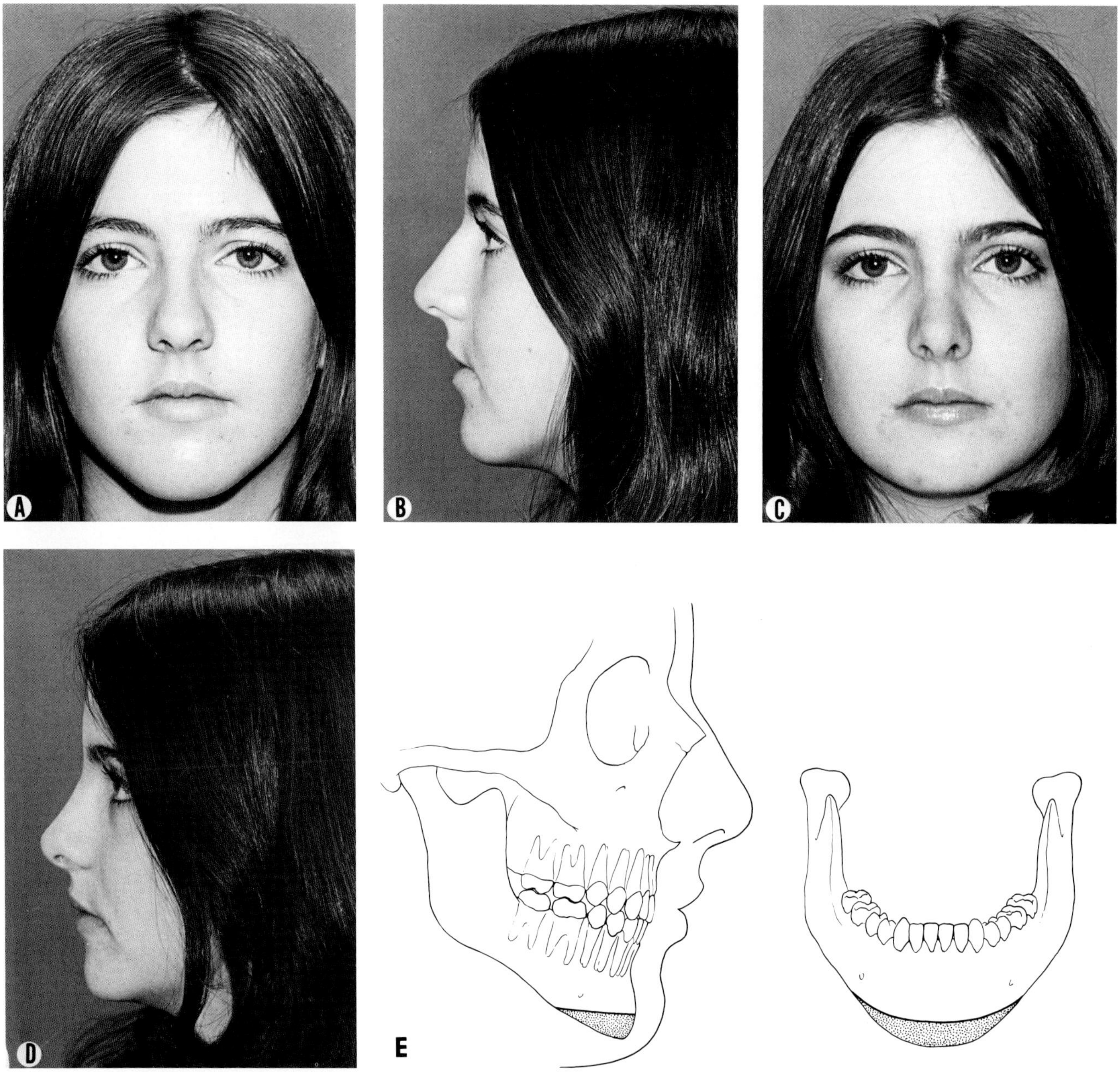

Fig. 2. (A, B) Preoperative appearance. (C, D) Postoperative appearance. (E) Diagrammatic plan for reduction genioplasty.

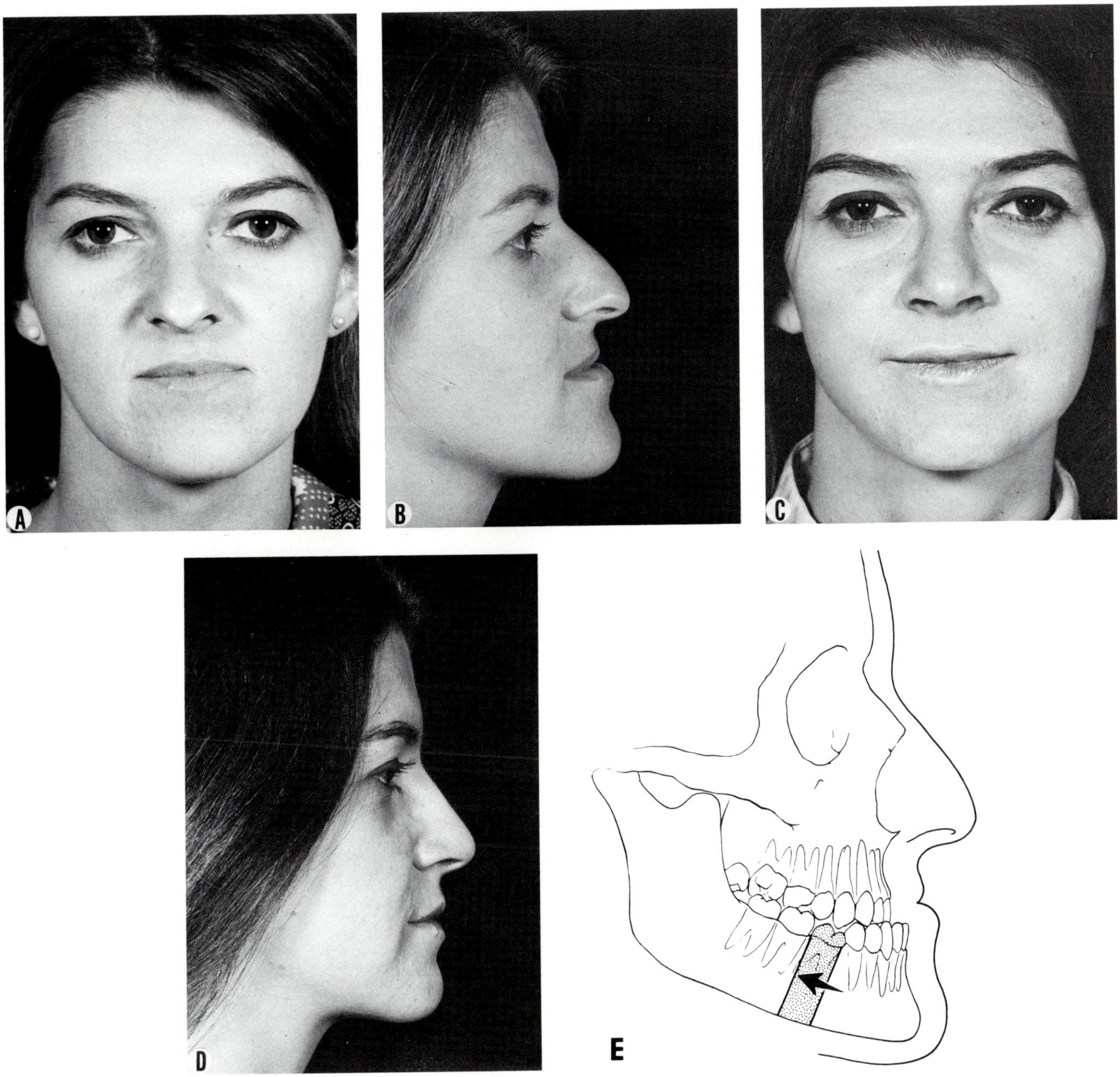

Fig. 3. (A, B) Preoperative appearance. (C, D) Postoperative appearance. (E) Diagrammatic plan for retracting mandible.

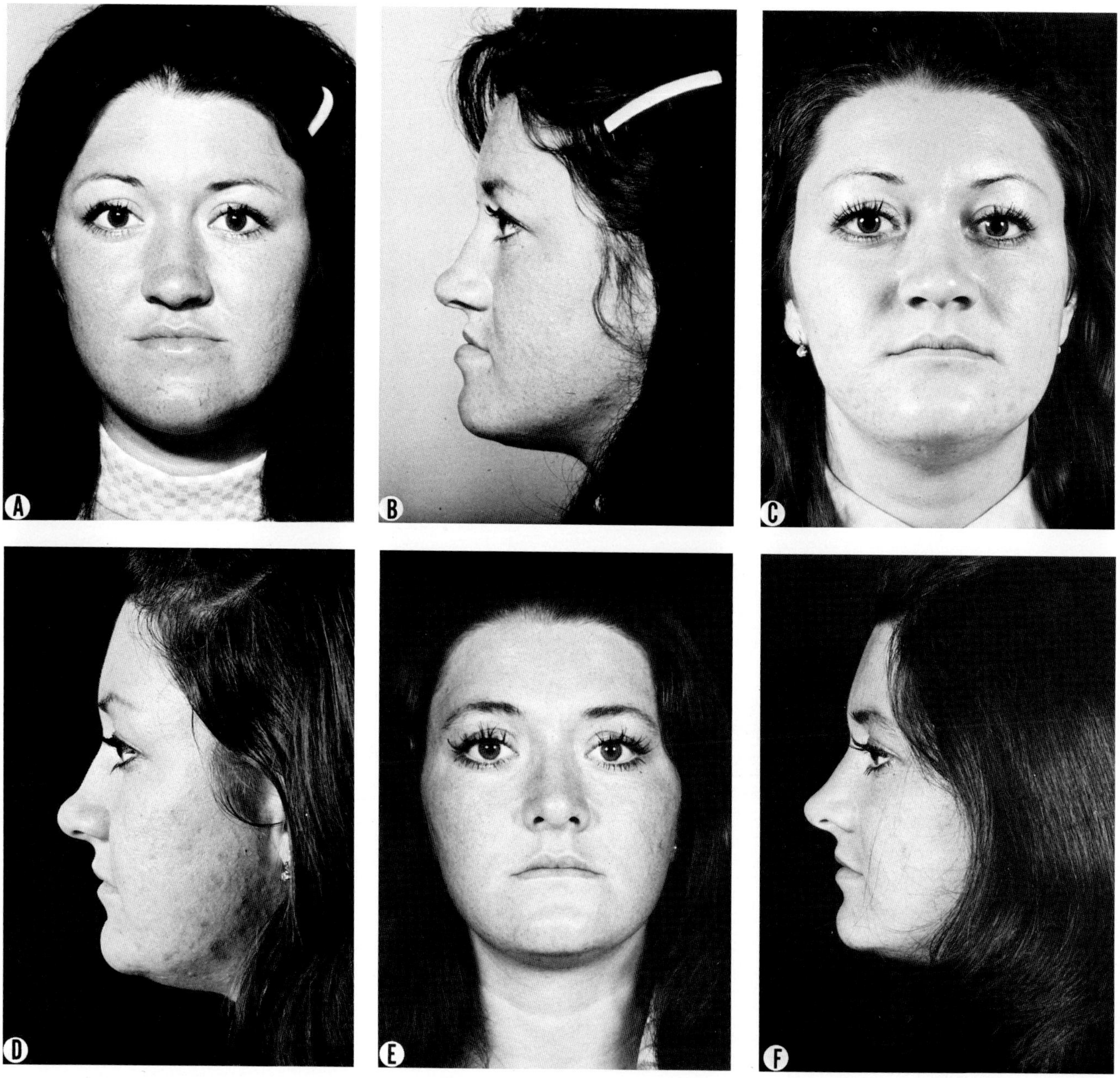

Fig. 4. See legend on facing page.

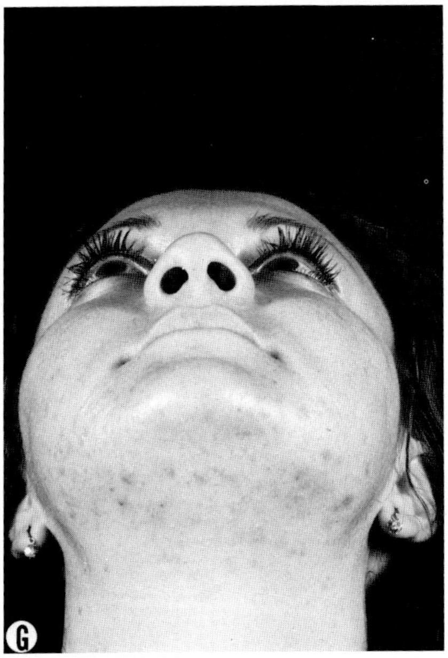

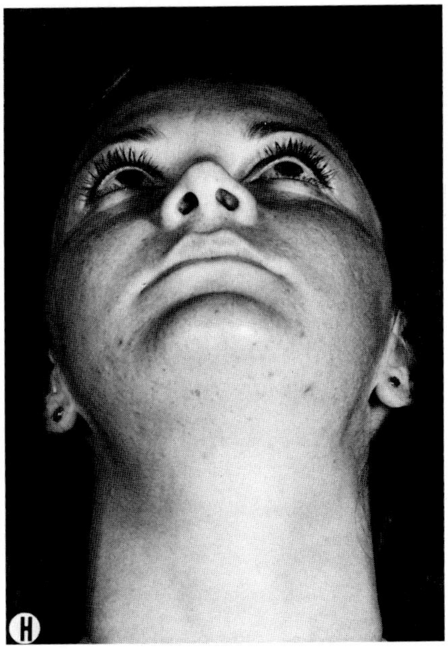

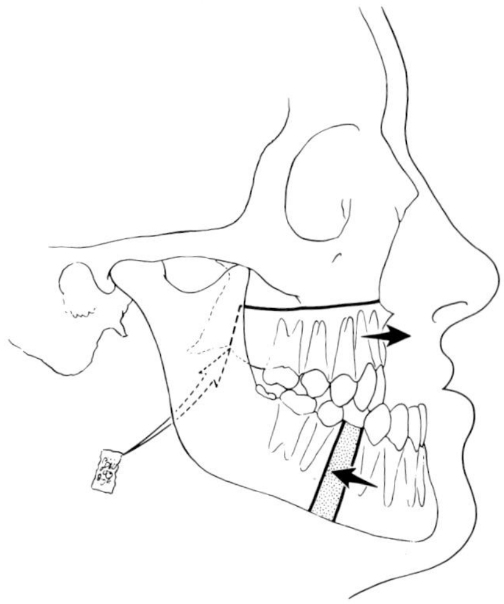

Fig. 4. *(A, B) Preoperative appearance. (C, D) Postoperative jaw surgery, preoperative rhinoplasty. (E, F) Postoperative appearance following jaw and nasal surgery. (G, H) Postoperative basal view showing effect of modified Weir procedures and tip configuration. (I) Diagrammatic plan for advancing maxilla and retracting the mandible.*

lower facial relationship, but the nasal deformity had become more pronounced due to splaying of the alar bases as a result of the maxillary advancement (Fig. 4C and 4D). Overall facial balance was achieved by rhinoplasty performed five months later to narrow the body and reshape the nasal tip (Fig. 4E and 4F). Modified Weir procedures were performed as part of the rhinoplasty to narrow the nasal base (Fig. 4G and 4H).

Case 5

A 21-year-old woman sought treatment to decrease the "prominence" of her maxillary teeth and improve the contour of her face. Clinical and cephalometric analysis disclosed vertical maxillary excess, Class II malocclusion, excessive exposure of the incisor teeth, a contour deficient chin and a lack of prominence in the midfacial region. Her maxillary anterior teeth were positioned 7 mm anterior to the mandibular anterior teeth. The nose was deviated, had a prominent dorsal hump and a small nasolabial angle (Fig. 5A–D).

The treatment for the jaw deformities was to reposition the anterior maxilla superiorly 7 mm and the posterior maxilla superiorly 9 mm which would facilitate forward and superior movement of the mandible (Fig. 5I). This shortened the facial height and improved the upper lip line-tooth relationship. With the maxilla raised, the mandible came forward helping to correct the Class II malocclusion and the contour deficient chin. Raising the maxilla increased the prominence of the cheeks and caused splaying of the alar bases (Fig. 5E and 5F).

Several months later rhinoplasty was performed to correct the nasal deformity. Although it reduced the dorsal hump and rotated the nasal tip, there was still some external deviation and splaying of the nasal base (Fig. 5G and 5H).

Case 6

A 34-year-old woman desired corrective surgery for severe jaw and nasal deformity. Clinical and cephalometric analysis revealed severe mandibular retrognathism, Class II malocclusion, proclination of the anterior maxillary teeth, and lip incompetence. The nose had a large bulbous tip with excessive projection. There was a moderate-sized dorsal hump (Fig. 6A and 6B).

The plan of treatment for the jaw deformity was to surgically reposition the four anterior maxillary teeth superiorly and upright the teeth to improve the upper lip-tooth relationship. The four anterior mandibular teeth would be moved

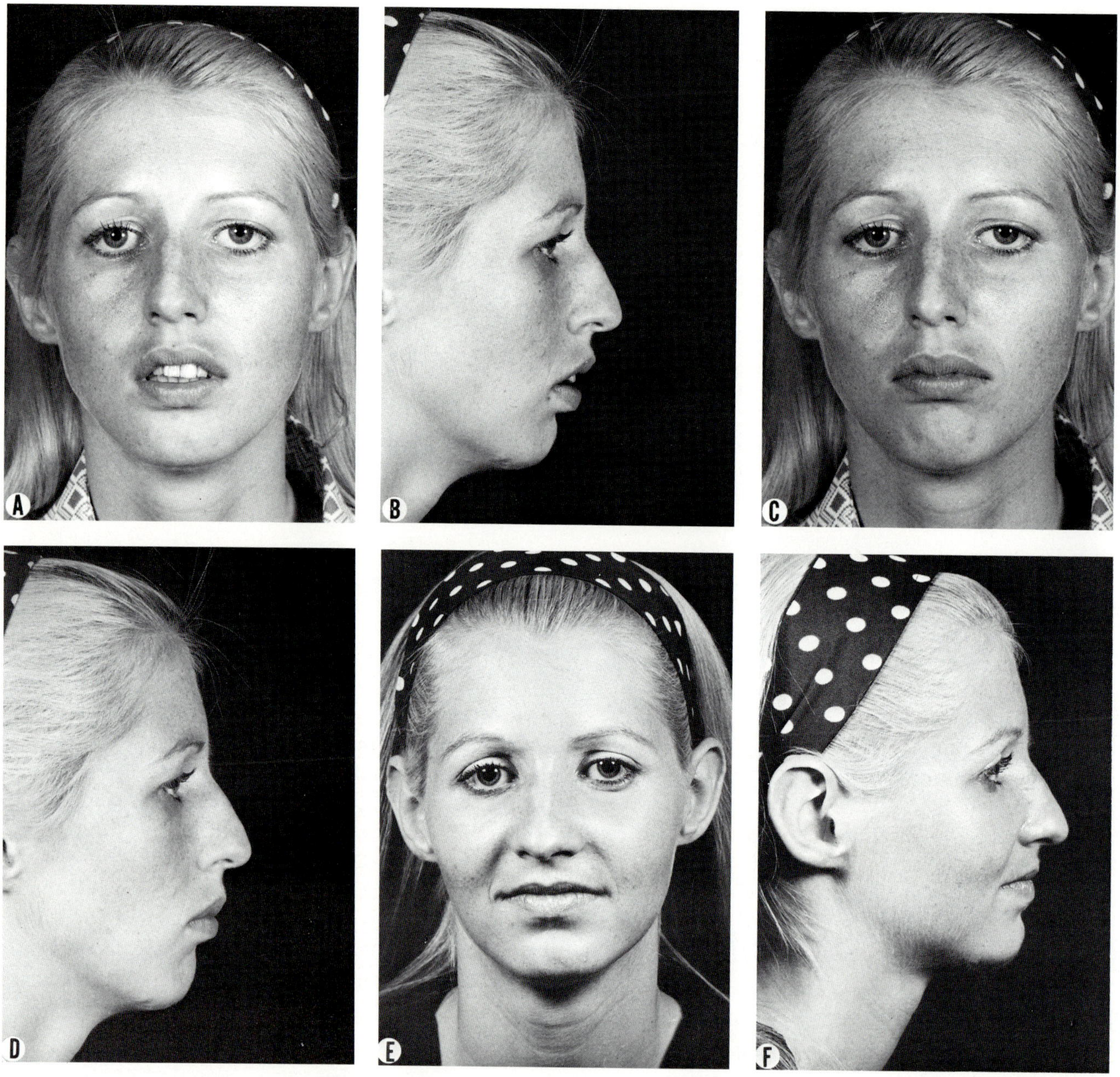

Fig. 5. See legend on facing page.

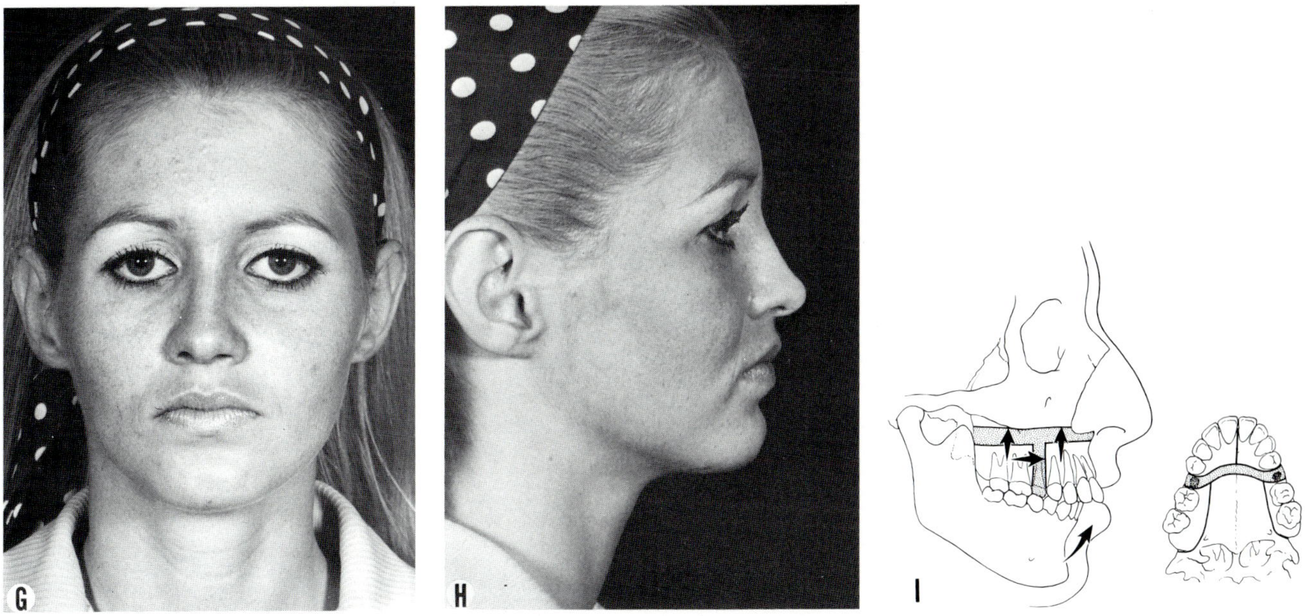

Fig. 5. (*A, B*) *Preoperative appearance with lips relaxed.* (*C, D*) *Preoperative appearance with lips forced close.* (*E, F*) *Postoperative appearance after jaw surgery with splaying of alar bases.* (*G, H*) *Postoperative jaw surgery and rhinoplasty appearance.* (*I*) *Diagrammatic plan showing repositioning of maxillary segments and autorotation and advancement of mandible.*

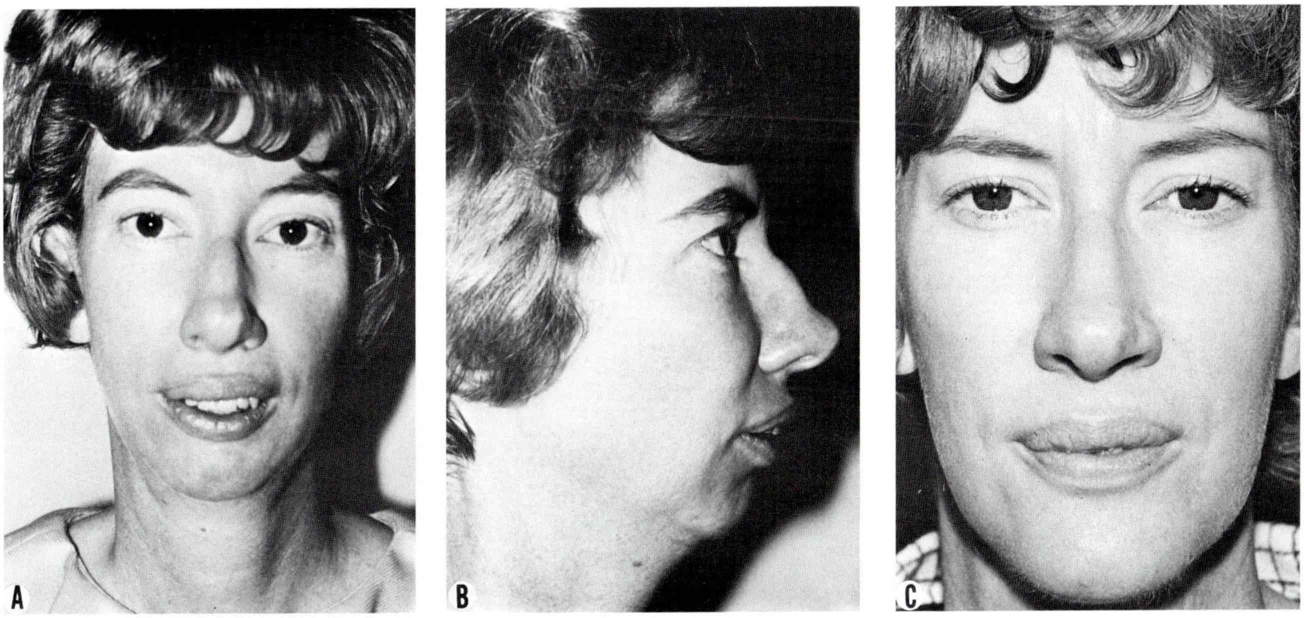

Fig. 6. *See legend on following page.*

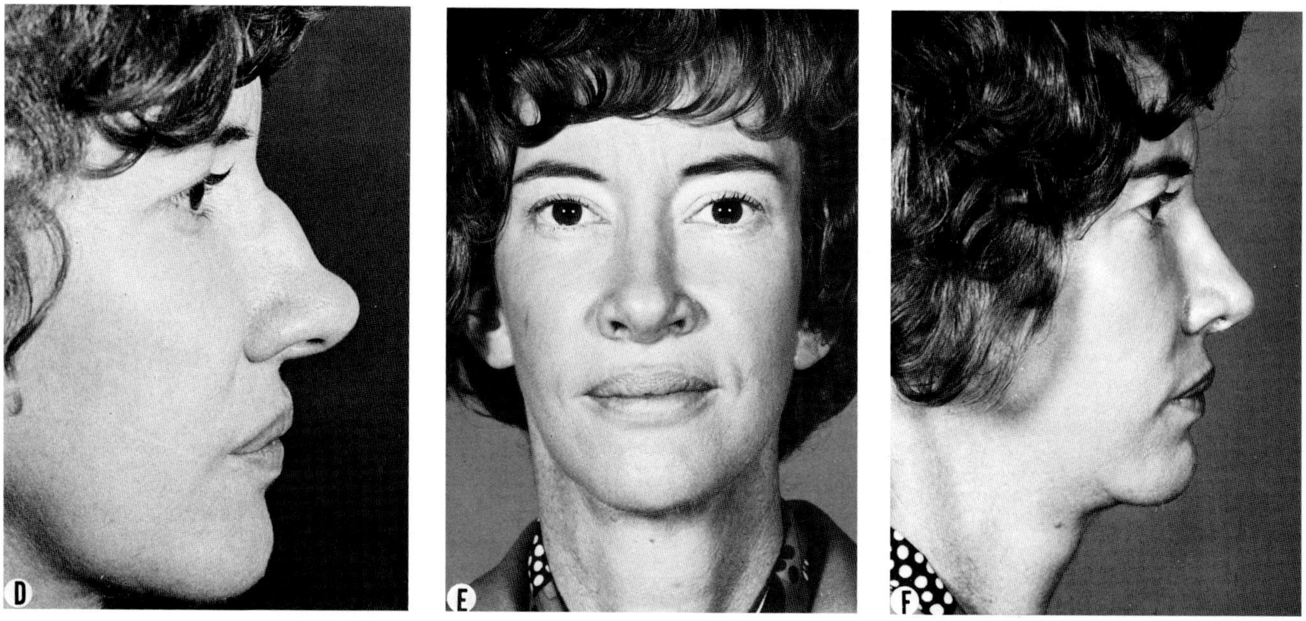

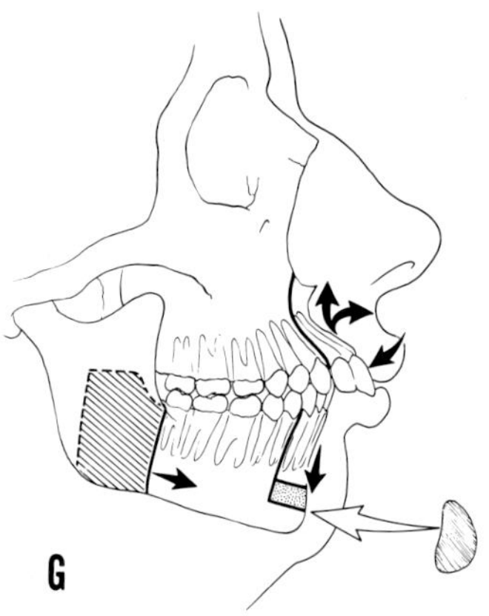

Fig. 6. *(A, B) Preoperative appearance. (C, D) Appearance following jaw surgery. (E, F) Appearance following jaw surgery and rhinoplasty. (G) Diagrammatic plan showing the repositioning of the anterior maxillary and mandibular segments, bilateral saggital mandibular steotomies and insertion of a silastic implant.*

inferiorly to level the lower arch, the mandible advanced 13 mm by bilateral saggital splitting osteotomies of the mandibular rami, and the chin augmented with a 10 mm silastic chin implant* (Fig. 6G).

After the jaw surgery was completed, the need for rhinoplasty was more apparent (Fig. 6C and 6D). Three months later the rhinoplasty was performed. In addition to routine hump removal and tip remodelling, a portion of the columella was resected to decrease the nasal tip projection. Although this was successful, it resulted in a bowing of the alar rims which could have been avoided with modified Weir procedures (Fig. 6E and 6F).

* Oral surgery was performed by Dr. Noel G. Stoker, Visalia, California and Dr. Bruce N. Epker, Fort Worth, Texas.

Correction of Deformities of the Base of the Nose

Kenneth H. Hinderer, Pittsburgh, Pa.

Corrective surgery of the base of the nose must be designed to correct any deformity resulting from trauma, infection or surgery, and prevent complications following septorhinoplastic procedures.

Normal nasal function depends upon proper anatomic relationship. It is the purpose of this paper to bring out the etiology of this deformity, the mechanism of its formation, and the structures involved. With this understanding, the surgical correction is based on undoing or reversing the process of its formation.

Since the nose is prominently placed in the center of the face, it is subject to frequent and varied types of trauma. The trauma may cause a variety of deformities, resulting in a change in the relationship of the structures to each other.

Surgical Anatomy

The nasal pyramid consists of four main structures: the bony pyramid, the cartilaginous vault, the lobule, and the septum. These structures are intimately associated with one another.

Corrections of deformities of the base is more than a localized problem. It involves many structures and their relationship to each other, namely, the caudal end of the septum, the membranous septum and its attachments to the medial crura, the maxillary spine, the prespine fibers, the lobular cartilages and their attachments to the upper lateral cartilages (Figs. 1, 2).

The semi-rigid portions of the nasal pyramid are the upper lateral cartilages which are fused to the dorsum of the cartilaginous septum and are referred to as the roof cartilage or wings of the septum. The terminal end or caudal border of the upper lateral cartilage is not fused to the septum, but is attached only by a fibrous band or aponeurosis. It is flexible and acts as the movable part of the valve. The septum is the fixed part of the valve. The lobular cartilages are horse-shoe shaped, which gives configuration to the nostrils. In normal position the upper margin of the lobular cartilage overrides the caudal end of the upper lateral cartilage.

During inspiration, the caudal portion of the lower lateral cartilage everts outward while the cephalic portion inverts inward creating pressure upon the caudal end of the upper lateral cartilage. In this manner the lobular cartilage acts as an accessory part of the valve. Each cartilage makes up the semi-rigid lower two-thirds of the nasal pyramid and is encased in its own fibrous envelope. These fibers decussate and form fibrous bands or aponeuroses which joins them together, yet allows freedom of movement between the neighboring cartilages. The most distinctive of these are:

1. The fibrous band of the cleft that joins the terminal end of the upper lateral cartilage with the septum giving flexibility to the valve.
2. The fibers between the caudal margin of the upper laterals and the cephalic margin of the lower laterals in the intercartilaginous space.
3. The fibers that join the caudal end of the septum with the cartilages of the medial crura.

Pathophysiology

The importance of these cartilaginous envelopes and their fibrous attachments to each other allows a flexibility that is of utmost importance, namely, the control of velocity, resistence and the direction of the inspired air currents. There may be a flattening of the bony dorsum from injury with dislocation of the lower border of the cartilaginous septum from the chondro-osseous joint. Thus, with the loss of height of the bony and cartilaginous vaults, there will be a downward pull on the membranes between these cartilages with changes in the

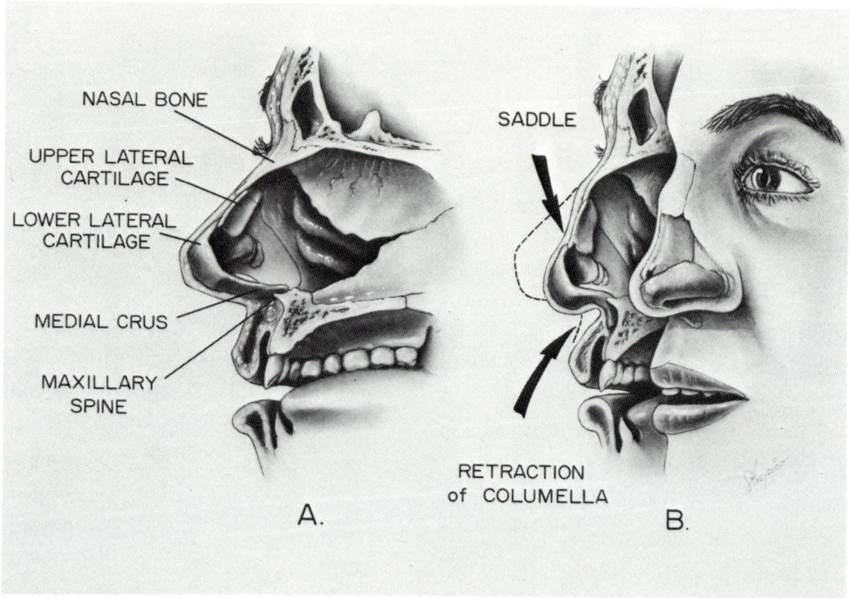

Fig. 1. (A) Represents the interior of the normal nose. (B) Represents the change in relationship of the cartilaginous structures, indicating that many structures of the base of the nose are involved.

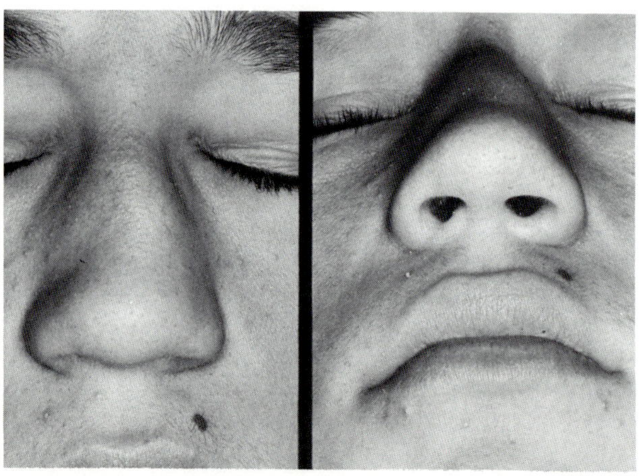

Fig. 2. Clinical picture of deformity as shown in illustration with wide base of nose and retracted columella.

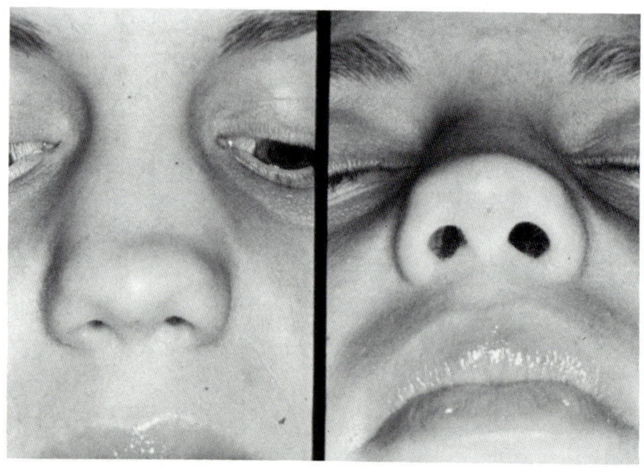

Fig. 3. Saddling and widening of base of nose from posttrauma injury.

contour of the nose which alters the relationship of these structures. This resultant alteration of shape and contour of these cartilages changes the control of the inspiratory and expiratory air currents. The etiology of the valve, septal, and lobular deformities is:

1. Early injury to the premaxillary structures with poor development of the maxillary spine area, usually occurring before the age of three or four.
2. Injury—posttraumatic—at any age with subluxation of the caudal end of the septum with retraction of the columella.
3. Infection—chrondritis, septal hematoma or abscess with loss of support with characteristic saddling, sinking, or sagging of the cartilaginous vault.
4. Previous surgery with over enthusiastic removal of cartilage during a submucous resection.

These deformities cause altered shape of the nose and are affected by excess scar tissue with a downward pull on the aponeuroses between the cartilages resulting in a stiffness that causes increasing difficulty in breathing (Fig. 3).

Clinical Findings

Clinically, the deformities that result will cause: retraction of the columella; decrease in the length of the columella; deformities of the columella due to subluxation of the caudal end of the septum; widening of the base of the nose; change in the shape of the nostrils from elliptical to round; saddling of the cartilaginous vault.

Respiration starts and ends at the tip of the nose. After supplying oxygen to all cells of the body and carrying off the products of metabolism—mainly CO_2—this process must be done with a minimum of effort. However, if the mobility of the structures of the nose are affected by injury, its function is changed. Over a period of time, there is an increasing effort on the part of the patient to obtain adequate oxygen. The struggle to breathe is usually overlooked as the secondary organ of breathing—the mouth—gradually takes over. A study of blood gases indicate varying degrees of hypoxia, with symptoms usually not associated with these deformities.

Many variations of normal anatomy do not interfere with function, but when the normal control of inspiration or expiration through either nostril is abnormal, these variations become pathological.

Foman (1948)[1] wrote "Today's techniques have been developed to such a degree that the rhinologist can with the greatest assurance, clear the airway by re-alignment, unbuckling or removing part or all of the deflected septum. The feeling of confidence is lacking however, when it comes to restoration of function." This is still the opinion of many nasal surgeons, but one must consider the concept of the type of surgery performed. When one is familiar with the method of handling the tissues of the valve region, as the removal of the caudal end of the upper lateral cartilage with its mucosal covering as one of the steps in the shortening of the nose such as performed in the typical Joseph rhinoplasty.

In reviewing the function of the os internum or valve area, Van Dishoeck,[2] after extended research on pressure and flow studies of the nose by rhinomanometry, concluded "The fact that the ostium internum plays a major part in regulating the pressure on inspiration, shows that breathing difficulties in many instances are not caused by septal deviation and hypertrophic turbinates, but by an abnormally built vestibule or ostium internum. In these cases, submucous resections and conchotomies are inefficient if not preceded by regulation of the vestibule and os internum."

Thus, surgery of this region requires handling of all the structures of the base of the nose and restoration of the proper relationship to each other by reconstruction of the caudal end of the septum, the spine area and the valve. Mobility of these structures must be restored to obtain maximum function.

In order to approach all of the deformities, a sequence of steps should be followed that will adequately expose all of the involved structures. It is surprising that when all planes are undermined and freed, all parts of the nose show a tendency to revert to their original position without the necessity of stylizing the nose. With extensive undermining there is no need to use sutures until the excess bone, cartilage and scar tissue is removed. Only then is the necessary suturing performed to hold the tissues in proper alignment supplemented by the internal and external splints.

After adequate history regarding the patient's symptoms, such as headaches, head colds, nasal allergy, difficulty in breathing, chest pain, fatigue, etc., the nasal deformity is evaluated. The type of nose—the large tension nose, the twisted nose, the flat, broad nose, etc. We are especially interested in this paper in deformities of the base of the nose that affect the airway such as the narrow elliptical nostrils that may indicate collapse of the alse on inspiration; the flat broad nostril with a wide base and round or oval nostrils; the twisted nose that follows the contour of the septal ridge along the dorsum. The nose should be examined externally and internally, with or without a nasal speculum. To check septal deviations, the interior of the nose should be examined thoroughly for obstructions, impactions and any variations that may obstruct breathing, and to examine the relationship of the upper lateral cartilages to the septum. Most important is the columella—the retracted columella, or any deformity caused by the long caudal end of the septum extending into the columella with distortion of the medial crura.

Experience indicated that the approach to the septal structures, the exposure of the spine area, the handling of the lobule and surgery of the upper lateral cartilages are the most important steps in repair of the base of the nose.

Surgical Approach to the Maxillary Spine Region

After adequate preoperative medication, local anesthesia is the method of choice, although some surgeons prefer hypotensive general anesthesia. The method of application is described in many books and basically is topical application of cocaine flakes on an adrenalin moistened cotton applicator. Next, the nasal pyramid is infiltrated with Xylocaine 2 percent with 1:50,000 adrenalin, or as some prefer Xylocaine 1 percent with 1:100,000 adrenalin for black anesthesia.

In many patients, such as retracted columella, prominent spine, wide base of the lobule with a dependent lobule, there is a marked scarring with attachment of the naso-labial structures to the maxillary spine. Mobility must be obtained by surgically freeing this area by sufficient undermining to free the tissues of the base of the nose. This allows narrowing and rotation especially in the retracted columella or dropping of the tip of the lobule.

Textbooks on anatomy describe the terminal ends of the medial crura as ending about at the junction of the middle third of the columella (Fig. 6).

However, the findings in numerous complete dissections reveal that the medial crura do not end at this point, but continues downward to diverge on either side of the maxillary spine and then continues laterally for several millimeters along the floor of each nostril.

The fact that the medial crura are consistent both in length and position suggested that they could be dissected free from their attachments to the nasal spine and used surgically in the correction of deformities of the base of the nose.

The procedure includes separating the medial crura by blunt dissection and elevating the skin lateral to the terminal ends of the cartilages allowing these structures to swing free from their attachments and used to bunch the base of the lobule in front of the spine.

Mattress sutures of 3-0 plain catgut will change the nasolabial angle from 75° to 95° or 100° thus making it possible to use the normal cartilages of the columella to correct its deformity.

The hemi-transfixion incision is the procedure of choice for adequate surgical approach to the region of the maxilla-premaxillary area and to the terminal ends of the medial crura (Fig. 4).

In most cases, after anesthesia the Cottle clamp is applied to exert traction toward the left nostril. The incision is then carefully made on the right side of the septum about 3 to 5 mm cephalic to the caudal end of the cartilage. The membranes are elevated over the end of the cartilage and carried down the left side of the septum. Elevation must be sufficient to free the septal tissues to permit their advancement.

To establish mobility of the tissues in this area, the pull from contraction of scar tissue must be eliminated by undermining the subcutaneous and deep tissues to free them from the spine and face of the maxilla.

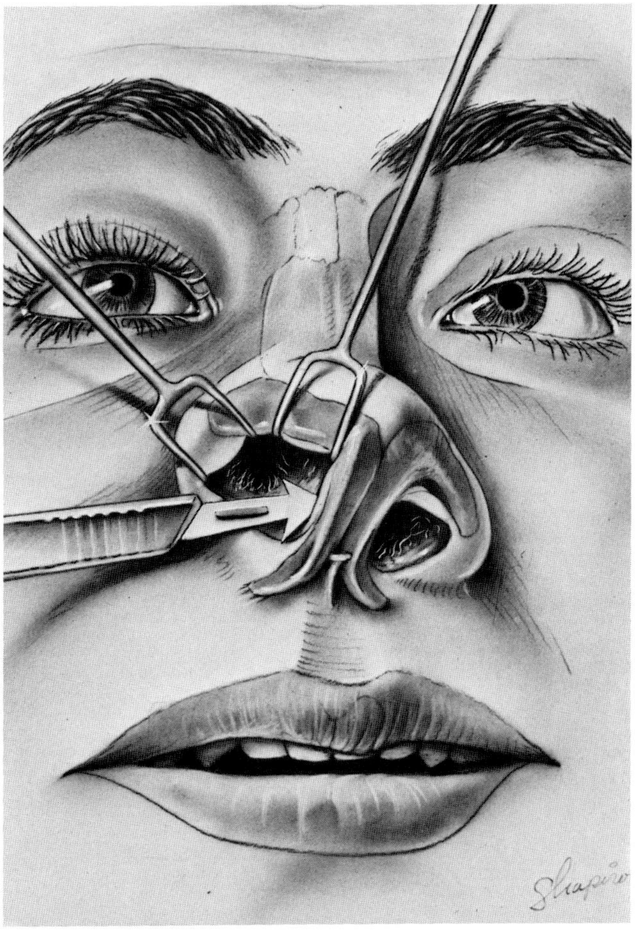

Fig. 4. Hemitransfixion incision indicating approach to the spine area, the terminal ends of the medial crura and face of maxilla.

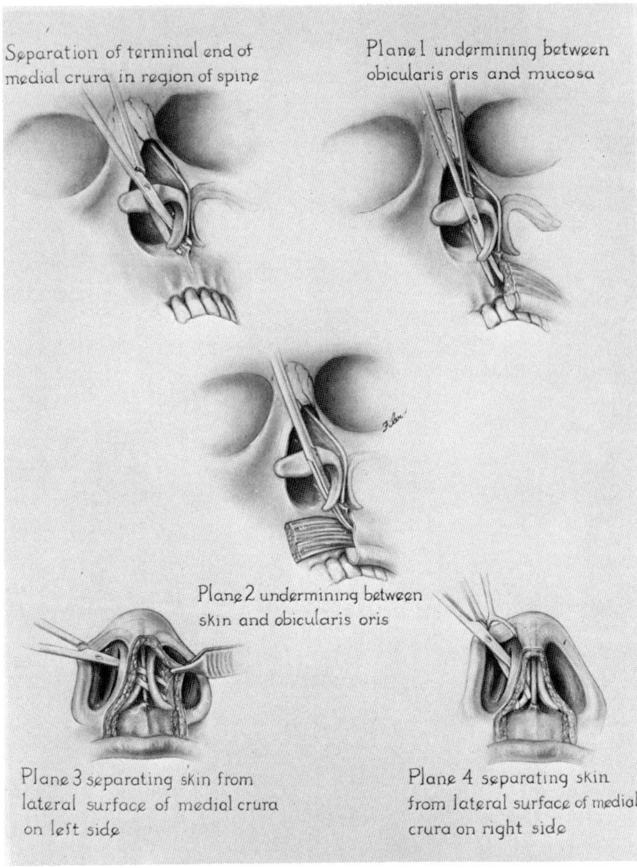

Fig. 5. Undermining of the structures of the base of the nose indicating sequence of steps to free and expose all structures by the Four Plane procedure. This approach will handle all types of deformities of the base of the nose.

Sufficient undermining is accomplished in five stages where the four planes are used to free the structures of the base of the nose, bunch them and seat them in front of the spine to prevent postoperative widening of the base of the nose and retraction of the columella (Fig. 5).

The first step is insertion of the tip of the Knapp scissors into the lower end of the hemitransfixion incision. With small spreading movements the area between the membranous septum and between the terminal ends of the medial crura. This procedure is used to obtain mobility of the base of the columella and as the method to approach to Plane 1.

The undermining is continued to the area between the orbicularis oris and the buccal mucosa and carry it extensively from left to right as far as the naso-alar folds.

Plane 2. In order to get a sliding action of the tissues on each side of the orbicularis oris, it is necessary to undermine the area between the skin of the upper tip and the orbicularis oris.

Plane 3. Separating the vestibular skin from the lateral surface of the medial crura on the left side entering through the hemitransfixion incision.

Plane 4. is separation of the vestibular skin from the lateral surface of the right medial crura as shown in Plane 3.

In the procedure of separation of the vestibular skin on the left and right side done in Plane 3 and Plane 4, the undermining must be carried to the ends of the cartilages where it diverges on each side of the spine where basal bunching sutures are used to narrow and seat these structures in front of the spine (Fig. 6).

With complete freedom of structures following the above procedures, it is necessary to proceed further with correction of the deformity of the lobule and reconstruction of the nasal valve.

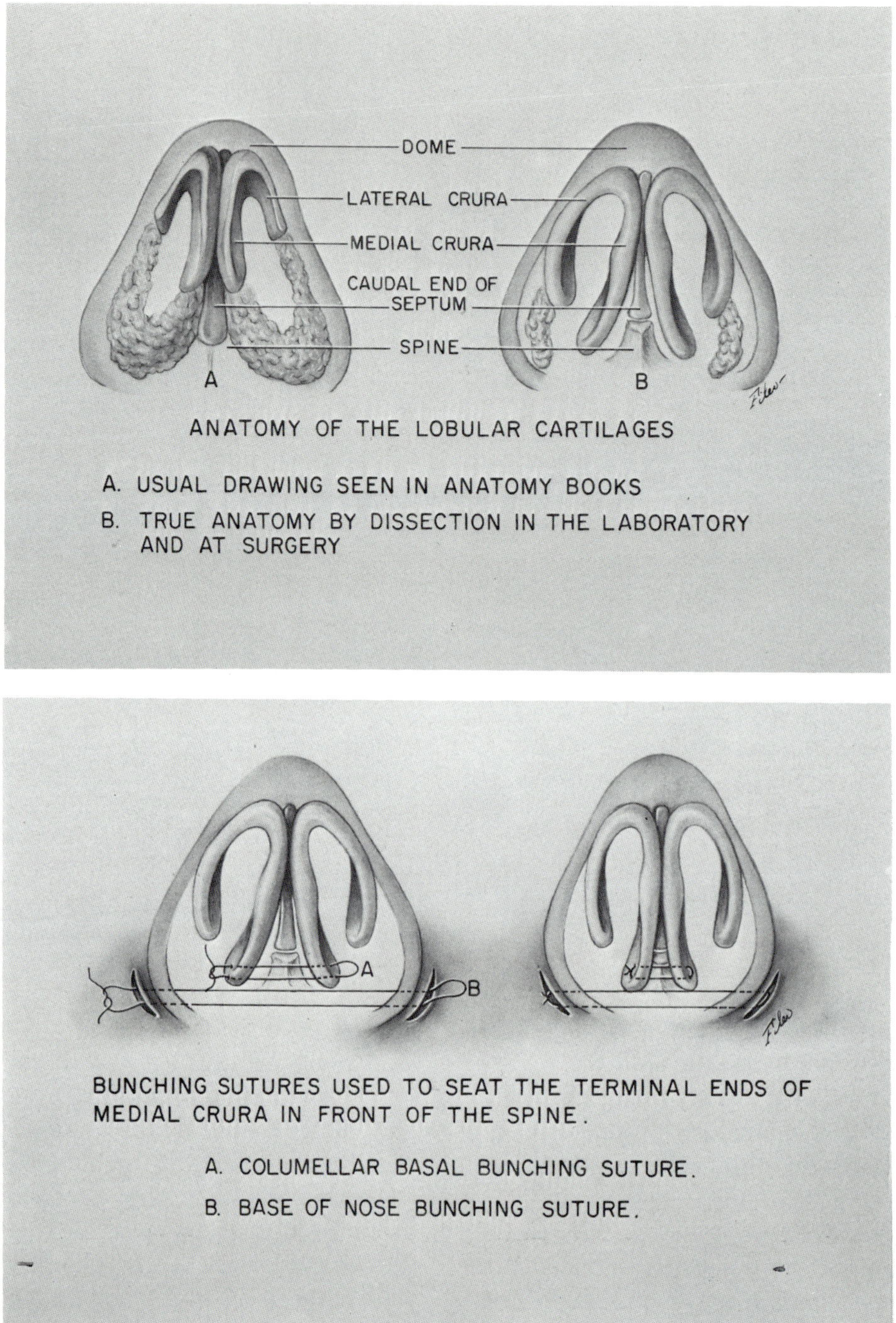

Fig. 6. (Top) Anatomy of the lobular cartilages. (A) Usual drawing seen in anatomy textbooks. (B) The true anatomy as shown by dissection in the anatomy laboratory. (Bottom) (A) Columellar basal bunching suture. (B) Base of the lobule bunching suture. Bunching sutures used to seat the terminal ends of the medial crura in front of the spine.

Corrective Surgery of the Nasal Valve

The nasal valve, first described by Mink in 1903 is the narrow passage between the lower or caudal margin of the upper lateral cartilage and the septum. It controls the respiratory air currents changing them from a column of air to a sheet of air. The relationship of the upper lateral cartilage to the septum is very important as the upper lateral cartilage must be capable of movement with respiration and the shift of the position of the head in sleep.

The etiology of a valve deformity is any injury that causes flattening of the nose or deviation of the nasal pyramid and septum from the midline (Figs. 7, 8).

The valve is part of the nose and surgery of the valve is one of the steps in the overall correction. The structures that make up the valve are intimately connected with the anatomy of the base of the nose. Thus, it is necessary to dwell on this area that is so important to nasal function. The lobule is an accessory part of the valve and surgery of the valve must be based on the recognition of this close anatomical and physiological relationship.

Surgery for restoration of the valve function is tedious and time consuming, but it is a rewarding procedure. It is done early in the operation when the anesthesia is good, the field is dry, and the patient is not restless. It follows the corrective surgery of the septum, the base of the nose with exposure of the spine with freeing of the tissues. The approach to the valve area is through the intercartilaginous incision following extensive elevation of the tissues over the dorsum. The skin over the lobule is undermined widely through the intercartilaginous incision with a curved Foman upper lateral cartilage scissors. The alar margin of the nostril is retracted and the caudal border of the upper lateral cartilage is grasped with a thumb forceps. A sharp curved iris scissors is used to tease and elevate the mucosa from the under surface of the upper lateral cartilage. The subcutaneous and muscle tissue that lies over the upper lateral cartilage that controls mobility of the valve is freed and pushed upwards. The mucosa is carefully preserved as well as the canopy of the muscle tissue. When both sides of the terminal end of the upper lateral cartilage has been denuded, the deformity is studied to determine the amount of cartilage to be excised (Fig. 9).

Next, the lobular cartilage is exposed through a slot or rim incision which is delivered to study the amount of cartilage to be removed for narrowing and projection of the lobule. Only the cartilage is removed from the cephalic border of the lobular cartilage with preservation of the vestibular skin of the cephalic border.

No mucosa is excised as the mucosa is dissected free from the cartilage, as it has a tendency to contract, but there is an adequate lip of mucosa remaining after this submucosal removal of a strip of cartilage from the cephalic margin of the lower lateral cartilage. It will be noted that a lip of mucosa is preserved at the time of removal of the caudal margin of the upper lateral cartilage. The strip of

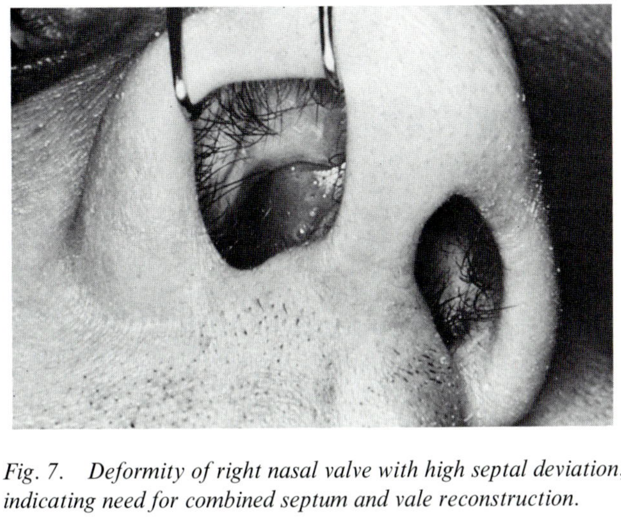

Fig. 7. Deformity of right nasal valve with high septal deviation, indicating need for combined septum and vale reconstruction.

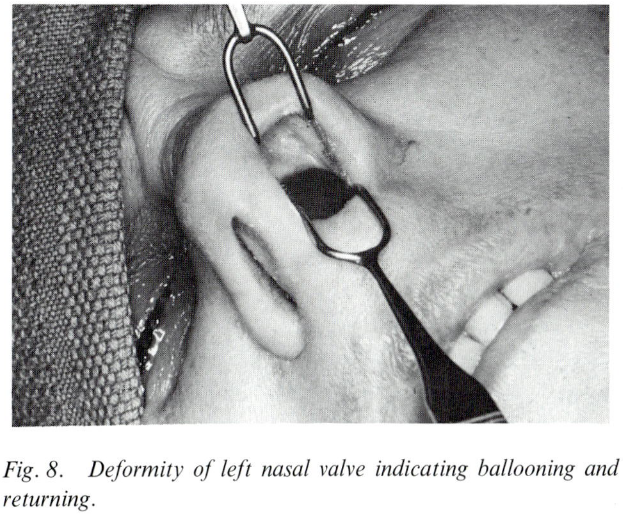

Fig. 8. Deformity of left nasal valve indicating ballooning and returning.

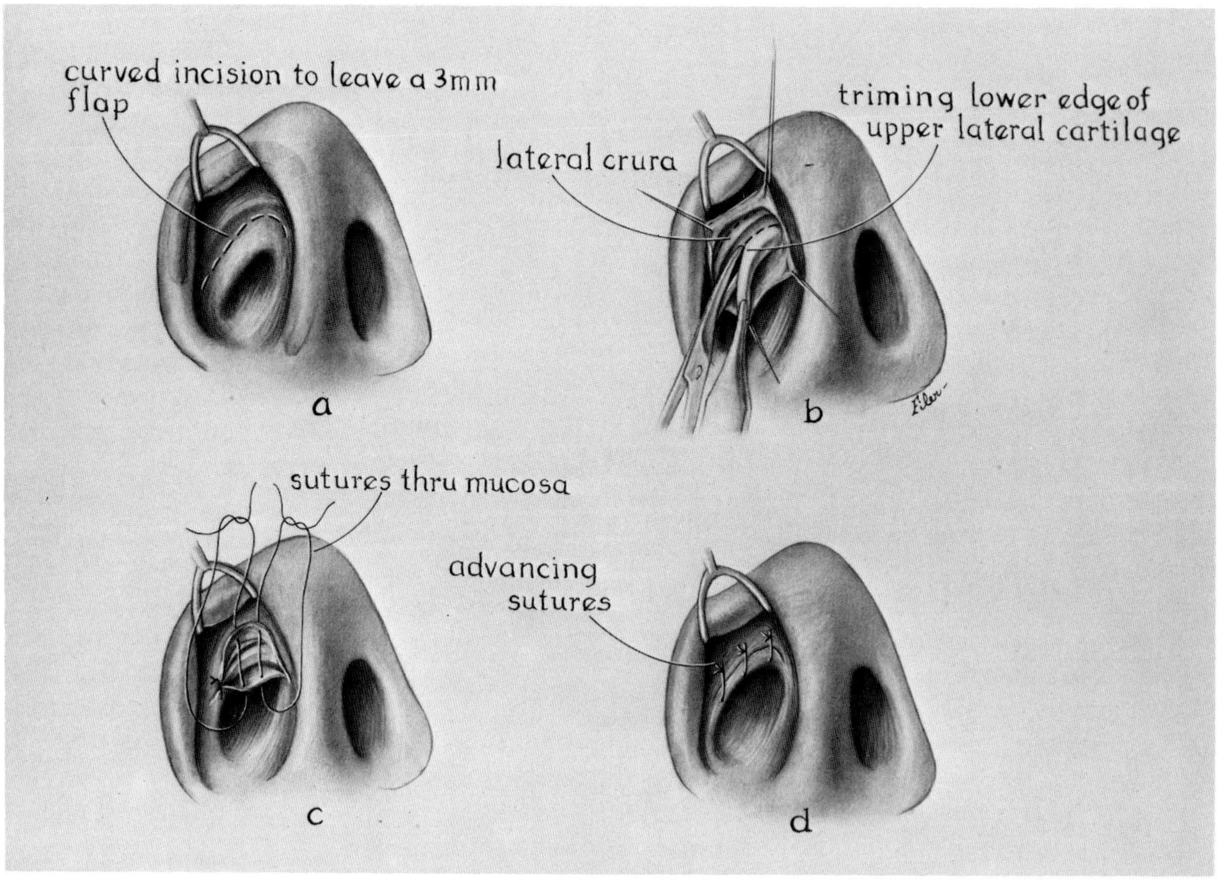

Fig. 9. Reconstruction of the nasal valve. (A) The intercartilaginous incision made with a 15 Bard Parker knife 3 mm caudal to the rim of the upper lateral cartilage. (B) Caudal edge of upper lateral cartilage excised with preservation of the 3 mm flap. A 3 mm flap is preserved in removing the cephalic border of the lobular cartilage. (C) The mucosal flaps are sutured with advancing sutures of 3-0 plain catgut inserted parallel with the septum. (D) Sutures in place.

mucosa along each margin of the intercartilaginous incisions when sutured with a 3-0 plain catgut advancing suture as indicated in Figure 4 C and D will correct or prevent any tendency to saddling of flattening of the cartilaginous vault postoperatively. A 3-0 plain catgut in a curved needle is used. The first suture is inserted inferiorly into the lip of mucosa on the cephalic margin of the lobular cartilage. These orthopedic sutures are inserted parallel with the septum and will advance the upper lateral cartilage and prevent any undue saddling of the mid-third of the nasal dorsum.

However, these advancing sutures are not put into place until all work is done in all parts of the nose. No sutures are used until all steps of the opertion are completed. At this time all parts of the nose are freely movable and will fall into position without tension before any sutures are inserted.

In addition to the surgery of the valve and the lobule, it is necessary in most cases to correct deformities of the bony pyramid by medial and lateral osteotomies with mobilization by infracture. When all of these structures are mobilized and the pull of the scar tissue corrected it is possible to visualize how the basal structures fall into proper relationship. It is necessary to hold these structures in alignment by:

1. Columellar basal bunching sutures.
2. Basal bunching suture with 2-0 chromic catgut.
3. Insertion of cartilage or bone in the septal envelopes.
4. Suturing of the hemitransfixion with 3-0 plain catgut.
5. Suturing of the intercartilaginous incisions by 3-0 catgut.

6. Intra nasal packing or internal splinting.
7. External splinting with adhesive tape supplemented by a dental wax mold.
8. Pressure dressing over the eyes for 12 to 18 hr.

Summary

Correction of deformities of the base of the nose concerns procedures, not only to correct defects present as a result of injury or surgery, but also to prevent later consequences of extensive septorhinoplasty procedures.

Deformity of the base of the nose creates a poor appearance, but more importantly, it is an indication of poor function. Correction of deformities of this area is more than a localized problem. It involves many structures and their relationship to each other, namely, the caudal end of the septum, the membranous septum and its attachment to the medial crura, the maxillary spine and the prespine fibers, the lobular cartilages and their fibrous attachments to the upper lateral cartilages. All of these structures are connected to each other by strong fibrous and muscular attachments which cause changes in their relationship resulting in poor control over inspiratory air currents. Characteristic deformities are saddling of the dorsum, retraction of the columella, widening of base of the nose, shortened columella, with round or oval nostrils. This deformity also involves the nasal valve which must be reconstructed at the same time.

Extensive undermining to free the involved structures forms the basis for surgical correction of this typical deformity.

The author has devised a method of reconstruction of the valve as well as the "four plane" procedure which mobilizes all of the structures for restoring the proper relationship. With adequate undermining and with the use of bunching sutures, the need for battens or struts are eliminated and the mobility of the structures of the base of the nose will be restored.

References

1. Foman et al: Plastic repair of the obstructing septum. Arch Otolaryng (Chicago) 47:7:29, 1948
2. Van Dishoeck HAE: Inspiratory nasal resistence. Acta Otolaryng (Stockholm) 30:431–439, 1942
3. Mink PJ: The nose as a means of breathing. Presse Otolaryng Belge 21:481–496, 1903

The Cleft-Lip Nose (Septo-Rhinoplasty and Combined Lip Repair)

Richard T. Farrior, Tampa, Fla.

Secondary nasal deformities for both the unilateral and bilateral cleft-lip will continue to be seen despite many improvements in the initial management of the deformity, including modern repair of the lip and nasal base, early orthodonics, and bone grafting. There will continue to be nasal deformities as nothing to date is done to overcome the existing mesodermal deficiency. The pathological embryology and the possible disturbances of growth potential by the necessary primary surgery remain contributing factors. Management of the residual nasal deformity presents a more difficult and serious problem and a greater challenge than secondary repairs of the lip.

The importance of the secondary nasal deformity in the cleft lip patient cannot be overemphasized regarding both esthetic appearance and disturbed nasal physiology. Altered nasal respiration and obstruction also affect speech. The surgeon's attention must be directed towards correcting the involved structures and his approach based on the study of the development of the defect, the influences of the primary surgery, and a critical analysis of the structures involved in the particular secondary deformity.[5] There is a tendency among rhinoplastic surgeons to neglect nasal physiology in their efforts towards ideal appearance.[7] The problems are more complicated in the cleft-lip nose but I do not believe too much emphasis can be placed on the need for correcting the variety of septal deformities and abnormalities of the nasal vestibule as seen in this deformity.

The Unilateral Cleft-Lip Nose

In the original publication[5] the operation as outlined contained several original techniques and these will be reviewed briefly here, but correction of the combined deformity requires the incorporation of many proven and well-known nasoplastic and septoplastic procedures[5,7,9,11]. Each deformity must be individualized and the required surgery performed including a complete rhinoplasty and septal reconstruction when indicated.

All phases of the operation, either for the unilateral or the bilateral deformity, may not be required in a particular case but if necessary they can all be performed in one sitting, including the necessary secondary lip repairs.

In 1954 I began using the techniques referred to here and this was published as a thesis in 1962.[5] This article for the unilateral cleft-lip nose was an in-depth study and review of the pathogenesis, analysis of the resulting deformity, and a critical review and comparison of previously published techniques. It is not the intention to review again these aspects of the problem, but I would refer the reader to this publication. The bibliography includes some additional references and the present paper makes a comparison with the bilateral cleft-lip nose deformity.

The Bilateral Cleft-Lip Nose

In comparing the unilateral and bilateral cleft-lip nose deformity (Figs. 1, 2 and 8) it is noted that the bilateral problem is compounded by the mesodermal mass which is lacking in all three compo-

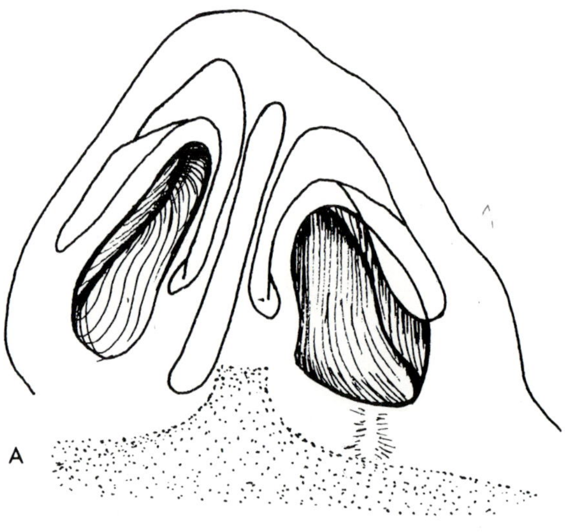

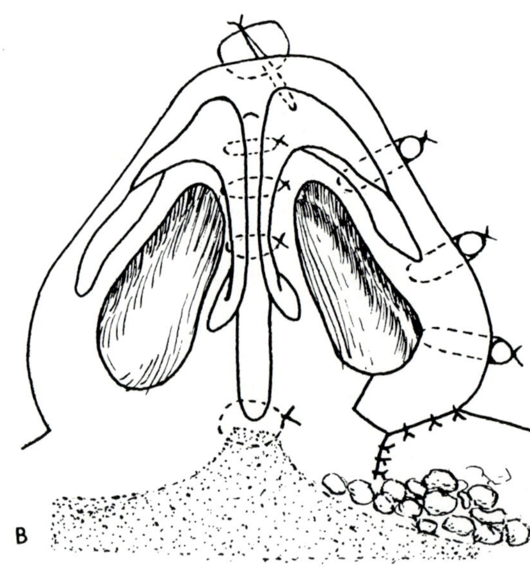

Fig. 1. (A) The pathological anatomy which must be corrected is: (1) caudal displacement and the abnormal relationship of the lower lateral cartilage on the involved side; (2) the alar attachment at the naso-facial and naso-labial areas; (3) the floor of the nostril including oronasal fistulas; (4) position of the columella and caudal margin of the septum; (5) the underlying maxilla beneath the alar attachment; (6) septal deflection and dislocations, anterior and posterior; and (7) additional associated nasal and lip deformities as indicated. (B) illustrates the repositioning and slight overcorrection of the lower lateral cartilage and reconstruction of the other components. The use of autogenous grafts over the face of the maxilla beneath the alar attachment is emphasized.

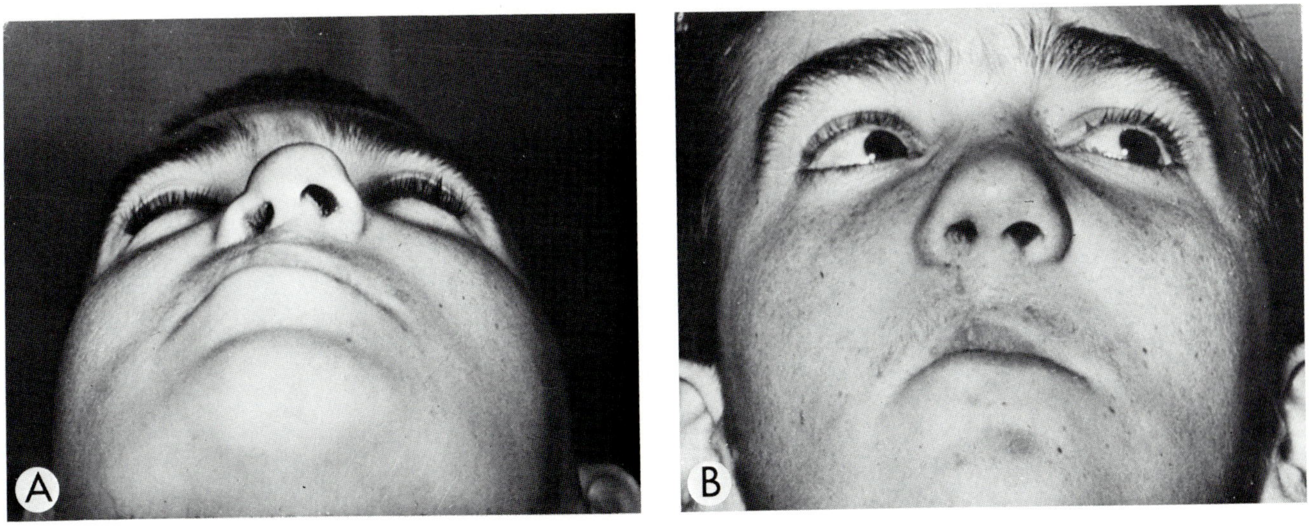

Fig. 2. (A) The preoperative picture demonstrating the anatomic distortions and underdevelopment of the maxilla. (B) Postoperative, demonstrating the repositioned alar attachment and balance of the lower lateral cartilages in the dome without surgery on the uninvolved lower lateral cartilage.

nents, or the two lateral maxillary masses and the medial premaxillary mass. The position of the premaxilla is less favorable than when attached to one side as in the unilateral lip. The premaxilla is more often better developed in the unilateral lip. The primordia of the nose and the globular process or medial mesodermal mass may well be involved in the bilateral cleft-lip nose. This would certainly seem more involved than in the unilateral lip.

To be considered in the original deformity and the resulting distortions which create the secondary deformity would necessarily be the width of the cleft of the lip and the palate and techniques used in the primary repair of these. Prior to approaching the secondary nasal deformity, what had been done regarding columellar lengthening, the use of a vomerine flap, repair of the palate, bone graft, etc.? It has been the author's impression both in the unilateral and bilateral cleft-lip that the lower lateral cartilage seems to be sufficient in substance but is simply distorted. Distortion is increased in the bilateral deformity, something which is readily understandable when the limited columella and prolabium are evaluated in the newborn (Fig. 8). All too often we still see that the entire premaxilla has been removed (Fig. 9). Perhaps an Abbe flap has already been performed before the nasal deformity is to be corrected. This may or may not have been done with an associated columellar lengthening.

Surgical Technique

The surgical technique for the unilateral cleft-lip nose has been previously published and is reviewed briefly in (Figs. 3–6). This may be modified in the case of nasal stenosis (Fig. 7), however, the other components are managed in essentially the same way. A reflection of the difficulties encountered in the repair of this deformity is seen in the literature as the published results show asymmetries and imperfections which the same surgeons by reputation would not get with other plastic procedures. In attacking these problems one must maintain an open mind, being prepared to use any one of the techniques already outlined in the indicated situations. The complete operation, as we have performed it, differs in three main respects from previously published articles for repair of the cleft-lip nose. There must be specific correction of the lateral and retrodisplaced area beneath the lateral alar attachment associated with underdevelopment of the maxilla. I use an autogenous implant over the maxilla in a single operation. The method of presenting the lower lateral cartilage is different from others in that the entire dome and lateral crus of cartilage are completely presented free of both surface and vestibular skin. The method by which the alar cartilage is repositioned, both in the dome and over the lateral aspects of the upper lateral cartilage, is unique. The approach to the lateral

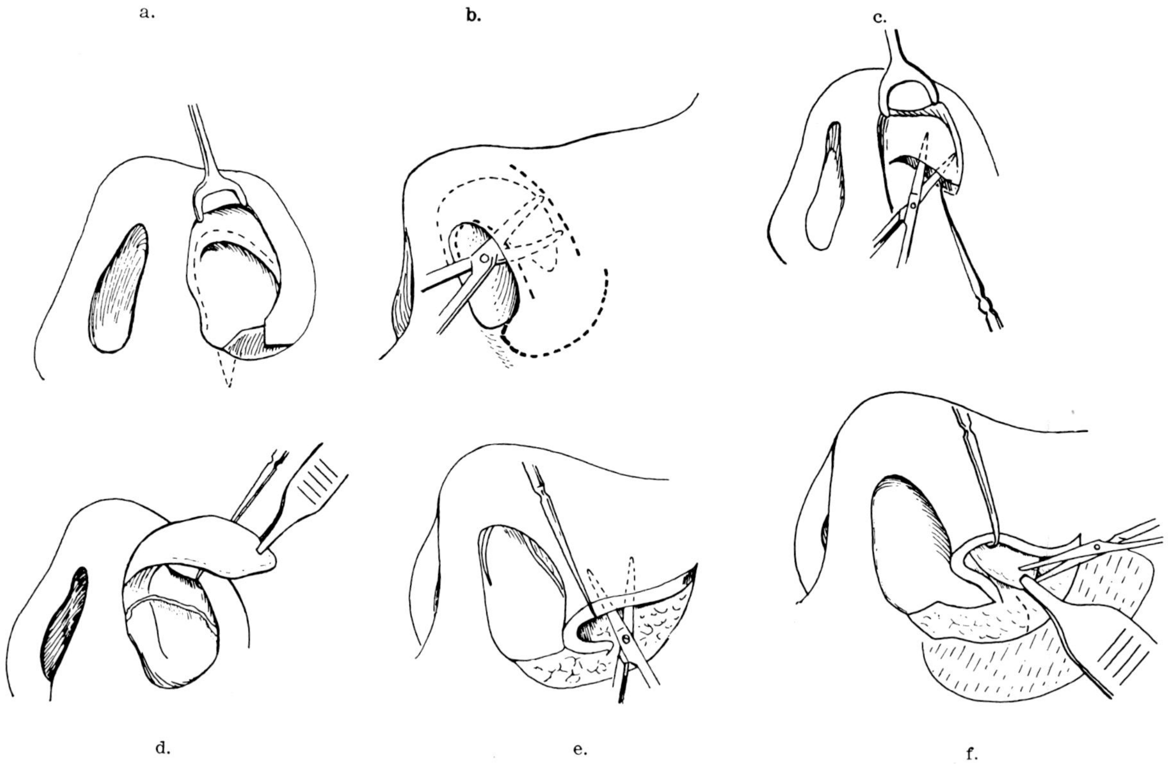

Fig. 3. Summary of the Author's Technique. For the unilateral cleft-lip nose, the lower lateral cartilage is presented completely free of both vestibular and surface skin and is separated at its lateral attachment. The lateral alar skin surfaces are separated so that they may be rotated on themselves with repositioning in a sliding plane. The lateral thickening is corrected by removal of intervening fibro-adipose tissue.

alar attachment at the naso-facial function has not been described in the cleft-lip nose particularly as regards to separating the two skin surfaces of the ala through this lateral incision. This lateral incision is further used for insertion of an implant over the underdeveloped maxilla and for thinning the thickened lateral ala.

General Considerations

When the complete operation is performed in combination with a total rhinoplasty it is preferable to wait until after adolescence before performing the surgery. In general girls may be operated on earlier than teenage boys, both because of the advanced physical development and because the nose need not have reached complete development to produce a pleasing cosmetic result. If only the nasal base and anterior septal cartilage is to be repaired, this can be performed in the older child and it is the option of many that the sooner the repair is accomplished the less severe distortion of the involved structures will result with continued growth. In line with the thinking related to the abnormal pull and malposition of the structures involved, it would seem desirable to correct the deformity at as early age as possible.[5,16] Establishing an adequate airway and realining the displaced structure should favor more normal growth rather than disturb growth. If the combined external nasal and septal deformity is producing significant obstruction to the airway and disturbing normal nasal physiology, it is desirable to correct the obstruction at an early age to prevent the characteristic facies of the child with chronic nasal obstruction.[7]

In carrying out the complete operation, the sequence may be altered to the individual surgeon's preference but in general considerable taking apart must be completed before any putting back together is done. Several stages of the operation directly influence the results of related or adjacent areas. Unless one structure is freed the others will not conform maximally to the new position. Correction of the lip, oronasal fistulae, and other associated

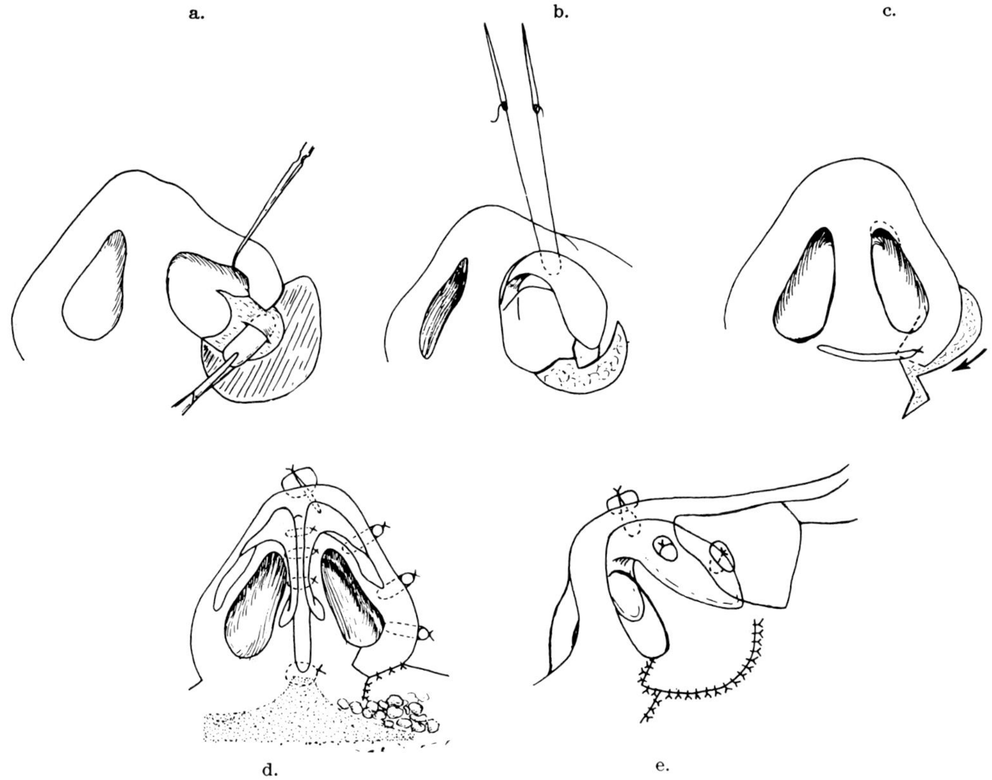

Fig. 4. Summary of the Author's Technique. The maxillary implant may be inserted through the same exposure. The repositioned lower lateral cartilage is sutured in the dome in slight overcorrection to the uninvolved side. Laterally, it is rotated and sutured over the upper lateral cartilage in a more normal position also correcting the infolding.

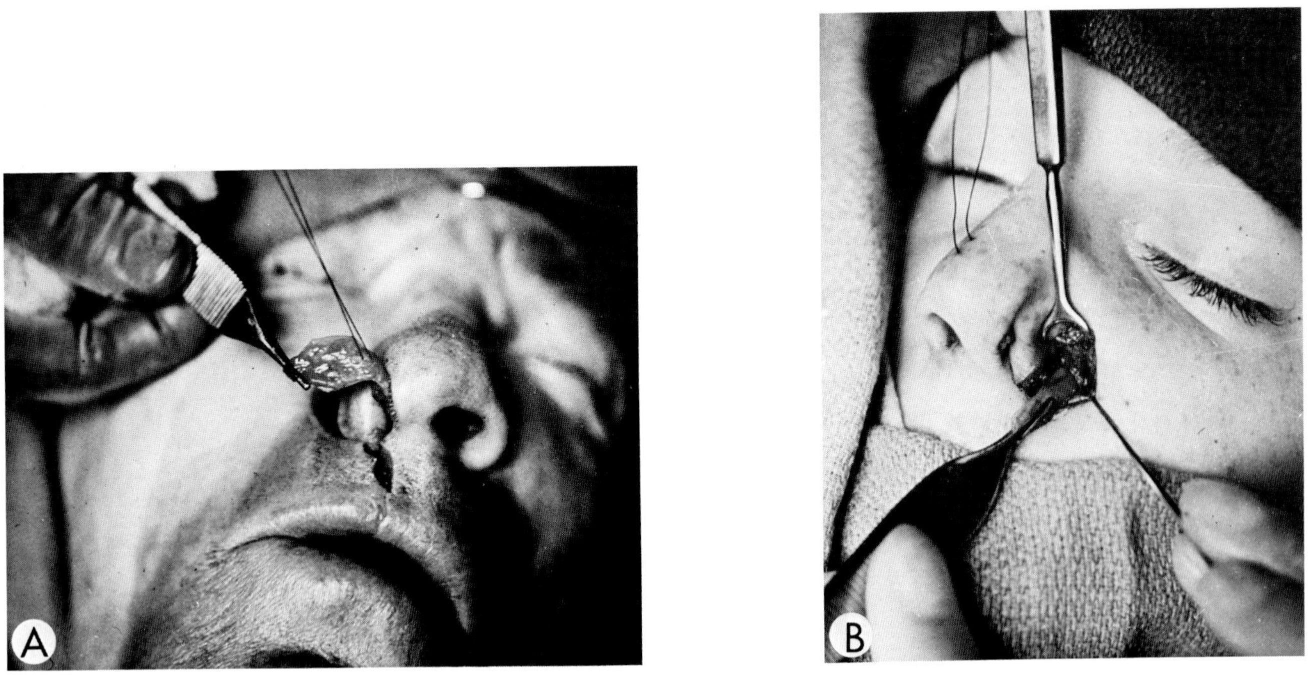

Fig. 5. (A) Demonstrates the presented lower lateral cartilage free of surface and vestibular skin. (B) Insertion of autogenous bone through the lateral alar incision.

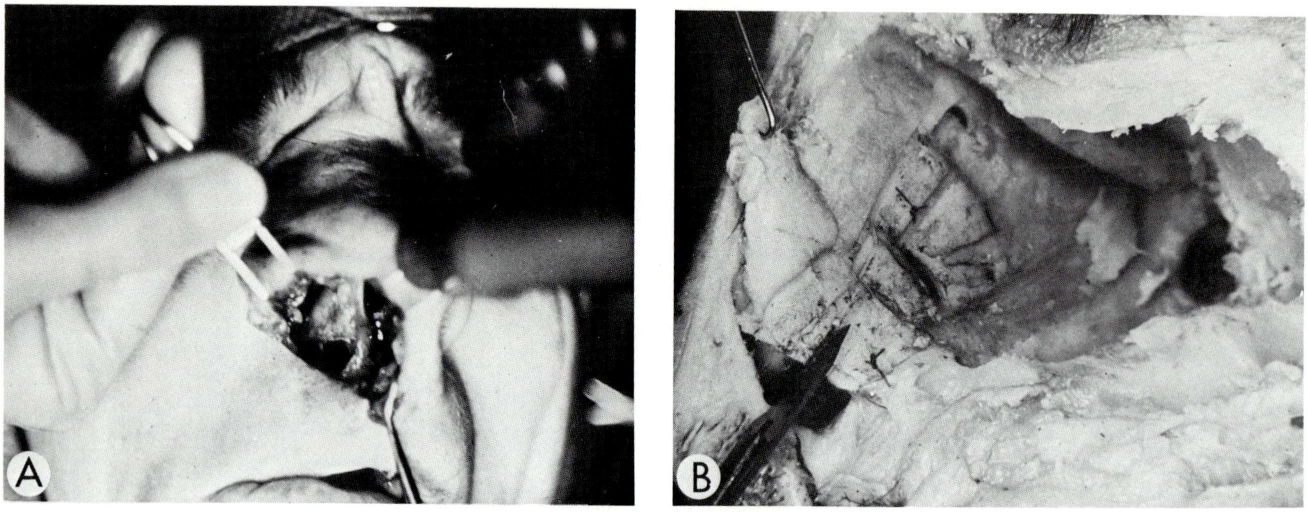

Fig. 6. *(A) Caudal displacement into the uninvolved side is classic. The author reports consistent posterior septal spurs to the involved side. A large spur on the side of the cleft is demonstrated here. (B) In the cleft-lip nose advanced septal reconstruction techniques are essential particularly of the anterior or caudal nasal septum. This is a cadaver dissection showing resuturing and cross-hatching of the caudal septum and reconstruction posteriorly.*

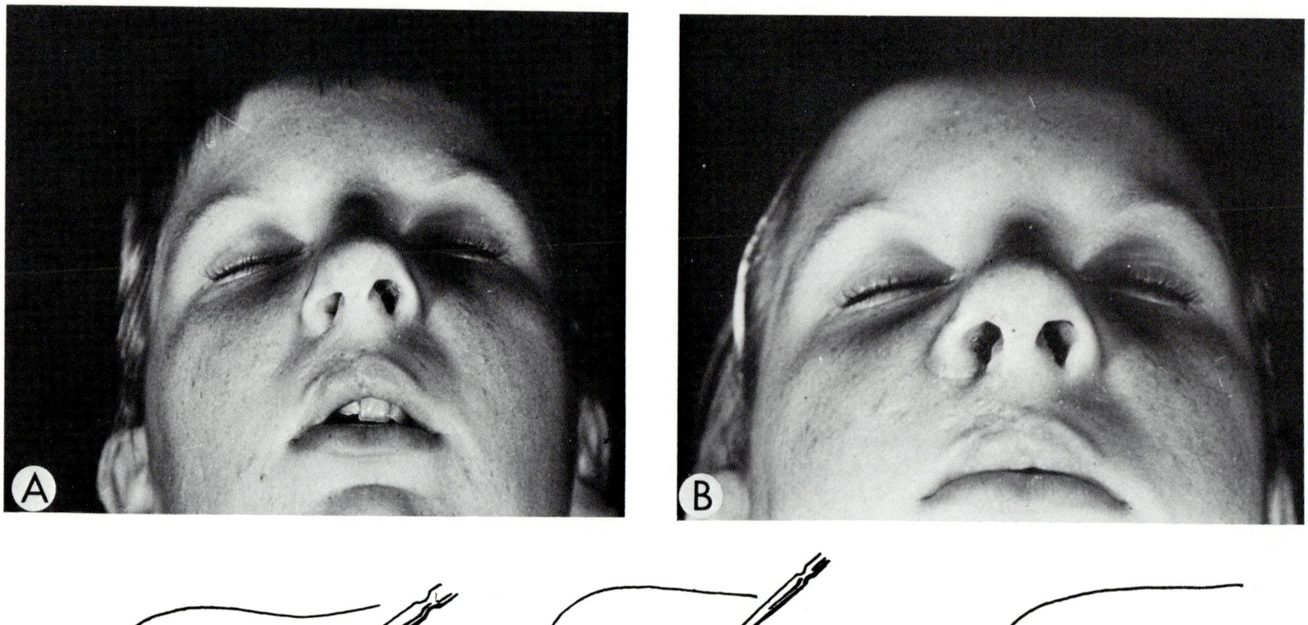

Fig. 7. *(A) Stenosis of the involved nostril. (B) Postoperative correction and lateral displacement with a V-Y closure. (C) Surgical technique.*

deformities calls for individualization and imagination but in general should be taken apart with those of the nose for the most satisfactory exposure and best final result.

Summary of Technique for the Unilateral Cleft-Lip Nose (Figs. 3–7)

1. The lower lateral cartilage is completely freed of both external and vestibular skin extending from the medial aspect of the dome to the lateral extent of the cartilage. This exposure is accomplished by eversion through the intercartilaginous incision and through an extended alar margin incision.

2. The lateral alar attachment is freed in the nasolabial and nasofacial groove. Through the freed margin the two surfaces of the ala are separated and excessive fibro-adipose tissue removed. This procedure, combined with (1) above, not only allows respositioning but aids in correction of the infolding at the lateral aspect of the limen vestibuli. No incision is made in the mucous membrane in this area.

3. The dorsal nasal hump is removed prior to any septal surgery and saved for use as an autogenous implant.

4. The septal reconstruction is now accomplished. The surgeon must be prepared to meet any number of abnormalities about the premaxilla and at the nasal floor, particularly if an anterior fistula exists, or if a complete cleft of the palate is present. The full complement of reconstructive septal procedures for removal and repositioning of the nasal septum, particularly along the anterior and caudal margins, should be familiar to the surgeon. All removed septum is used as an autogenous implant.

5. Through the alar attachment incision the periosteum over the maxilla about the lateral and inferior pyriform rim is elevated to receive the implant.

6. The routine medial and lateral osteotomies are carried out bilaterally. The lateral osteotomy on the involved side is performed through the lateral incision and site of the previous periosteal elevation.

7. The alar cartilage is now repositioned by utilizing a bolster suture which passes through the cartilage only on the vestibular side, slightly lateral to the abnormal dome. When the suture is passed through the dorsal skin the recessed dome on the cleft side is pulled into a slightly over-correct position relative to the normal dome. The medial crus on the involved side is further splinted to the medial crus of the uninvolved side and to the nasal septum. The vestibular skin is then sutured with mattress sutures to the repositioned cartilage.

8. The lateral wing of the lower lateral cartilage is placed so as to override the inferior margin of the upper lateral cartilage in a normal fashion to prevent narrowing and infolding.

9. The alar attachment is repositioned at a height and angle matching the uninvolved side. The separated alar surfaces allow necessary rotation in two planes for the production of normal contour about the new alar margin.

10. The autogenous bone and cartilage implant is placed about the pyriform rim especially beneath the new alar attachment. This raises the attachment away from the face of the maxilla in a ventral direction, thus overcoming the underdevelopment of the maxilla in this area.

11. Sutures are passed through the vestibular skin, lower lateral cartilage, and external skin and tied over small bolsters, as necessary for maintaining the new position of each component.

12. The lateral defect is now closed by advancing the cheek and lip downward and medialward. This is accomplished as an advancement flap in cases when the lip is completely sectioned for revision.

13. When narrowing of the nostril is required, a section of the nasal floor is removed. If the nostril must be enlarged, the author's "V-Y" incision and closure is utilized.

14. The bolsters used and the intranasal packing are of cellulose cord sponge. When osteotomies are done, a routine rhinoplasty splint is modified so as not to produce excessive pressure over the bolsters.

The Bilateral Cleft-Lip Nose

The philosophy and the techniques, where applicable, are also used in the bilateral cleft-lip nose. These techniques in particular are the method of

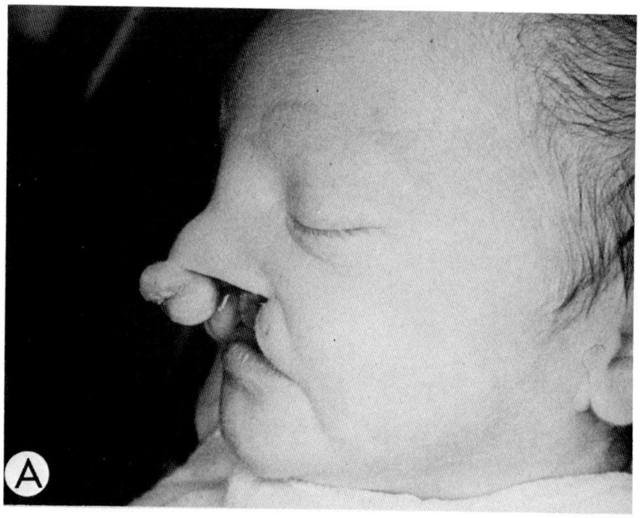

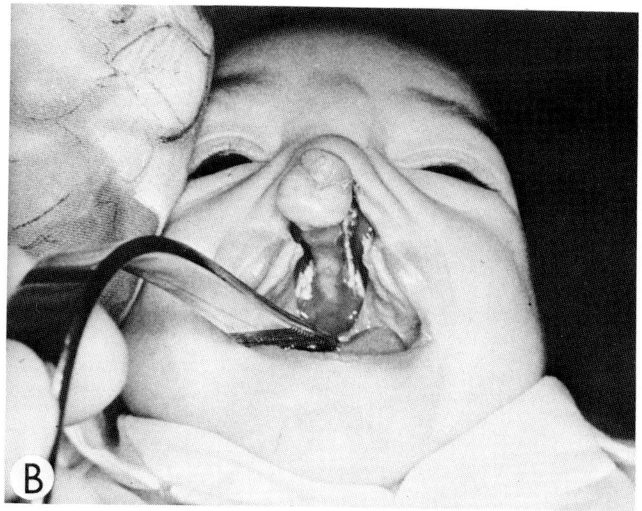

Fig. 8. (A) Severe bilateral cleft lip compounding the problems by mesodermal deficiency medially as well as laterally. (B) The management of the premaxilla and columella influence secondary surgical procedures.

presenting and repositioning the lower lateral cartilage, the use of implants over the maxilla to build up the nasal base, the alar-facial incisions and repositioning as described above.

To say the least, the operation is more complex for the bilateral deformity. More often it is necessary to use some modification of the Abbe flap (Figs. 9–12). The peri-alar cresentic excision may be utilized to advance the lateral lip thereby reducing the size of the necessary Abbe flap and also serve the purpose of assisting in narrowing the nasal base (Fig. 12). In the severe deformity in the older patient prosthetic devices are often required. This may be due either to the severity of the deformity which prevented some aspects of primary repair or to overenthusiastic primary repair (Fig. 11).

In the repair of large, bony defects in the older patient, autogenous cancellous bone remains the implant of choice (Fig. 13). I would discourage the use of synthetics, even silicone, in the nose and about the nasal base.[8,9]

Septal Reconstruction

As mentioned, all advanced rhinoplasty and septoplasty techniques may need to be incorporated in a particular case. In my experience, several simple developments have occurred through the years in septal reconstructions but these can only be briefly mentioned here. I would say that in general, with improved techniques, the septum may be more and more thoroughly taken apart but at the same time less and less tissue is removed. The excision of angulated portions of the septum may be more vigorously carried out if the mucous membrane is left attached to one side of the septum (Fig. 6). Intranasal splinting with polyethelene plates has proven helpful both in maintaining the new position of the septum and in preventing postoperative synechiae. In the cleft-lip nose, particularly the unilateral cleft-lip nose, particular attention must be given to the anterior or caudal septum. This is often dislocated and must be freed from the existing anterior spine and maxillary crest (Fig. 6). When resutured in position one suture should be passed between the cartilage and the pedestal of the anterior spine to prevent dislocation off of the spine. Sutures passed between the cartilage incisions for angulations also prevent overriding or dislocation. The use of draw sutures through the dorsal skin, as well as into the columella, are helpful either in positioning and maintaining position or in holding the position until the completion of operation and proper nasal packing and splinting. Should there be a loss of support, the dorsal draw suture may be passed out through the dorsum of the nose and tied over a bolus to be held in position for seven days. If necessary, removal of the caudal septum and repositioning as a free graft or columellar strut may be done. All efforts should be made to gain tip projection by the procedures outlined, however, columellar struts

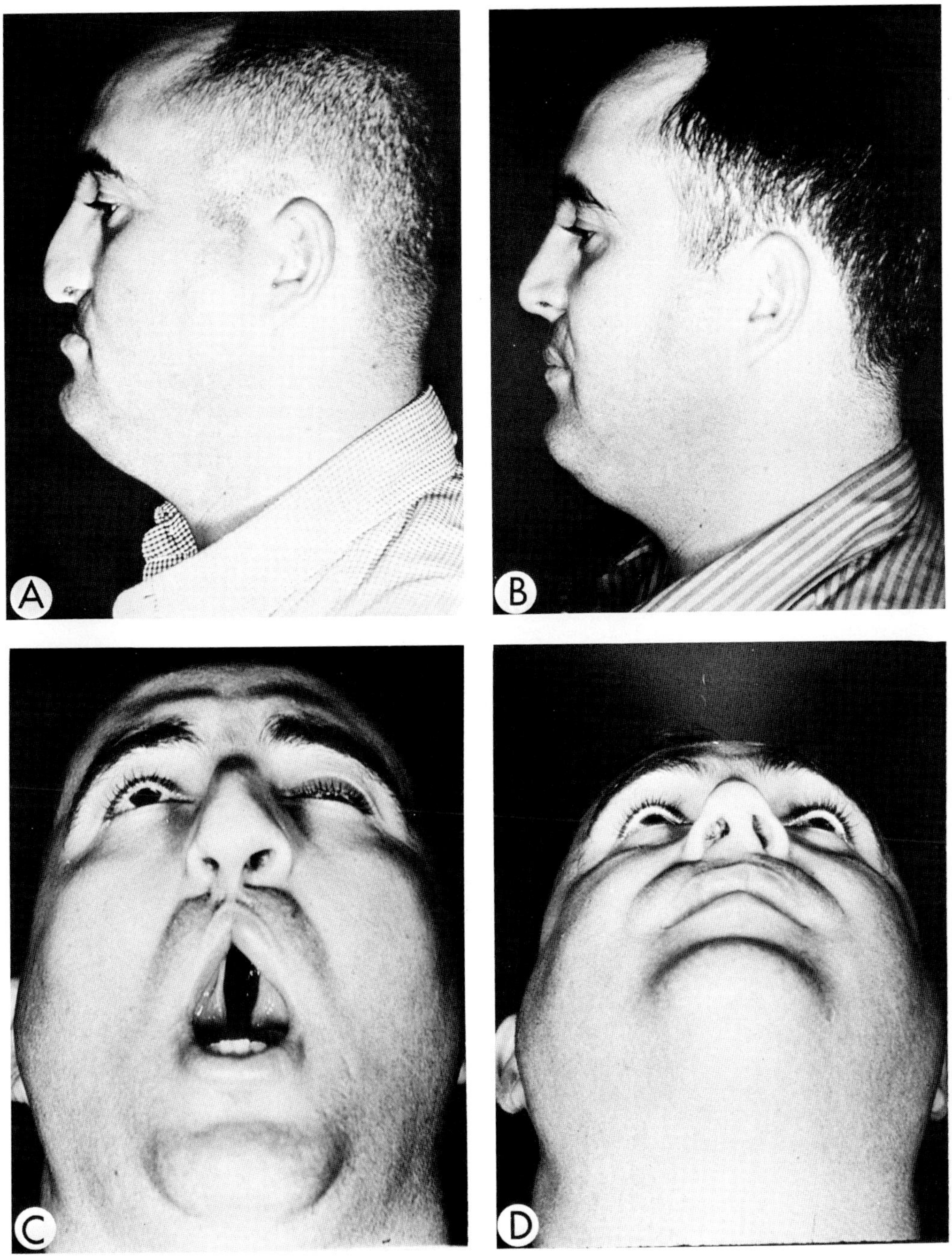

Fig. 9. *(A) Classic deformity of the bilateral cleft-lip nose with previous resection of premaxilla. (B) Postoperative profile following the composite operation with reconstruction of the lip utilizing an Abbe flap and combined septo-rhinoplasty. (C) Basal view showing the unrepaired cleft palate and stenosis of the right nostril. (D) Basal view showing tip projection and symmetry following exposure and repositioning of the lower lateral cartilages. An asymmetrical Abbe flap was utilized to correct the stenosis on the right and will require minimal secondary correction.*

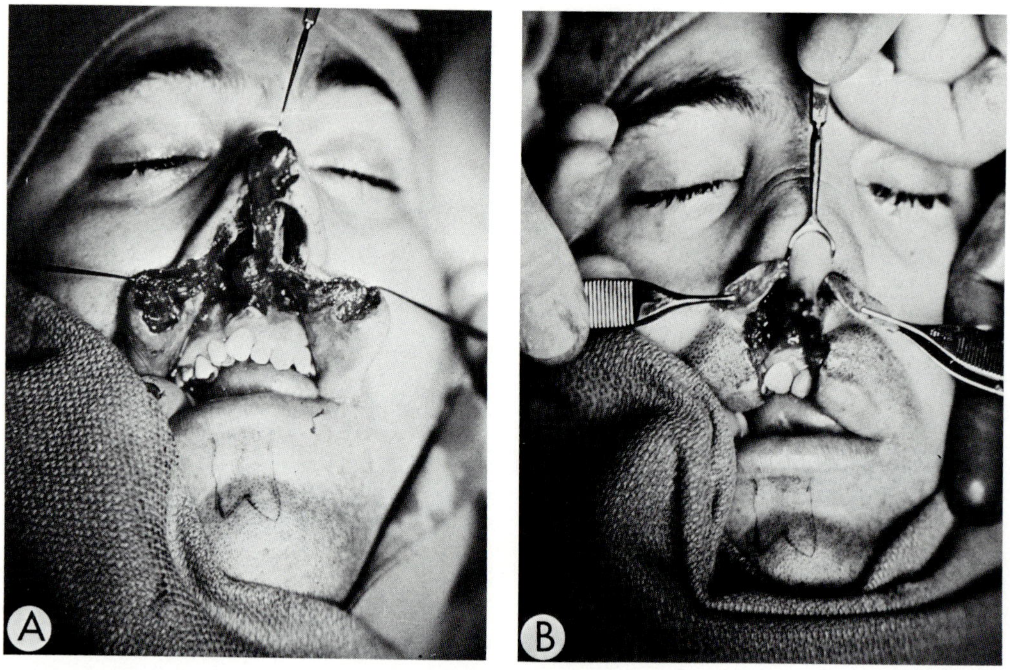

Fig. 10. (*A*) *Operative exposure on the patient shown in Figure 9. Exposure and take-down for approach to the nose and the complete septo-rhinoplasty. Note the outlined asymmetrical Abbe flap.* (*B*) *Complete freeing and presentation of the lower lateral cartilages before repositioning.*

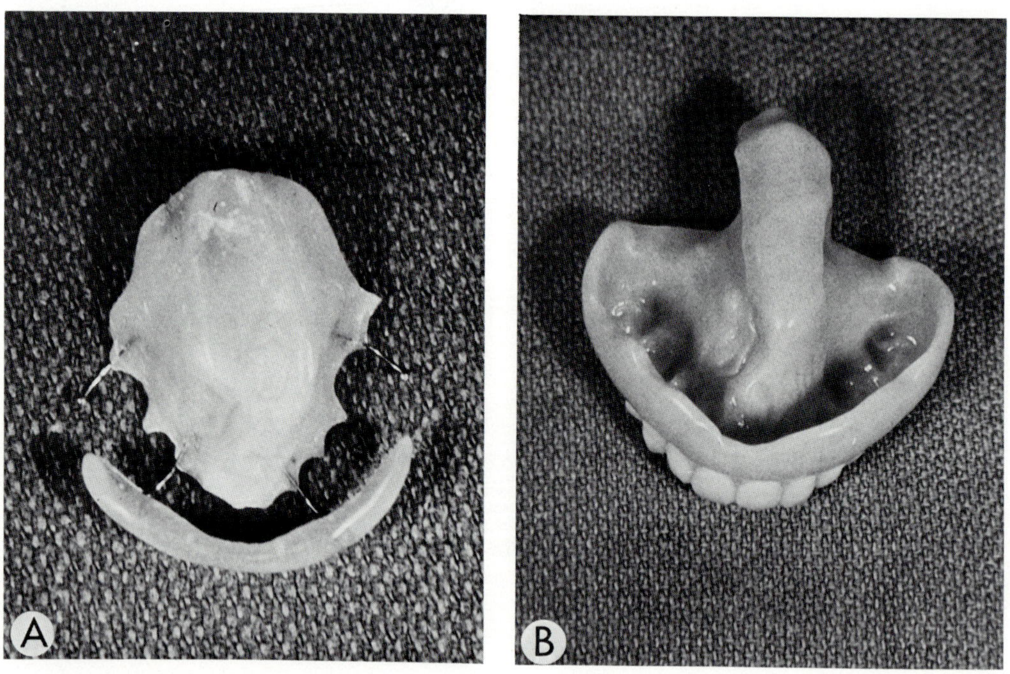

Fig. 11. (*A*) *Temporary prosthesis and pusher.* (*B*) *Final overlay prosthesis which assisted in projection of the lip. The bone graft was essential for creating an adequate nasal base.*

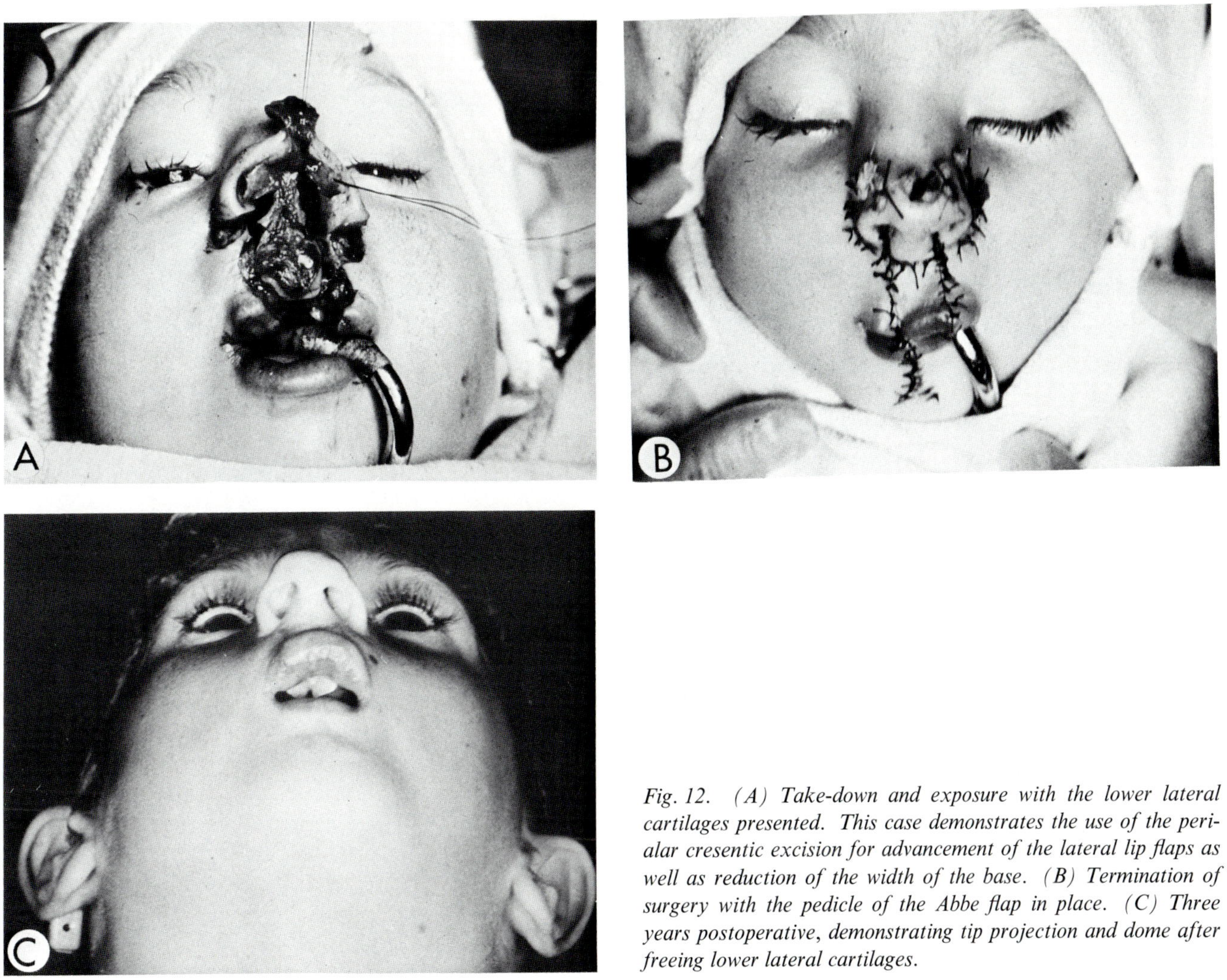

Fig. 12. *(A) Take-down and exposure with the lower lateral cartilages presented. This case demonstrates the use of the perialar cresentic excision for advancement of the lateral lip flaps as well as reduction of the width of the base. (B) Termination of surgery with the pedicle of the Abbe flap in place. (C) Three years postoperative, demonstrating tip projection and dome after freeing lower lateral cartilages.*

may be required. I prefer not to have to use implants in the nasal tip and dome itself.

Additional Surgical Procedures

In the original publication it was the intent and major effort was made towards balancing the two lower lateral cartilages in the unilateral cleft without operating the uninvolved lower lateral cartilage. More often now, particularly in the older patient, to obtain better tip projection and definition the uninvolved lower lateral cartilage is also operated. The excised cephalic margin of the uninvolved cartilage makes ideal implant material should the operator interpret that the involved cartilage is deficient. This implant has been described by Millard.[11]

Columellar struts and struts for support of the medial crus are more often used as a secondary procedure after the composite synchronous operation. Chrondo-cutaneous composite grafts from the ear can be utilized to add both lining and support. Variations in the use of this material have been described by Musgrave,[12] Rees,[13] and Walter from Germany.[17] The classic columellar lengthening procedures utilizing the skin of the prolabium may be incorporated with the combined procedure in the bilateral cleft-lip. The modifications of Brauer,[1] Cronin,[2] and Stark[15] may be incorporated and offer advantages.

A comparison of our original operation with that of McIndoe and Rees was made in the original article on this subject.[5] Since that time, Rees[13] has

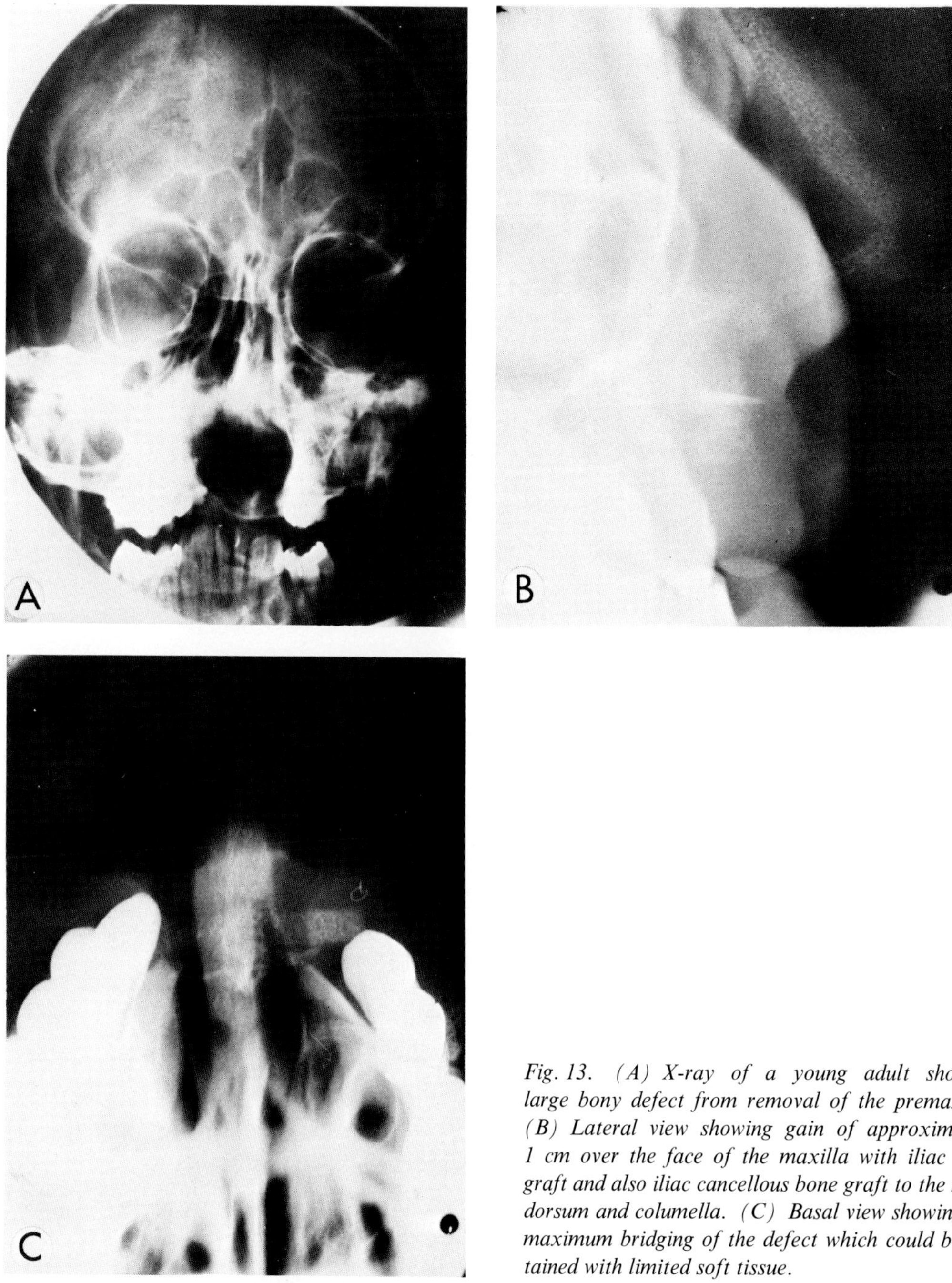

Fig. 13. (A) X-ray of a young adult showing large bony defect from removal of the premaxilla. (B) Lateral view showing gain of approximately 1 cm over the face of the maxilla with iliac bone graft and also iliac cancellous bone graft to the nasal dorsum and columella. (C) Basal view showing the maximum bridging of the defect which could be obtained with limited soft tissue.

made an addition with the use of a free graft laterally where a raw surface is created. In his rotation of the lower lateral cartilage Rees leaves the vestibular skin attached as opposed to our procedure where the cartilage is completely freed of vestibular skin. Following our technique, most often the skin of the vestibule can be utilized and may even be redundant, not requiring therefore the use of the free graft.

Our objective has been to avoid external excisions except for the occasional removal of a cresent in the unilateral nose immediately beneath the dome. This is hidden at the alar rim. The only other external incision is about the alar-facial attachment. External incisions have been advocated by many in the past and this has been previously reviewed.[5] Musgrave[12] has advocated this when there is severe discrepancy between the two sides or in the near bifid nose. Some type of external incision is used in the columellar lengthening procedures mentioned above. Dingman[3] feels that the skin can be adequately repaired and that one should not fear using external incisions. He apparently uses them freely when he feels that this would provide the best approach.

In advancing the lower lateral cartilage, I was carrying my draw suture through the dome of the nose over to the normal structures on the opposite side for support but did not mention specifically including the uninvolved upper lateral cartilage as has been done by Reynolds and Horton.[14]

Conclusions

The secondary nasal deformity associated with the unilateral and bilateral cleft-lip remains a challenging problem. Surgical repair requires imagination and the incorporation of all proven surgical techniques regarding septo-rhinoplasty and management of the nasal base. The composite operation performed as a single procedure, I believe, offers advantages primarily in the improved exposure for attacking the entire nose-lip complex. This frees all components which facilitates repositioning, and with this exposure and freeing there are no unoperated involved structures which tend to recreate the distortion with healing. In these deformities, despite some recurring anatomic contributing factors, there is no standard surgical anatomy and therefore no standard procedure. The operative technique and the surgeon must remain flexible.

An argument is presented for the combined procedure for improving function as well as appearance. The operative techniques discussed are directed toward correcting the involved structures and based on the study of the development of the defect, the influences of the primary surgery, and critical analysis of the structures involved in the secondary deformity.

Even with improved primary techniques and bone grafting, there will continue to be secondary nasal deformities as a result of the tissue insufficiencies which result from the pathogenesis of the cleft-lip. In general, the author has found the lower lateral cartilages in both the unilateral and bilateral cleft-lip nose to be sufficient in substance but distorted by the underlying insufficiencies and abnormal traction.[5,16]

The nose remains a major challenge in secondary repair often much more than the lip, and produces the additional difficulties of improving nasal breathing as well as the esthetic appearance. I am sure that an in-depth study would reveal more problems and variables than answers. We must therefore use all available techniques to the present date considering the abnormal development and the possible disturbance of growth potential created by the primary surgical procedures.

Summary

The primary purpose of this publication has been to present operative techniques which will add to the surgeon's armamentarium when he is faced with the challenge of repairing this combined developmental and surgical deformity. The techniques presented differ from other primarily in the method of presenting and repositioning the lower lateral cartilage, the management of the lateral alar attachment, and the use of autogenous implants over the underdeveloped maxilla beneath the alar attachment.

References*

1. Brauer RO, Foerster DW: Another method to lengthen the columella in the double cleft patient. Plast Reconstr Surg 38:27–31, 1966
2. Cronin TD: Lengthening columella by use of skin from nasal floor and alae Plast Reconstr Surg 21:417–426, 1958
3. Dingman RO: 221 North Ingalls, Ann Arbor, Michigan, personal communication
4. Dingman RO, Walter C: Use of composite ear grafts in correction of the short nose. Plast Reconstr Surg 43:117–124, 1969
5. Farrior RT: The problem of the unilateral cleft-lip nose. The Laryngoscope 72:289–352, 1962
6. Farrior RT: Cervicofacial congenital anomalies. Amer Acad Ophth Oto, 1960
7. Farrior RT: Corrective surgery of the nasal framework (with emphasis upon septal surgery). J Fla Med Assn 45:276–289, 1958
8. Farrior RT: Implant materials in restoration of facial contour. The Laryngoscope 76:934–954, 1966

* A complete bibliography has been given in the previous publications of the author.[5–9] Additional references since these publications are included for the reader's convenience. This list is by no means complete.

9. Farrior RT: Synthetics in head and neck surgery. Arch Ophthal 84:82–90, 1966
10. Marcks KM, Trevaskis AE, Berg EM, Punchner G: Nasal defects associated with cleft-lip deformity. Plast Reconstr Surg 34:176–181, 1964
11. Millard DR Jr: The unilateral cleft-lip nose. Plast Reconstr Surg 34:169–175, 1964
12. Musgrave RH: Surgery of nasal deformities associated with cleft lip. Plast Reconstr Surg 28:261–273, 1961
13. Rees TD, Guy CL, Converse JM: Repair of the cleft lip-nose: Adendum to the synchronous technique with full-thickness skin grafting of the nasal vestibule. Plast Reconstr Surg 37:47–50, 1966
14. Reynolds JR, Horton CE: An alar lift procedure in cleft-lip rhinoplasty. Plast Reconstr Surg 35:377–384, 1965
15. Stark RB, Dehaan CR, Washio H: Forked flap columellar advance. Cleft Palate J 1:116, 1964
16. Stenstrom SJ, Oberg TRH: The nasal deformity in unilateral cleft lip. Plast Reconstr Surg 28:295–305, 1961
17. Walter, C: Composite grafts in nasal surgery. Arch Otolaryngol 90:662, 1969

Revision of Rhinoplasty

Lionello Ponti, Rome, Italy

The surgeon who sets about revising a rhinoplasty, performed by others, takes on a great responsibility and must then be sure to give the patient an appreciable improvement.

It is often very difficult to value the damage to be repaired. While the functional and aesthetic impairments due to malformations and traumas can be sufficiently realized, those caused by the surgeon are often unexpected.

The accurate diagnosis of the case is essential.

The nasal pyramid is to be examined with great care from both an exterior and endoscopic point of view.

Rhinoscopy

This examination aims at emphasizing possible retracting scars of vestibular skin as a result of alar cartilage and skin overextirpation.

Furthermore, we can observe marginal scars with irregular joint of cut borders with consequent deformation of alar cartilages.

We can find synechiae between the septum mucosa and turbinates, as a result of a wrong osteotomy.

A nose, originally straight on the outside, may become deviated after a rhinoplasty because the osteocartilaginous septum was deviated in a more internal plane.

Once the hump is removed, this plane is reached and, after performing the osteotomy, the bones are jointed on the medial line, resulting in a crooked nose.

It is advisable to check if a septum revision has been carried out. In that case, one should make sure whether the residual cartilage is substantial or partly absorbed or deviated.

Skin Examination

By this examination we can know if there are skin reddening areas, teliangiectasias or adhesions to lower planes. These complications are due to an imperfect cleavage plane for skin detaching or excessive removal of periosteum.

Inspection is to be made to know whether the columella is falling forward or is retracted or it includes foreign bodies (cartilaginous or heterologous grafts).

The skin of the third lower section of the nasal pyramid may look very thickened, inelastic and globose, rich in sebaceous glands. That is often due to excessive subcutaneous fibrosis which replaces the removed alar cartilages.

The objective examination is then completed by palpation, enabling the evaluation of adhesion degree, tissue elasticity, cartilage and bone irregularities.

Evaluation of Osteotomy

The lateral osteotomy may be incomplete, only unilateral or performed at too high a level.

One or both bones may be polyfragmented, with irregular surface, or partly lacking, or else they may be featured by a greenstick fracture. In that case the nose root looks wide and, immediately underneath, too narrow. Moreover, the bones may be separated leaving between them an empty space where the septum can be raised (syndrome of "open root").

The medial osteotomy may be wrongly performed resulting in an inclusion of a bone section into the septum or vice versa. This defective situation can be felt as a step corresponding to an internal depression.

Nose Dorsum

The nose dorsum may be irregular from an inadequate septum or triangular cartilage modelling or due to a thick subcutaneous fibrosis—the so-called "supratip"—at the third lower section of nasal pyramid.

This defect is due to a poor modelling of septum cartilage or to the fact that the skin, being particularly thick, rich in glands and not very elastic in this area, does not take a proper cicatricial retraction.

Alar Cartilages

The most frequent and serious mistakes are those concerning the nasal tip.

The lateral crura may be irregularly resected or, sometimes, wholly removed giving rise to a pointed nose with respective collapse of nostrils and various asymmetries.

The medial crura are generally left in a normal position but, at the dome level, they are wrapped by a layer of close fibrous tissue.

The vestibular skin corresponding to the lateral crura, which is largely removed, is irregularly thickened and having retracted scars, especially at dome level, reducing the respiration capacity. The retracting scars and subcutaneous fibrosis lead to asymmetries and rounding of the nasal tip.

Once the diagnosis has been specified, a general evaluation, from the artistic point of view too, is taken into account. In other words, we want to see if we can improve the nose aspect, in addition to the rectification of errors.

All technical and artistic difficulties are to be explained to the patient who, obviously, is ready to blame the effects of the operation on the surgeon and, therefore, should not expect more than what can be offered to him.

In rectifying other people's errors, the surgeon should avoid making others of his own; thus, after settling a definite operative plan he must act with extreme caution and delicacy.

According to our experience, we advise operations as follows:

Imperfect Skin Undermining

After performing the intercartilaginous incision, the new elevation shall be carried out trying to stick to the perichondrium and periosteum as much as possible. Great attention shall be paid to adhesions between skin and osseous plane, where skin is particularly thin.

To avoid a new adhesion at the end of the operation, it may be useful to interpose a thin cartilage layer.

For skin detaching, it would be better to use Ragnel scissors than lancet.

Irregular Osteotomy

In this case both medial and lateral osteotomy are to be performed again. It is often advisable, mainly when deviated noses are involved, to separate the upper lateral cartilages from the septum.

The bones, after being properly modelled, are fractured again at frontal-nasal articulation, trying to obtain a satisfactory coalescence between the bones themselves.

Sometimes, the nasal bone of frontal section is too large, not enabling the nose narrowing. In such a case the bone bulk is carefully reduced by means of a sharp, bone-scooping forceps.

If the bone coalescence does not occur due to deviation of ethmoidal and vomerine plane, the latter shall be fractured by a blunt forceps.

Once the osteosynthesis is performed, a loss of osseous substance caused by previous, excessive removal can take place. In that case the lost substance is replaced by osseous or cartilaginous grafts.

Nose Dorsum

The septum cartilage and the triangular cartilages making up the nose dorsum generally seem wrapped by a thick fibrous layer, which is to be removed, while the cartilages are to be modelled.

If the cartilaginous septum is deviated, it is to be rectified, while for the osseous septum the use of a dislocator will be sufficient to take it back on the median line.

If the upper lateral cartilages, too, are considerably deformed by deviation, it is advisable to suture them to the septum by a mattress stitch of Dexon.

Nose Tip

The nose tip revision is the most delicate operative phase. We perform a marginal incision and, by an accurate detaching, we take off what remains of the lateral crura from the skin.

Even if the cartilages are missing, we go through this operative phase, by incorporating the fibrous tissue which has replaced the cartilages into the vestibular skin.

The detaching is then pursued above and before the medial crura in such a way as to set free all the cartilaginous structure of the nose tip or what remains of it.

By a hook we extract the nostril dome and, following the I.B. Goldman technique, we dissect it on both sides including the cartilage and vestibular skin into the incision.

By this way we achieve the separation of medial crura from the lateral ones. If cartilages are left, we free them from fibrosis and model them properly. On the contrary, if one or both cartilages are missing or insufficient we replace them by free cartilaginous grafts. We use the cartilage of the patient himself or, failing it, cartilage of fresh lateral crura taken from another patient.

These grafts are fastened to the vestibular skin corresponding to lateral crura by one or more mattress stitches with cat gut and, then, modelled.

The medial crura are freed from the fibrous tissue and then examined. If they are flabby, hypertrophic, or missing, they may be stiffened by a strip of septum cartilage introduced between the crura or, at least, between the two skin pieces, thus becoming prominent enough to give a satisfactory tip projection.

This support is fastened by one or more sutures of cat gut which is passed through the medial crura and the graft itself.

After checking the removal of all the excess fibrous tissue from the skin covering the nose tip and after adjusting the cartilages properly, the marginal incision is sutured and the columella is set in the septum.

If the columella is still retracted, it may be integrated by a further cartilaginous graft to be located, for all its length, in front of the medial crura.

When, despite these contrivances, the nose tip is still too turned-up for an excessive removal of lateral crura and upper lateral cartilages, free grafts of mucosa or skin or cartilage and skin are to be utilized.

The mucosa can be taken from a lower turbinate and the skin from the retroauricular area.

The composite graft, suggested by Dr. Claus Walter[1] to repair serious mucosa and cartilage removals, proved very useful.

The graft removal is carried out in the retroauricular area. In addition to attached skin, the incision includes the amount of cartilage required to fill the loss of nasal substance. This cartilage, always attached to the skin, may be modelled and dissected as needed.

In the nasal fossae the skin is separated in the middle above the septum and cartilage is arranged where needed. The graft is sutured and, then, retained by a proper splinting.

When there are anterior perforations of septum and full lateral crura, the perforation can be successfully closed by using, as pedicled, composite flaps, half of lateral crura, each sutured at perforation level.

The above is only part of the measures a surgeon can adopt to improve a rhinoplasty uncorrectly performed.

It is to be stressed that, in such cases, in spite of everything, a perfect result cannot be achieved.

Summary

Prior to performing revision surgery of a previous rhinoplasty analysis of the problem should be carefully executed. Both the physiologic and the cosmetic deformities must be evaluated. All aspects of the nose including the skin, cartilage and bone are to be examined. Autogenous auricular grafts may be required and the technique is discussed. The surgical limitations of revision surgery in rhinoplasty should be outlined to the patient in detail.

References

1. Walter Claus: Survey of composite grafts. Otolaryngologic Clinics of North America, October 1972

Face

Aging Face: Revisions and Complications (Panel)

Walter Berman:

"Everyone who does much surgery for rehabilitation of the aging face has problems." Slides were presented to illustrate his "extended lift," which involves a great deal of skin undermining, the dissections often joining in the midline of the upper neck. The resulting sheet of scar tissue serves to hold the overlying skin firmly. The importance of placing flap tension in the scalp area, rather than on the auricle was emphasized. Loss of hair in the temporal area can be a problem postoperatively, and is best prevented by avoiding too superficial dissection. He distinguishes two layers of postoperative edema; the first is smooth and resolves in one week, the second layer then becomes apparent, and appears lumpy due to localized accumulations of clot or lymphedema. This will always resolve spontaneously, but occasionally one might wish to aspirate such an area to hasten resolution. An occasional small skin slough can occur at the periphery of the flap. In most cases these will heal spontaneously and satisfactorily without grafting. The problem of ectropion was illustrated. As follows with the discussion of other panelists, suggestions for avoidance and treatment were presented.

Crowell Beard:

The removal of too much skin from the upper lid is a far more serious problem than when it occurs with the lower lid. The lagophthalmus which is associated with the problem is very troublesome. The treatment is never entirely satisfactory, because of the unique thinness of the upper lid skin. Penile skin most approaches the texture of upper lid skin, but is not available in most cases. Postauricular skin is too thick, so probably best to settle for a split-thickness graft. The problem of ectropion was discussed in detail. He thought that the operation was much safer when performed with local rather than general anesthesia. With the wound open, the patient is instructed to gaze upwards with the mouth open. The precise amount of overlapping skin is noted and resected. Ectropion can be corrected with a free graft of upper lid or postauricular skin. A technique for correction of ectropion with an upper lid transposition flap was demonstrated. Vigorous massage of the ectropian lid was thought to be of value. Fortunately, skin necrosis is a rare complication of blepharoplasty surgery, but requires a split-thickness graft when it occurs. Ptosis of the brow was considered. Dr. Beard, as an ophthalmic surgeon, preferred the direct approach rather than through the temporal rhytidectomy.

Pierre F. Fournier:

As an opening remark, Doctor Fournier offered this advice, "prevention of complications is more satisfactory than their cure." In discussing the face-lift, he advised that one should be certain that the patient has not been taking salicylates preoperatively. Superficial dissection or excessive tension contribute to skin sloughs. He prefers knife dissection to scissors, believing that less trauma and a thicker skin flap thus results. He did not believe that any lasting result occurred with the mini-lift; "mini-lift, mini-result, maxi-complications." The most common complication encountered in his experience with chemexfoliation was hyperpigmentation, often interspersed with areas of hypopigmentation. Most cases improve with strict avoidance of direct sunlight to the facial skin. "Round" or "Pig" eye is the most common complication of blepharoplasty, and can be prevented by avoiding excessive resection of lower eyelid skin. The upper lid resection should be limited to the central, granular appearing zone. He demonstrated the use of the periorbital fat as a filler for glabellar wrinkles; "the poor man's silicone." He mentioned Dr. Lintilhac's operation for reduction of the supraorbital ridge as well-suited for correction of the "deep set" eye. The rare case of retrobulbar hematoma is simply treated with removal of the lower lid sutures to relieve tension. In his experience with two cases, it is impossible to isolate a definitive bleeding point.

Richard P. Ariagno:

The proper placement of the rhytidectomy incisions was considered in detail. Examples of poorly planned incisional scars were presented, well illustrating the problem of concealment encountered by the patient. The anterior limb runs transversely across the temporal area to give access to the brow. It should be high enough that hair bearing skin remains below the line of closure following the resection. Inferiorly, the closure should be tucked under the lobule without tension. A technique was described for augmenting the lobule when necessary to assure scar camouflage. The postauricular incision is placed high on the pinna rather than in the sulcus, as the scar invariably tends to drift down postoperatively. The posterior limb is placed entirely within the occipital scalp. The problem of chemexfoliation scars was presented. These respond best to intralesional and systemic corticosteroid therapy. Maintaining proper rapport with the patient is of utmost importance during this period of slow regression and prolonged therapy.

Richard C. Webster:

In discussing the prevention of "scleral show" and the "hound dog eye" (his term in describing the combination of scleral show and mesial and inferior displacement of the lateral canthus and lateral half of the free border of the upper lid) he demonstrated the flap suspension technique for lower lid blepharoplasty combined with M-plasty and roughly hourglass excision upper lid blepharoplasty. The M-plasties are used to prevent excessive extension of incision lengths. The hourglass excision of upper lid skin allows for tailored and appropriate excision of the common mesial or nasal excess as well as the lateral excesses of upper lid skin. The lower lid flap is pulled externally and superiorly by appropriate excision of skin at the level of or just above and lateral to the lateral canthus. The superior edge of the flap thus exerts and upward and lateral push on the free border of the upper lid and lateral canthus. For this procedure to work effectively, it is wise to design the upper blepharoplasty so that closure of its wound will exert a superior pull on the lateral extent of the lower lid blepharoplasty wound. Still further safety is afforded by an eyebrow or temple lift. Correction of the three deformities produced in standard blepharoplasties by variations on the flap suspension technique were demonstrated. Doctor Webster emphasized that face-lifting, both cheek and neck lifts, and cheek-neck temple lifts, may be performed successfully with less undermining and more superficial undermining with the wounds closed more tightly than in those maneuvers carrying out radical or wide undermining. Undermining just far enough forward and downward to get to the "rolling or mobile fat," combined with plication of the platysma to the sternocleidomastoid fascia, has given adequate results with avoidance of danger to the facial nerve because of the very superficial undermining possible. Morbidity from hematoma and partial or full-thickness slough is minimized because the flaps are short. As much as two to four pounds of pull have been exerted on the tightest parts of the closures in the scalp just anterior to and posterior to the ear. The scalp wound is approximated with stainless steel staples, and Davis and Geck 6-0 mild chromic continuous suturing with very tiny bites for closure of the cheek flap to the ear, this edge being tailored so that no tension is applied to the ear. The vertical wound on the posterior surface of the ear or in the sulcus is not sutured. The point that Dr. Webster makes is that there are two major variations in facelifting, one the wide undermining with closure under less tension and the other with much less undermining but with a tighter skin closure. In both cases, blepharoplasty and facelift, he presented what he considers to be safer surgery than the usually taught procedures. He stated that each surgeon might weigh for himself just how much risk he is willing to subject his patient to in this almost totally elective surgery.

Augmentation Mentoplasty Using Polyamide Mesh

G. Jan Beekhuis, Detroit, Michigan

Many patients who are to undergo rhinoplasty require a simultaneous correction of chin retrusion. Unless there is major malocclusion, the preferred method is to augment the mental area by the use of a graft or an implant.

Among the autogenous grafting substances used are iliac bone, and rib cartilage. Unfortunately these materials require an additional site of surgical incision, with the risk of associated morbidity that unnecessarily complicates an otherwise relatively simple cosmetic procedure. Homogenous cartilage has been used with various rates of success.

A multitude of implant materials have been utilized.[1] All synthetic alloplastic implant materials have the advantage of being readily commercially available and of being easily sterilized. In the mental area there is a moderate amount of soft tissue to cover over the implant material, and problems with host rejection or with extrusion therefore have not been frequent. For these reasons, in the last few years, for chin augmentation most surgeons have been using alloplastic implants—the commonest being methylmethacrylate (acrylic) and silicone rubber—solid or sponge.

The methylmethacrylate implant[2] is well accepted by the host, there being a minimum of subsequent infection or rejection. The disadvantage is that the acrylic is an extremely hard substance difficult to sculpt; it does not consistently conform to the shape of the mandible, and therefore one corner or the other may become more prominent, giving rise to asymmetry; when inserted under the periosteum the graft rarely shifts, but, when placed directly above the periosteum, deviation and late displacement occur rather frequently.

The solid silicone rubber implant[3] is much easier to sculpt, but when inserted through the intraoral route, perhaps has a slightly higher incidence of infection and extrusion than that of methylmethacrylate.

In the last few years there have been several reports[4–6] of bone resorption under plastic chin implants. Although the exact clinical significance of this result has not yet been fully determined, it is a cause for concern. Possible causes for bone resorption could be relative to the hardness of the implant material, its size, and its position in regard to the periosteum. For these reasons many surgeons now are placing the implant material on top of the periosteum, although, unfortunately, the implant is less stable and more likely to be asymmetric or subject to displacement.

Some of these problems are overcome by the use of fine-cell silicone sponge,[7] especially when it is introduced in multiple small pieces. Unfortunately, the incidence of postoperative infection with silicone sponge is higher than that with the other above-mentioned implant materials.

About 6 years ago I[8] first used polyamide mesh implants in correcting saddle nose deformities, and the results were better than those from any other type of implant material used. The mesh implant material has a number of advantages that seemed to be applicable to augmentation mentoplasty. For the past 3 years now I have been using polyamide mesh as the implant material of choice.

Technique for Augmentation Mentoplasty

Preoperatively the patient washes the face and neck thoroughly with an antiseptic soap. Next, a sedative is administered intravenously, as the surgical procedure always is performed with the patient under local anesthesia. The polyamide (Supramid Extra) mesh is autoclaved, and then is fashioned to the appropriate size and shape (Fig. 1).

A marking pen is used to outline on the skin the proposed position. Invariably an external route

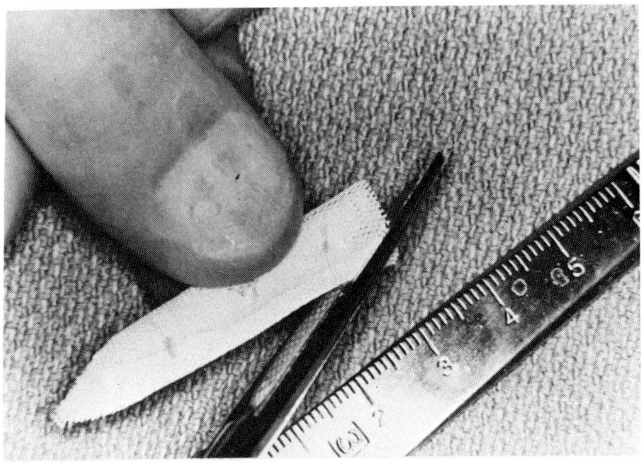

Fig. 1. The autoclaved polyamide mesh is rolled firmly, sutured through and through, and trimmed to the appropriate size and shape.

of entry is used. A small incision approximately 1 cm in length is made underneath the mandible, where, when closed, it can be hidden in a natural fold of the skin. With double-edged scissors, a pocket now is made, in front of the mandible and external to the periosteum, to conform to the proposed shape and size of the implant (Fig. 2). Care is taken not to injure the mental nerve laterally. Excessive undermining is avoided; the pocket should be such that the implant will fit snugly and cannot be displaced. The implant is grasped with a hemostat and one end of the implant is inserted. The hemostat is removed; the opposite end of the implant is grasped and is inserted and then is correctly positioned. When bleeding has subsided, the incision is closed with a few tiny interrupted sutures. Only a small dressing is applied over the incision line. No other external dressing is necessary. Most patients were given a course of antibiotics.

Results

During the last three years I have used polyamide mesh for augmentation mentoplasty in 70 patients. In some patients there has been transient edema, collection of some serous fluid (which could be aspirated), and ecchymosis.

There have been no clinical signs of host rejection. No implant has had to be removed. There have been no major problems with asymmetry. There has been no postoperative displacement or extrusion of the implant or irritation of the mental nerve.

A number of other advantages to the use of this material in augmentation mentoplasty are worthy of mention. The polyamide mesh is extremely flexible and therefore can be inserted through a tiny incision and into a "tight-fitting" pocket. This means that there is less chance of bleeding and subsequent displacement, and there is no need of bulky external fixation dressings. The highly flexible implant material readily conforms to the shape of the underlying mandible (Fig. 3).

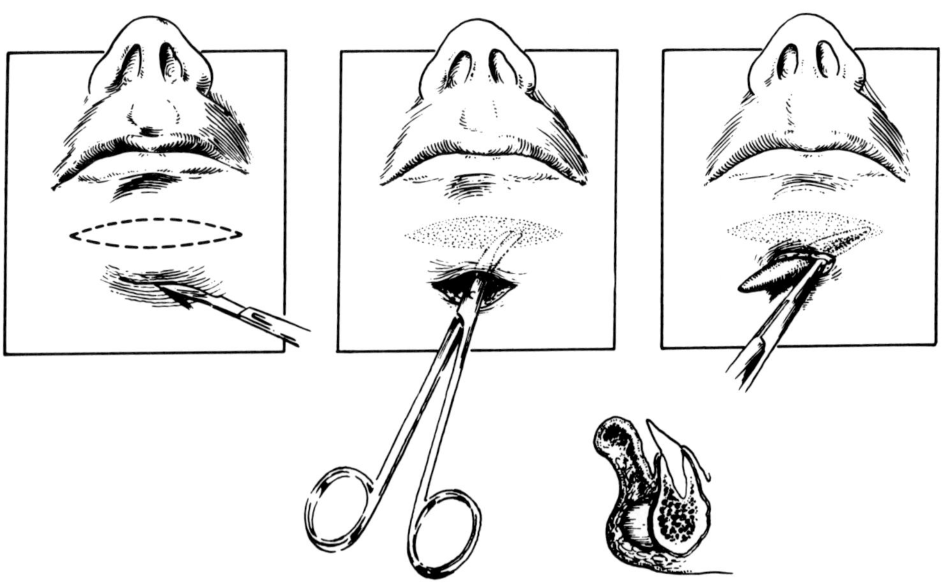

Fig. 2. The proposed position of the implant is outlined on the skin of the patient's chin. An incision about 1 cm long is made in a natural skin fold in the submental area. With double-edge scissors a pocket is made supraperiosteally to conform to the size of the implant. The implant is then inserted, and when bleeding has been controlled the incision is closed with a few fine interrupted sutures. No fixation dressings are required.

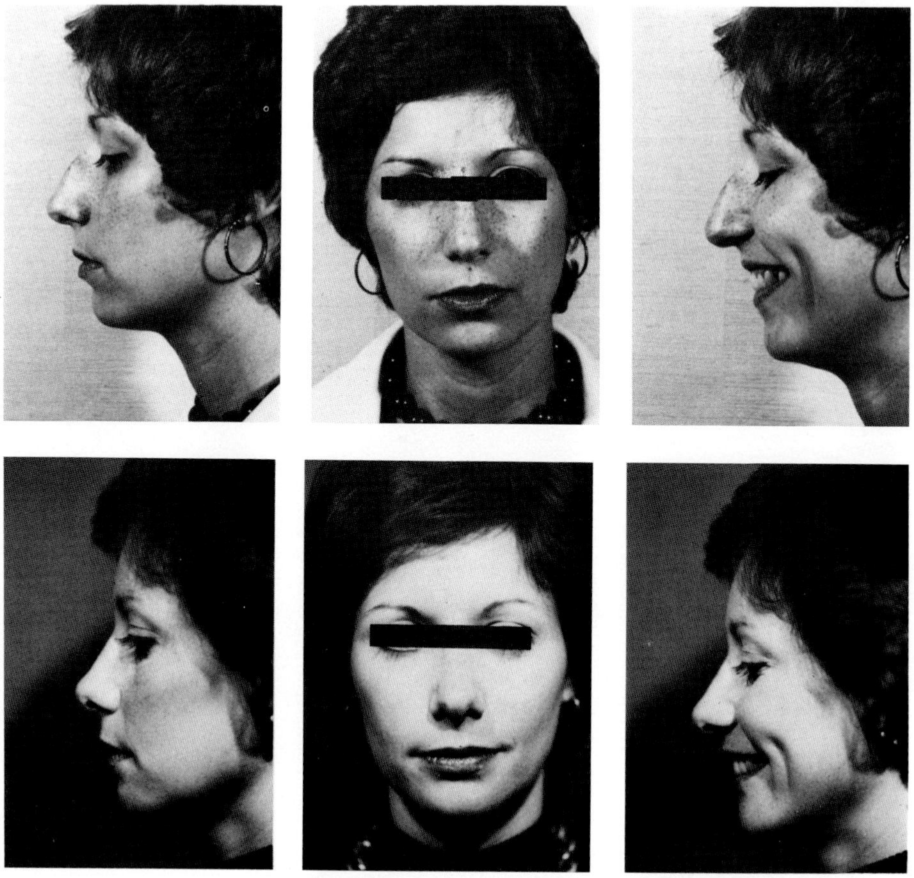

Fig. 3. Preoperative and postoperative photos of a patient who underwent both rhinoplasty and augmentation mentoplasty with the use of polyamide mesh.

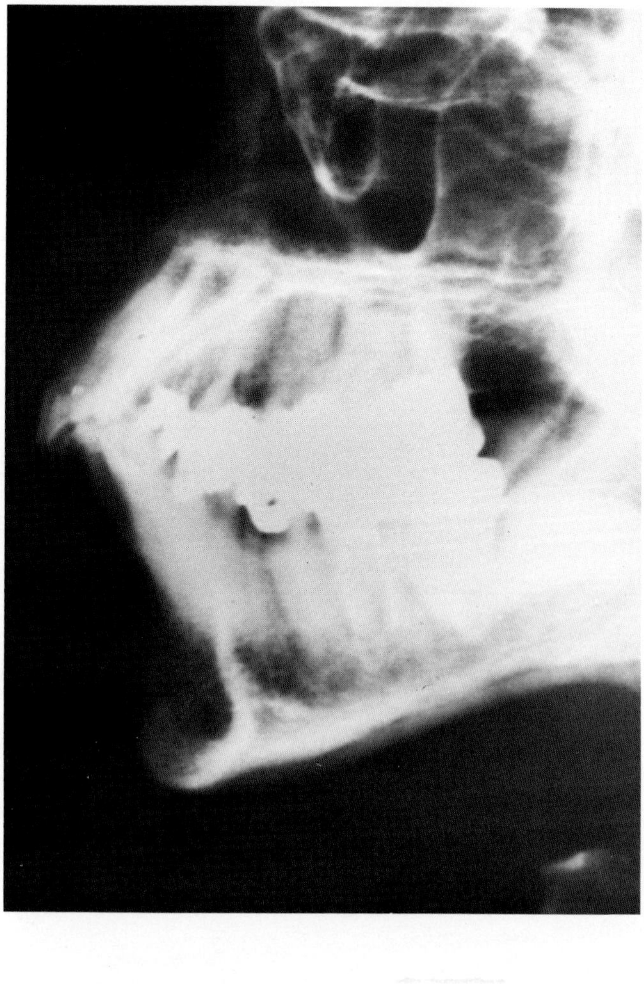

Fig. 4. Postoperative roentgenogram of patient's chin, which shows no evidence of bone resorption.

There has been minimal postoperative reaction and morbidity. Within a few weeks after the operation the mental contour has returned to normal, and even by palpation the implant appears to have blended into the normal tissues.

Because the material is mesh, and ingrowth of fibrous tissue occurs, the position of the implant becomes fixed, and it therefore feels almost like normal tissue; this also insures that it is not likely to become displaced even at a later time and even when subjected to trauma.

Roentgenograms of several of the patients were made at various times, and in no case was there evidence of bone resorption of the underlying mandible (Fig. 4). It is not known whether this absence of resorption is because of the softness and flexibility of the polyamide mesh or its supraperiosteal position.

References

1. Carlin GA: Personally fabricated chin implants. Plast Reconstr Surg 51:121–128, 1973
2. Rish BB: Alloplastic materials in the creation of facial contour. Arch Otolaryngol 72:212–218, 1960
3. Tresley IJ, Arenberg IK, Polterock J: Augmentation mentoplasty—reflections. Laryngoscope 82:2092–2102, 1972
4. Robinson MJ, Shuken R: Bone resorption under plastic chin implants. Arch Otolaryngol 27:116–118, 1969
5. Robinson M: Bone resorption under plastic chin implants. Arch Otolaryngol 95:30–32, 1972
6. Jobe R, Iverson R, Vistnes L: Bone deformation beneath alloplastic implants. Plast Reconstr Surg 51:169–175, 1973
7. Parkes M: Avoiding bone resorption under plastic chin implants. Arch Otolaryngol 98:100–101, 1973
8. Beekhuis GJ: Saddle nose deformity: etiology, prevention, and treatment; augmentation rhinoplasty with polyamide. Laryngoscope 84:2–42, 1974

Technique of Facial Chemosurgery

Pierre F. Fournier, Paris, France

As a means of facial rejuvenation and facial embellishment chemical face peeling is well accepted by a great number of plastic surgeons.[1,2] Early prejudices and fears are slowly giving way to confidence in this method of treatment. Dr. L. Winter[3] of Budapest, in 1949, first described the use of phenol for the removal of freckles. This technique consisted of applying the phenol to the skin and immediately, washing it off with alcohol. Various lay operators in Europe, and in the United States, began using this method of treatment. The lay operators differed from the original phenol application used by Winter, inasmuch as they left the phenol on the skin, undiluted, and covered this with adhesive tape. Litton in 1959 and Brown[4] in 1960 started researching this technique, independently of each other, approximately two years before Baker and Gordon[5] began their investigations. The first presentation to the American Society of Plastic Reconstructive Surgery was made by Litton in 1961.

Since the original presentation, there have been several articles reviewing the original work, and recently, Spira has reconfirmed the clinical and histological changes reported by the earlier authors.[6,7] Contrary to most beliefs, the technique of chemosurgery of the face is relatively unknown in Europe, and is performed by very few surgeons, or lay operators.

Three fears have prevented this treatment from becoming a part of the plastic surgeon's armamentarium: (1) fear of local tissue reaction resulting in permanent scarring; (2) fear of absorption of phenol through the intact skin with resultant systemic toxic effects; and (3) fear that the final result does not last long enough to warrant the patient going through with the procedure, or "the end does not justify the means."

Litton, who used this mode of treatment in a large number of cases over a 14 year period and the author no longer have fears of local or systemic reaction, if the method is used in a judicious manner. There have been two instances of local scarring in this series. The neck is not included in the treatment routinely, and the supraclavicular regions should be avoided if the neck is to be included. This area is more susceptible to unfavorable scarring, whether by knife or chemical.

Chemical Therapy

Indications for Chemical Therapy

The following are indications for such therapy. (1) Tired aged face, evidenced by abnormal wrinkles and loose skin of face neck; (2) postacne scarring; (3) telagiectasia; (4) pigmentations; (5) follow-up after scar revisions; (5) early senile keratosis and pigmentation; (6) bleach out split thickness skin grafts; (7) Post-irradiated skin.

Contraindications of Chemical Therapy

The following contraindicate therapy. (1) Redundant skin of the face and neck, especially where there is a large amount of subcutaneous fat; (2) Lower cervical areas that have been known to react unfavorably in some cases.

Advantages and Disadvantages

In some instances, this may be compared with the surgical face lifting procedure, and has the following advantages over the surgical technique and dermabrasion: (1) removes wrinkles of the forehead, eyelids, and around the mouth; (2) gives the entire face a clean, youthful appearance; (3) removes pigmentation (freckles, etc.); (4) can be done as an outpatient or office procedure; (5) no anesthetic is required (only premedication); (6) results are longer lasting.

The disadvantages of the chemical procedure are: (1) color and texture of the skin are different from the surrounding skin; (2) no absolute way of predetermining the permeability of skin to solution in each case; hence, limited amounts should be used at one time; and (3) no absolute way of predetermining if the patient's skin might have unfavorable scarring reaction.

Chemical Formula

1. Phenol (C_6H_5OH) is known as carbolic acid although its formula does not contain the carboxyl (COOH) group—characteristic of organic base or alcohol.
2. Glycerin
3. Distilled water
4. Croton oil. (from seed of *Croton tiglium*); irritating because croton resin causes vesiculation and sloughing. Phenol has to be used in a concentration of at least 50 percent to be effective. Pure phenol crystals are diluted to approximately 50 percent with glycerin and water. This controls the penetration power of phenol, limits its depth of action and the amount to be absorbed systemically. The croton oil is added in minute amounts purely as a skin irritant to cause a more thorough peeling effect. The penetration power of the phenol can be decreased or increased by varying its concentration and surface tension. Small amounts of oil will control surface tension. The penetration power is greater when the concentration and surface tension are lower.

Local Reaction to Phenol

After phenol is applied to the skin, there is an immediate reaction of keratolysis and keratocoagulation. There is a coagulation necrosis of the epidermis and, in some instances, it extends into the papillary layer of the dermis. Biopsy studies were taken in the following manner (Figs. 1–4):

1. Control biopsy before treatment. Epidermis of regular width with single layered basal cell stratum; fine-fibrillar thin stratum papillare of dermis; interwoven coarse bundles of stratum reticulare.
2. Forty-eight hours after treatment. Coagulation necrosis of epidermis, coalescence of fibers of stratum papillare; marked hyperemia inflammatory reaction; some coalescence of collagenous fibers of stratum reticulare.

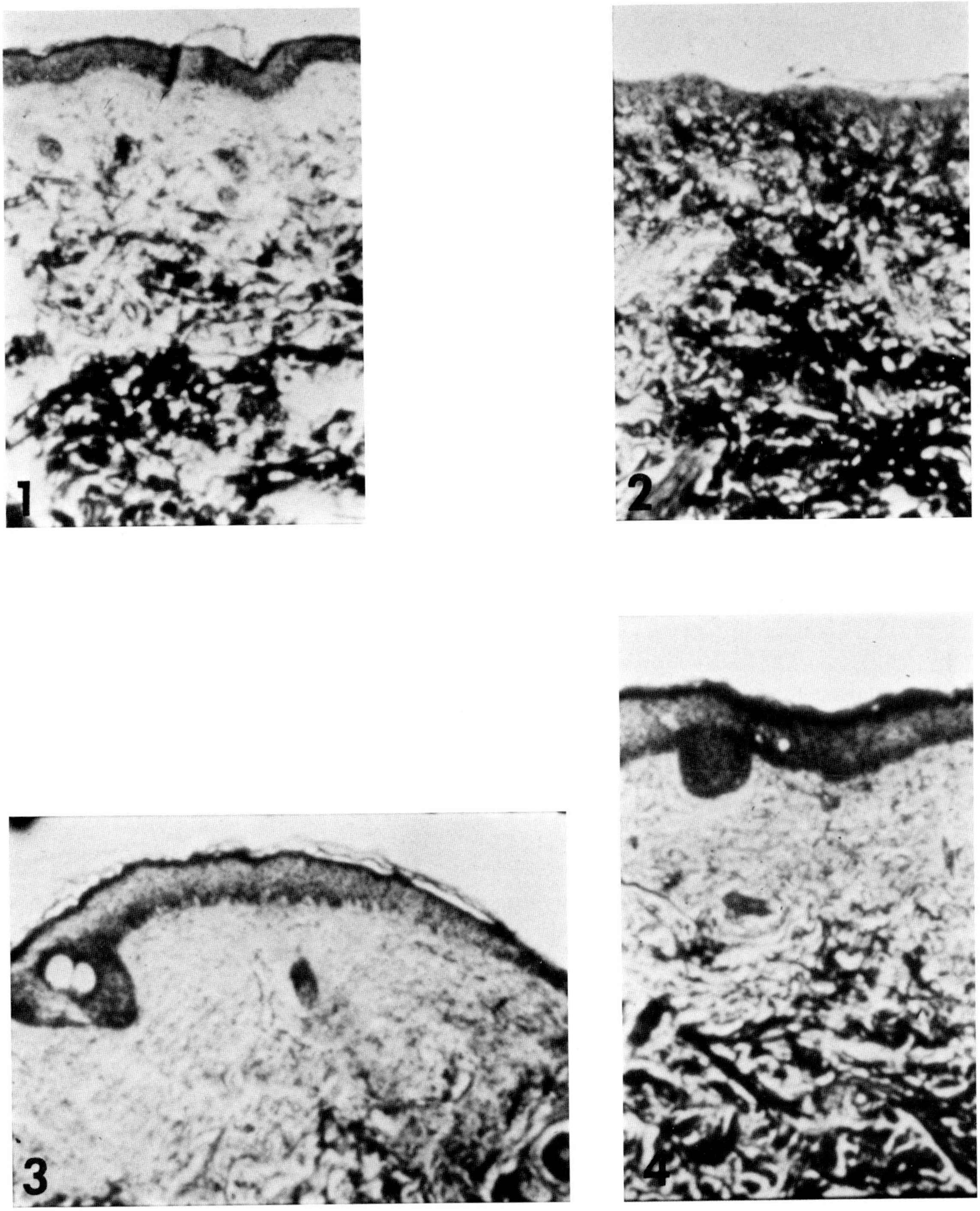

Figs. 1–4. Biopsies before treatment, 24 hr after treatment, 3 weeks after treatment, and 3 months after treatment.

3. Three weeks after treatment. Evidence of regeneration of epidermis, crowding and high cellularity of basal layers; widening of stratum papillare; significant increase in vascularity; increase in number and thickness of fibers[8] sclerosing edema; remnants of inflammatory hypercellularity; no significant changes in stratum.

4. Three months after treatment. Still remnants of activation of epidermis; marked widening of stratum papillare with increase of number and width of vessels; no remnants of cellular inflammatory reaction; stratum reticulare not shown, but without significant pathologic changes.

From these studies, it is felt that the significant histologic changes as a result of the application of phenol occur in the stratum papillae. These histologic findings (marked widening of stratum papillare with increase of number and width of vessels) are consistent with every one of the cases; whereas the changes in the deep layer of the dermis, i.e., lamination of collagenous fibers and thickening of elastic fibers are spotty in these cases and not necessarily consistent. The destruction of the basal layer of the epidermis and its reformation can account for the removal of pigmentations and the failure of their return at a later date.

The increased color and vitality of the skin can be explained in the changes in the deep stratum papillare such as the significant increase in vascularity which is normally the location of the vascular structures controlling the color of our skin. No one can predict just how long these histologic changes will last; however, it is possible to assume that since we have the formation of new structures their life span might be quite lengthy before they undergo degenerative changes.

Blood Phenol Studies

It is a well known fact that phenol is absorbed through the intact skin. In order to determine the safety of the amount used for this procedure, a study has been carried on wherein blood samples of 1, 3, and 5 hr intervals have been analyzed. Blood phenol is very accurately measured by the spectrophotometer. Litton's studies revealed that if 3 cc of a 50 percent solution of phenol were applied to the entire face, the following results were obtained: (1) One hour after application—0.68 mg percent phenol maximum; (2) two hours after application—0.19 mg percent phenol maximum; and (3) four hours after application—less than 0.1 mg percent phenol.

Application to half of the face revealed the following: less than 0.1 mg percent phenol with the exception of one case which had a 0.38 mg percent phenol level. To date there has been no toxic level established in man; however, there has been a case where 23 mg percent of blood phenol was reported in man after ingestion. This points out the relative margin of safety between 0.68 mg percent obtained on the entire facial application of a 50 percent solution of phenol, compared to the 23 mg percent blood level demonstrated in man 15 min after ingestion. Routine urinalysis at 5 and 24 hr intervals revealed a 4 to 9 mg percent phenol level. It is not necessary to use more than 2 to 3 cc of phenol for each procedure.

Systemic Reaction to Phenol

After the phenol is absorbed into the blood stream, it is rapidly conjugated with glycuronic acid, or sulphuric acid, and excreted by the kidneys, or detoxified by oxidation to hydroquinone, or pyrocatechin; or it can remain as free phenol in the blood stream and can be excreted as such by the kidneys. The signs and symptoms of phenol poisoning are usually those of a central depression, fall in blood pressure, headache, and/or nausea. There can be a direct toxic effect on the blood vessels and myocardium which usually causes the fall in blood pressure. Cardiac arythmias and tachycardia can occur if the solution is applied too fast.

Technique of Chemical Face Lifting

1. The advantages and disadvantages are discussed very carefully with the patient. It should be pointed out to the patient that this procedure is not any panacea and that improvement is variable, depending on the individual patient. All of the weak points should be discussed, and a release, which has been carefully prepared by an attorney, signed by the patient. This will minimize the chances of the patient taking legal action. It is important to have the patient write out the release in his own handwriting as well as signing the

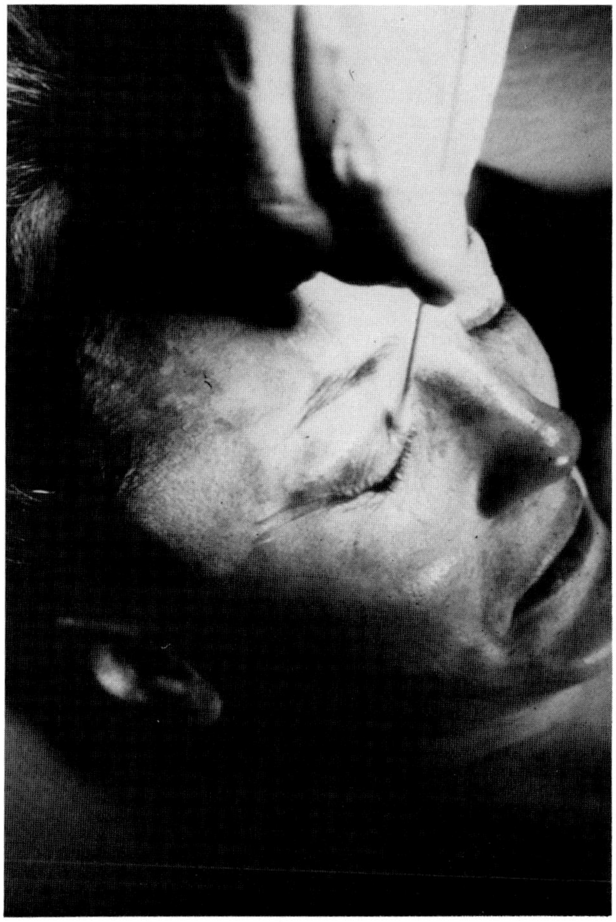

Fig. 5. Application of the solution on the forehead and upper eyelids.

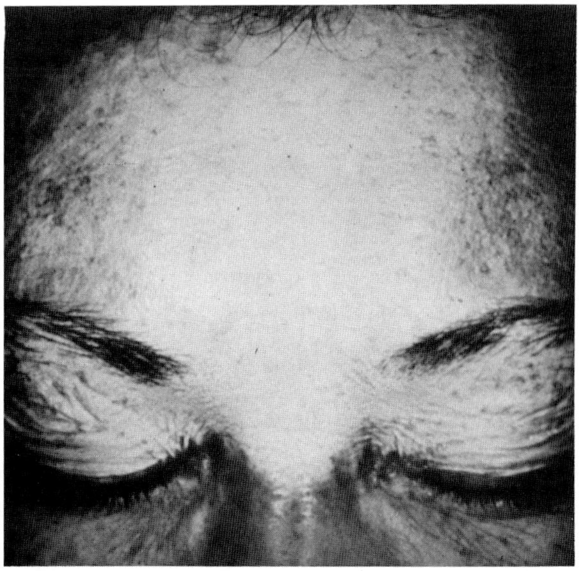

Fig. 6. View of the forehead and upper eyelids after application of the solution.

prepared release, so that he will not be able to claim he did not read the release prior to signing.

2. Careful photographic studies should be made before and after so that the results can be compared in an accurate manner.

3. The history of the patient should be checked for liver and kidney disease and previous sensitivity. We have found that the use of Innovar anesthesia has been successful in this treatment in as much as the Innovar provides analgesic and hypnotic effects for approximately 4 to 6 hr, which is usually more than enough time to provide adequate comfort following this application of the chemical.

4. The forehead and upper eyelids are usually done first (Fig. 5) and this area is cleaned well with ether. An orange stick is used, with the end moistened, in order to retain the necessary amount of cotton. The formula is unstable, so that it must be mixed thoroughly each time it is used. The phenol solution is then applied in small amounts to the forehead, and instant digital pressure is applied to counteract the stinging sensation. The skin turns white immediately on contact with the solution (Fig. 6). The pressure is held for 5 to 10 sec, and a new area is covered. The solution is applied freely over eyebrows, and the upper eyelids are also covered down to a level of approximately 4 to 5 mm above the eyelashes. The eyelids (which must be dry with no tears) can best be painted by a small cotton applicator, making sure there is no excess solution to cause eye damage.

The stinging sensation lasts for a few minutes and then almost completely subsides. The forehead and eyelids are then covered by means of small strips of adhesive tape. Approximately 3 layers of tape are applied to the involved area (Figs. 7–10). The stinging sensation becomes greater again after the application of tape and lasts for 1 to 2 hr. The tape is necessary so that the maximum chemical reaction will take place within the skin and minimal evaporation will occur. The patient is usually watched carefully for approximately 1 to 2 hr.

Forty-eight hours later, the tape is removed revealing a moistened surface containing exfoliation of surface skin and serum (Fig. 11). The surface is then cleansed with peroxide applicators

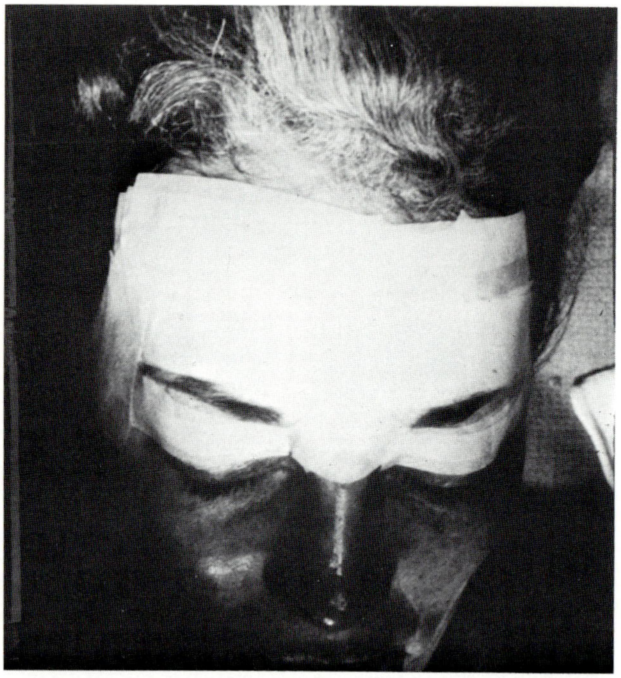

Fig. 7. Tape is applied to the forehead and eyelids.

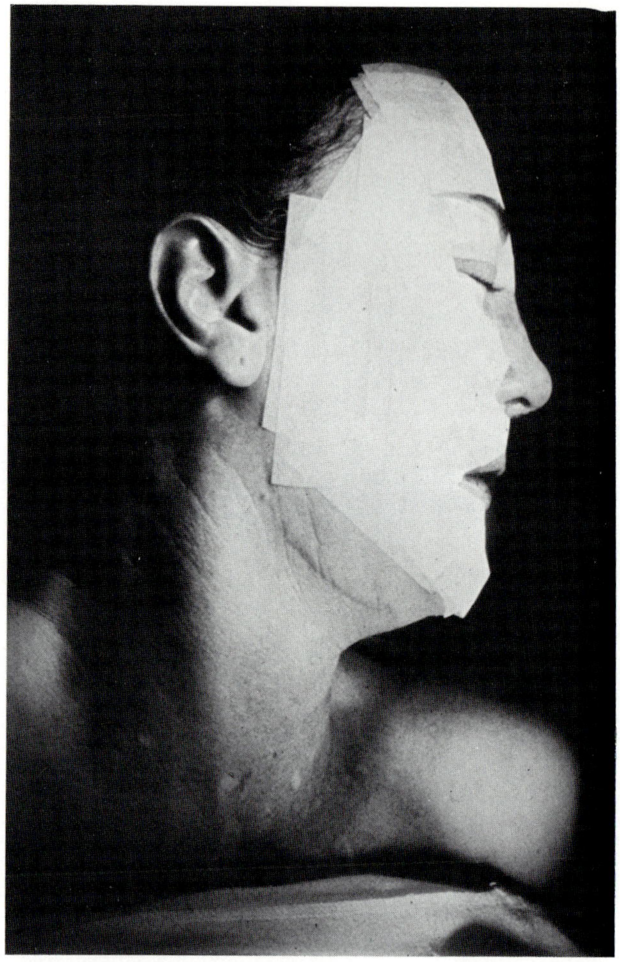

Fig. 9. No paper is applied on the upper neck.

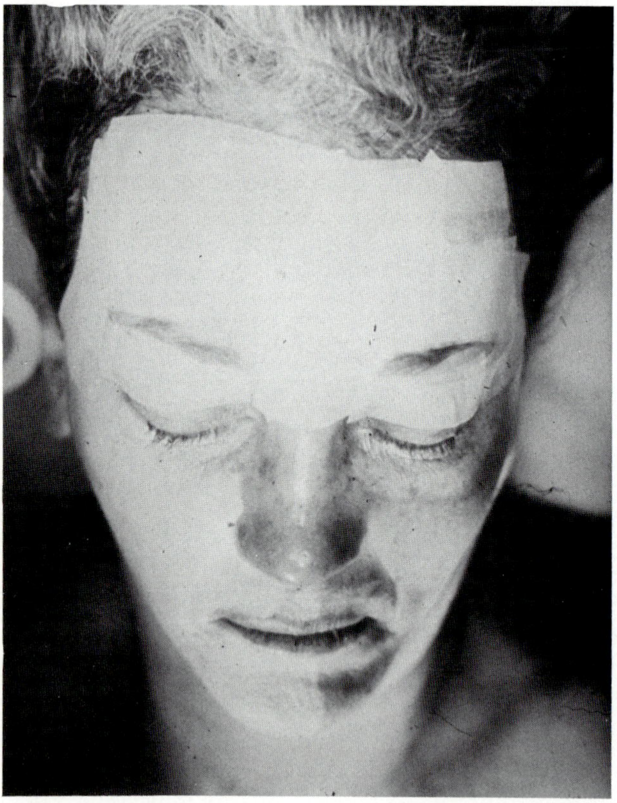

Fig. 8. The solution is applied to the middle of the face.

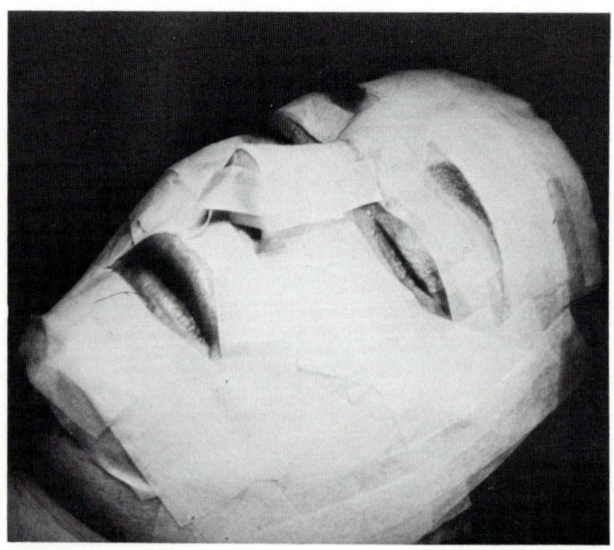

Fig. 10. The patient remains under the mask for 24 hr.

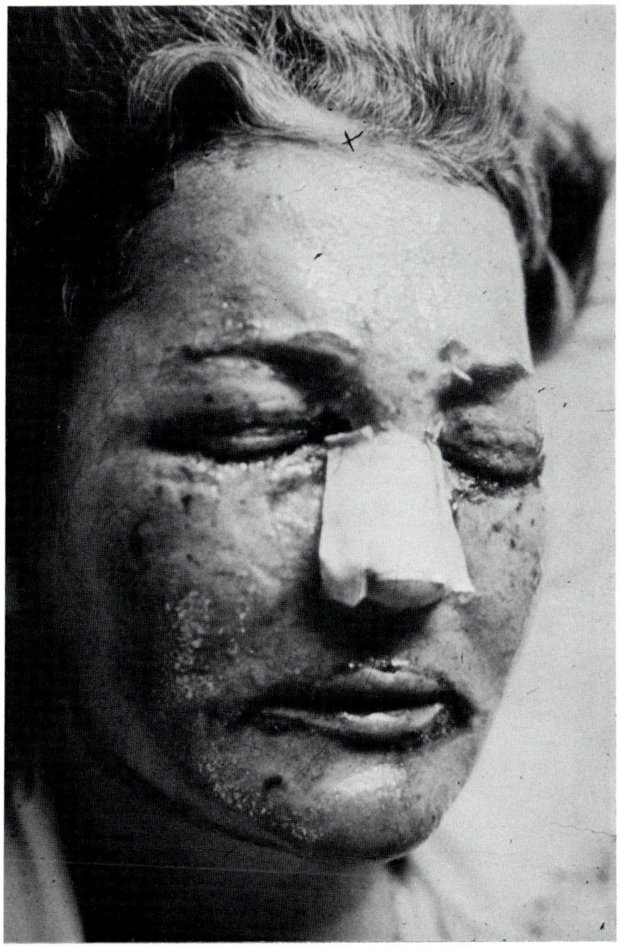

Fig. 11. View of the face when the mask is removed.

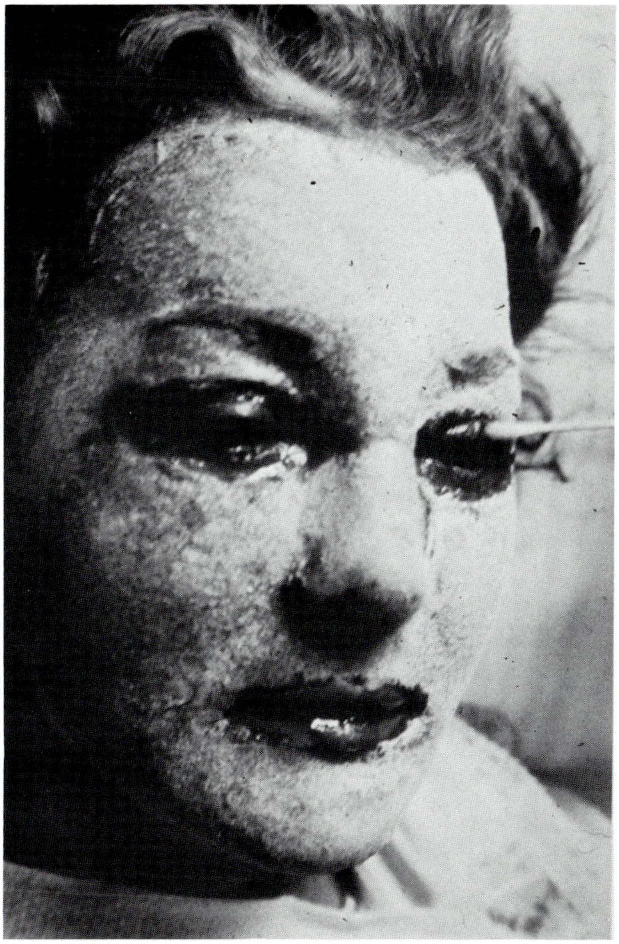

Fig. 12. Thymiol iodide powder is applied to the surface of the skin and paraffin oil is applied to the lids and mouth.

and thymol iodide powder is applied to the surface of the skin (Fig. 12). The patient is instructed to apply thymol iodide powder to the area involved at least three times a day. The patient is then discharged and returns to the office in approximately 3 days with instructions to place Vaseline over the powdered area approximately 3 times, beginning the night before the office visit. By the end of 5 to 7 days, the skin has usually completely healed and the powder mask is easily separated from the underlying tissue. The patient is then advised to use some type of skin softener for the next 2 weeks.

The same procedure is carried on for the lower face, being careful to avoid the vermillion tissue of the lip. The neck can be done in one stage, but here the operator has to be careful to keep the solution at a level just below the thyroid cartilage. The area above the clavicle and sternum is prone to develop scarring and, therefore, it is safer to avoid this region. In one case, a patient developed 3 small hypertrophic scars of the sternal and supraclavicular area. In most instances, we avoid doing the neck unless the patient insists.

Inasmuch as different regions of the face and neck are of different thicknesses of skin, a skin test is not accurate, since it would be impossible to check every section to be covered by the solution for strength and strength sensitivity. If the neck is done, do not use adhesive tape. This will have a tendency to lessen the reaction of the phenol and diminish the chances of scarring. On this region, surgical ointment (kip's surgical ointment) is applied after 48 hr instead of the powder. It is better to divide the treatment into 2 phases so that the upper and lower eyelids are done at different

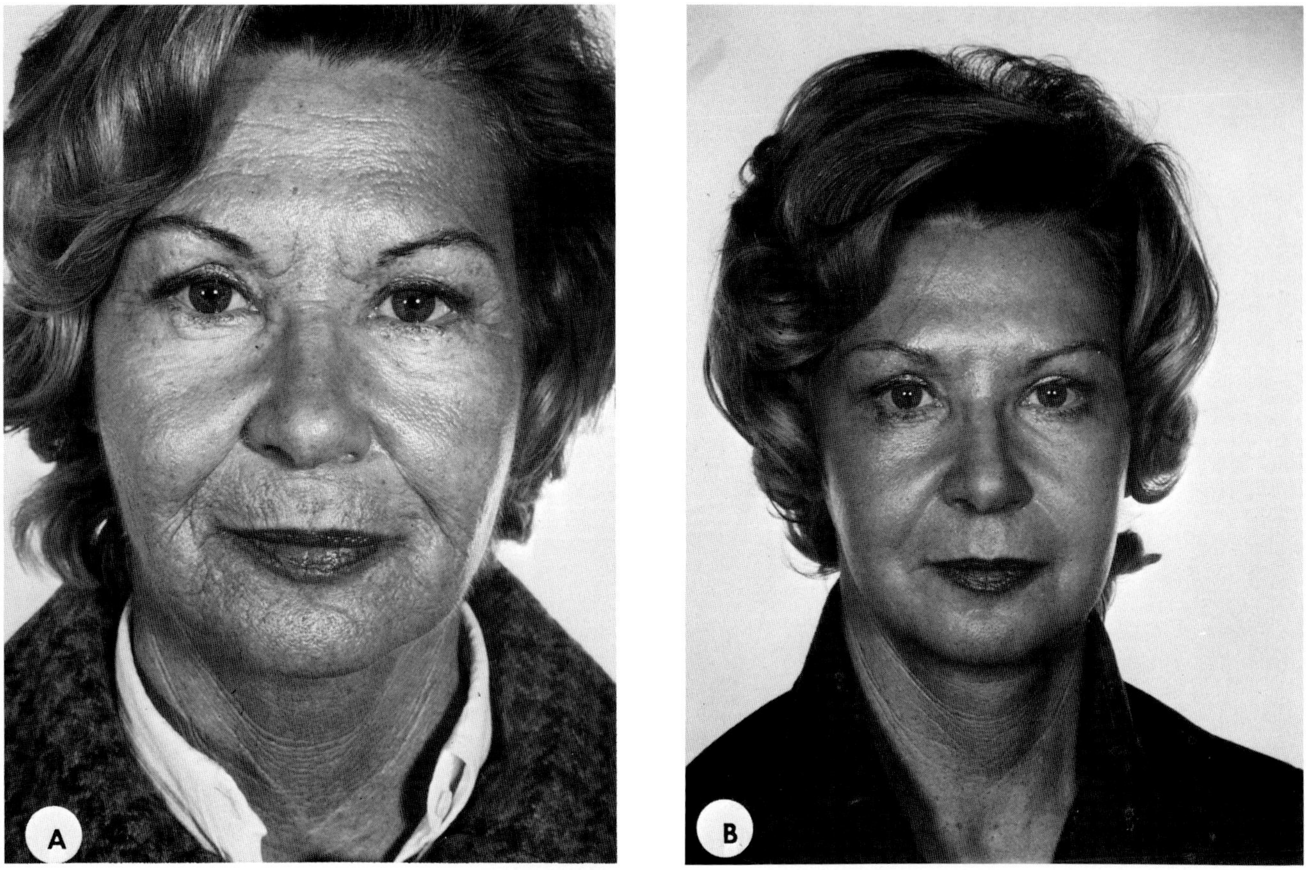

Fig. 13. (A, B) Result of chemical peel on wrinkles.

times to avoid simultaneous swelling if it is done as an outpatient. This will cause the patient to experience diminished vision from 2 to 4 days.

The word carbolic acid should not be used as a synonym for phenol, because this is very frightening to the patient.

Only rarely does the skin have the appearance of a granulated surface after 48 hr, and is usually more superficial than the appearance of a dermabrasive treatment at the same stage. The redness also diminished more rapidly than in the abrasive treatment, and usually by the end of 6 to 8 weeks, the patient has normal color. Instructions are given to avoid direct sun for a period of 3 to 4 months.

Remarks

The removal of freckles and telangiectatic areas has been very successful using this solution.

However, the treatment of postacne scarring is not any better than the present-day dermabrasive therapy, which, in my experience, has seldom rendered any improvement to exceed 30 percent. The use of this solution on hands and arms to rejuvenate the tissue has not proved to be satisfactory. The chemical treatment does not damage hair bearing areas, and is proven totally unsuccessful in the treatment of port wine stains, nevi, and other skin diseases, which have their basic pathology in the lower dermis. Patients are not light sensitive after this treatment (Figs. 13–16).

Conclusion

If the proper type of case is selected and the patient well prepared, the technique known as chemical face lifting can be a useful adjunct. The physician must be aware of the dangers of phenol, both locally and systemically, and should treat his

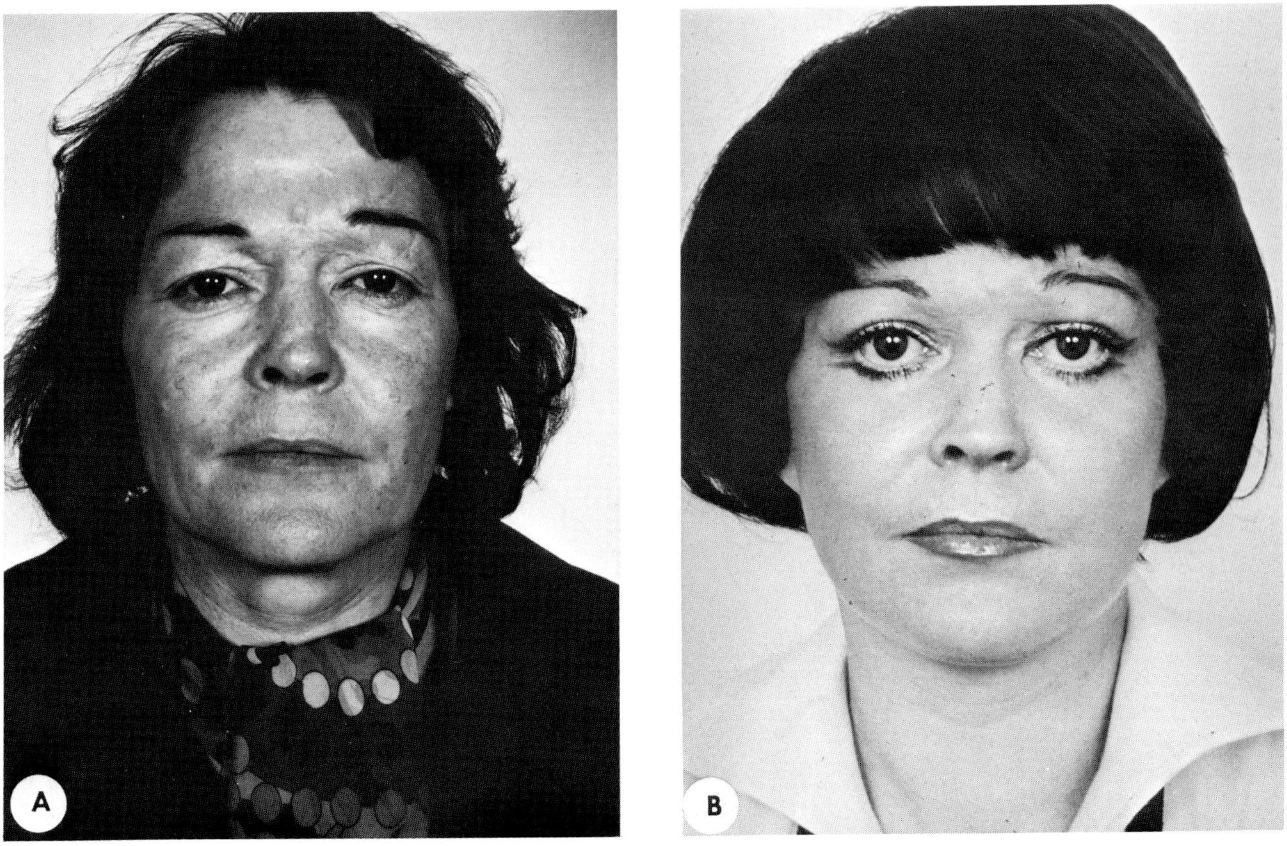

Fig. 14. (A, B) Chemical peel after face lifting and blepharoplasty.

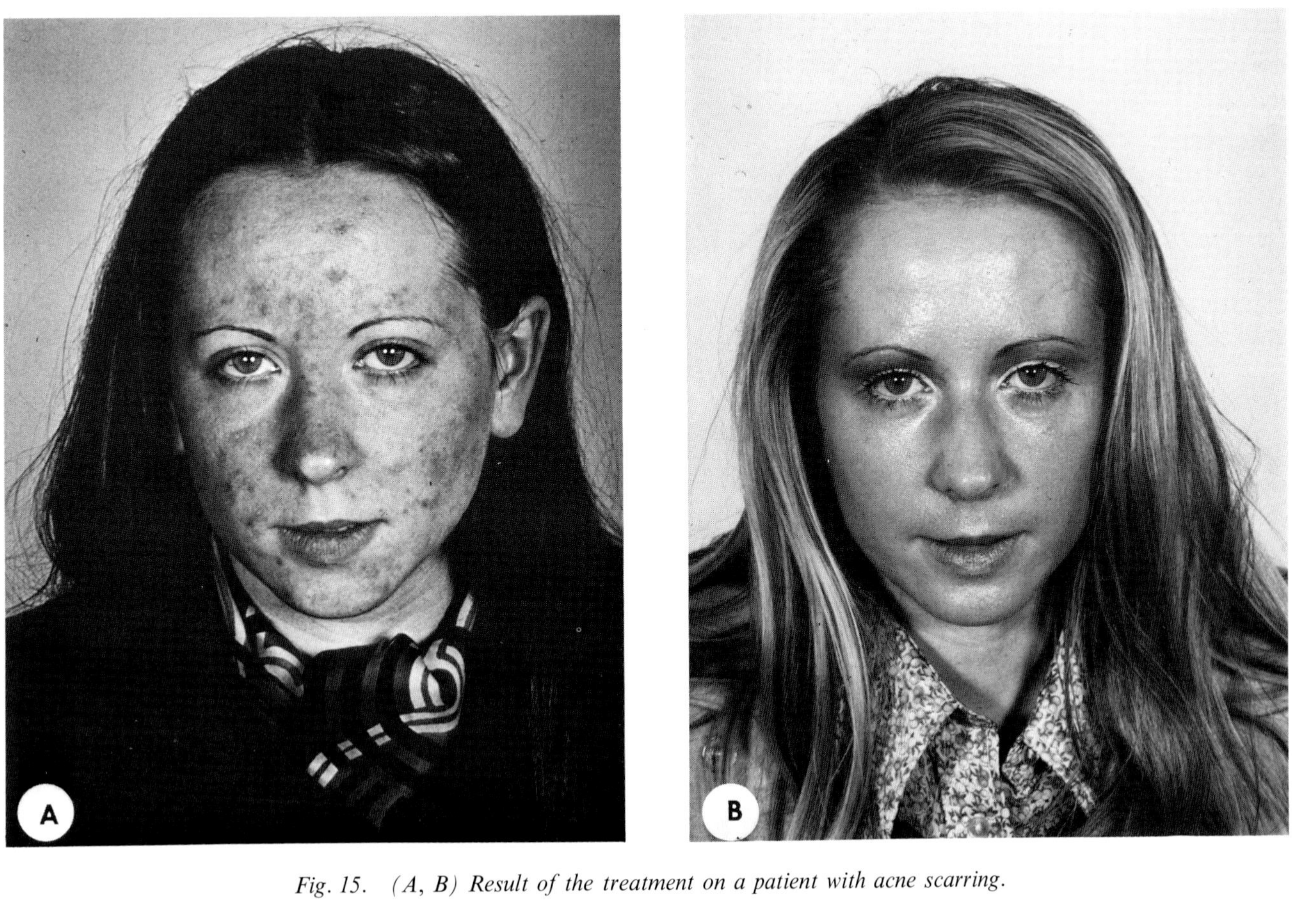

Fig. 15. (A, B) Result of the treatment on a patient with acne scarring.

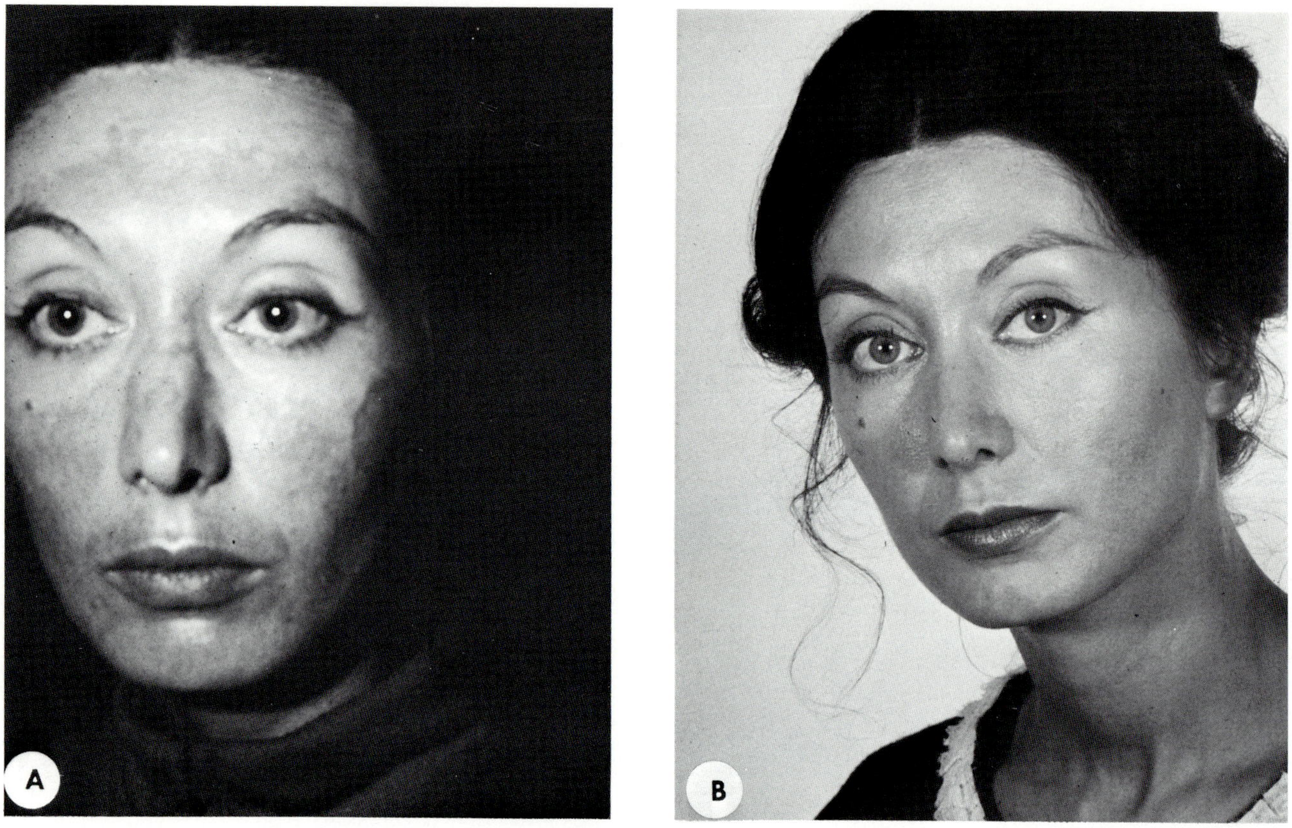

Fig. 16. (A, B) Before and after pictures from the treatment.

patient with minute detail in order to avoid complications. This is not the type of treatment that should be turned over to every physician for indiscriminate use, but should be kept in the hands of the physicians who have been trained in skin changes that are produced by such treatments. There are bound to be some failures and deleterious results when this is used by a large number of doctors, just as there are failures in every known operative procedure.

The long lasting results obtained in this treatment seem to be due to a formation of new structures in the basal layer of the epidermis and superficial layer of the dermis. Even though the results of this treatment are originally caused by an inflammatory reaction, the changes that occur are not just due to transient edema.

Summary

A solution containing phenol has been used and tested for many years by a great number of surgeons. This procedure is not meant to replace surgical face lifting in most instances, but can be used as an adjunct to surgery. The local and systemic effect of phenol has been discussed.

References

1. Litton C, Fournier P, Albert C: A survey of chemical peeling of the face. Plast Reconstr Surg 51:1973
2. Litton C, Portillo A, Fournier P: Chemical peeling. Transactions of the First Congress of the International Society of Aesthetic Plastic Surgery, Rio de Janeiro, Feb, 1972. The International Microfilm Journal of Aesthetic Plastic Surgery.
3. Winter JJA: Method of permanent removal of freckles. Brit J Dermatol Syphilis 62:83–84, 1950
4. Brown AM, Kaplan LM, Brown ME: Phenol induced histological skin changes. Brit J Plast Surg 13:158–169, 1960
5. Baker TJ, Gordon HL, Seckinger DL: A second look at chemical face peeling, Plast Reconstr Surg 37:487, 1966
6. Spira M, Sahl C, Freeman R, Gerow F, Hardy SB: Chemosurgery–histological study. Plast Reconstr Surg 45:247, 1970
7. Spira M, Gerow FJ, Hardy SB: Complications of face peeling. Plast Reconstr Surg 54:397, 1974
8. Baker TJ, Gordon HL: Chemical face peeling, an adjunct to surgical face lifting. South MJ 56:412–414, 1963

Extended Cervical-Facial Rhytidectomy

John R. Hilger, Tacoma, Wash.

Contemporary society has placed an increasing demand on those engaged in plastic surgery to modify and reduce the effects of aging. Correspondingly, the surgical correction of the aging face is escaping the harsh criticism of past decades[1–5] and is becoming more widely accepted. Present social standards with their increased emphasis on the youth culture have placed subtle pressure on older citizens wishing to compete for job opportunities in the modern business world. This has resulted in a broadening of the age categories requesting this type of surgery. In the past, patients usually were seen in the fifth, sixth, and seventh decades of life. Recently patients in the fourth decade have presented themselves in the surgeons office requesting corrective procedures. Their goal is to defer the process of aging rather than have a generalized correction at a later date.

Patients who have a major change in their lifestyle sometimes seek facial plastic surgery to assist them in obtaining a fresh beginning at a new juncture in life.[14] Additionally, patients who have had an alteration of female image by radical expirative surgery often welcome the improvement corrective surgery can offer, enabling them to recapture a more youthful facial appearance, improving and remodeling their distorted body image.

The average surgical patient approaches surgery with reluctance, anxiety, and uncertainity. In contrast, patients requesting facial plastic surgery often approach their surgical appointment with marked enthusiasm. Thus, an entirely different psychological attitude is expressed by this surgical group when requesting corrective assistance.

Correction of the aging face has been practiced for decades. Rather standardized techniques have evolved. Recent modifications in facial plastic surgery have been proposed by various authors[6–13] to enhance the aesthetics of surgical correction. This discussion presents an extended concept using a staged posterior cervical dissection technique. In advanced cervical pathology resection of cervical skin at the nape of the neck is utilized.

Photographic Analysis

Thoughtful analysis of the patient's problem demands a composite evaluation[11] of the area under consideration (Fig. 1). It also presumes adequate photographic analysis. This is extremely important in terms of forming a preoperative record for use before, during, and after surgery. Photographs of the rhytidectomy patient should be taken in five projections. The straight frontal projection and the lateral and quartering view of the face on either side are required. This presents a circumferential view of the facial area, allowing one to make accurate determinations for the forthcoming surgical correction. The photographs are enlarged on 5 × 7 in. (black and white glossy prints) thus accentuating the fine detail so important in facial analysis. Color photomicrographs are additionally made available. The photographic technique involves a single lens reflex camera system using the 105 mm lens. Photofloods offer uniform illumination.

A subsequent discussion with the patient for purposes of photographic analysis is extremely important. It helps form realistic goals in the patient's mind. It may assist by pointing out that the surgical ideal the patient has in their mind may be unobtainable, and if achieved, lacking in aesthetic quality.

Anterior Surgical Considerations

Particular attention is given the temporal area. The standard radical undermining of temporal hairbearing skin followed by excision with suturing under tension may produce alopecia in the area of the surgical scar.[16,17] This is distressing to both patient and surgeon. Regrowth may appear but often takes an extended period of time. In addition, the standard dissection with undermining and pullback of the temporal flap produces an elevation of the temporal tuft of hair, thereby raising the hairline. This is particularly disturbing to patients who have a high frontal hairline and those patients who have undergone a standard secondary rhytidectomy with subsequent further elevation of the temporal area. With these observations in mind, an increasing percentage of primary surgical candidates are treated by excision of a skin strip 1.5 to 2.0 cm in width from the temporal area. The skin margins are approximated without undermining using the interrupted suture technique and the autosuture stape device. Triangular excision of the cheek flap is completed in the preauricular area. If further frontal temporal effect is required the brow lift procedure is employed.[9,15]

The preauricular technique should include supratragal indentation of the preauricular incision to give a natural pretragal scar. The posttragal incision with concealment of the tragal scar can be alternately selected.

Posterior Surgical Considerations

The postauricular incision divides the junction of the ear lobe with the facial skin inferiorly thereafter rising superiorly on the conchal bowl approximately 1.0 cm from the auricular-mastoid crease. This incision is carried 1.0 to 2.0 cm superior to the external auditory canal on the mastoid skin. The incision then moves posteriorly into the occipital hair rather than descending anterior to the mastoid hairline. The latter approach narrows the auricular-mastoid skin pedicle making survival of the flap tenuous. In addition, it places an unsightly scar anterior to the mastoid hairline. This is particularly distressing to the patient who values flexibility in hair styling.

Undermining

The undermining is performed under local anesthesia[19] using the blunt scissor dissection technique. This produces a relatively bloodless field and minimizes the possibility of hematoma formation. The dissection extends to within one finger breadth of the oral commissure and joins the midline of the neck inferiorly. Dissection of the sternomastoid and mastoid area must be adequate to allow proper redraping of the flap. Hemostasis is controlled with proximal cautery and distal ligature of bleeding points.

A relative microgenia and a low lying hyoid bone may complicate the cervical problem in the aging face. In these instances, a submental lipectomy[18] and/or augmentation menoplasty may be indicated.

Flap Placement

It should be stressed that it is impossible to adequately predict the precise degree of skin excision prior to dissection and freeing of the cheek-neck flap. Freeing of the skin creates an entirely new dimension that influences the amount of skin to be excised and the tension to be exerted in the upward and backward pull. Techniques that use predetermined measurements to judge the degree of skin excision should be viewed with skepticism.

The anterior flap is rotated both anteriorly and superiorly thus closing the excised Burrows triangle in the preauricular area. A temporal tacking suture is utilized.

Proper positioning of the posterior flap is the single most important factor in obtaining uniform smoothness in the anterior cervical area. The posterior flap is securely held while a vertical incision (Fig. 2) is created at the skin-hairline junction. This is extended inferiorly for a short distance. The surgeon must accurately determine the precise location of the posterior tacking suture. If minimal deformity is present, the skin-hairline junction of the inferior flap is joined to the skin-hairline junction of the superior flap (Fig. 3, Point A).

In a greater percent of cases, the skin-hairline junction of the inferior flap is placed slightly posterior to create proper draping of the anterior cervical tissues (Fig. 3, Point B). Redundancy of the inferior flap is handled by the shirring technique or by Burrows triangular excision.

In cases of far advanced cervical sagging and typical wattle formation, the skin-hairline junction

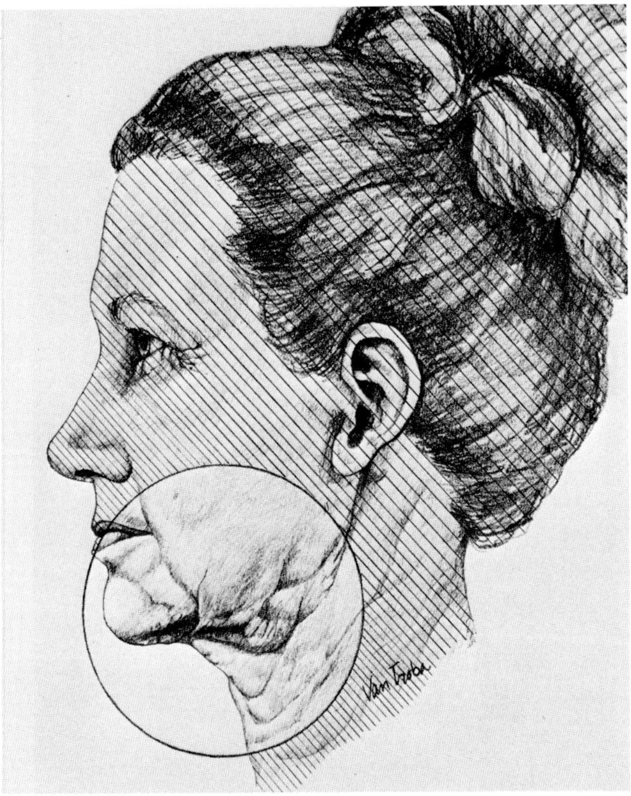

Figure 1.

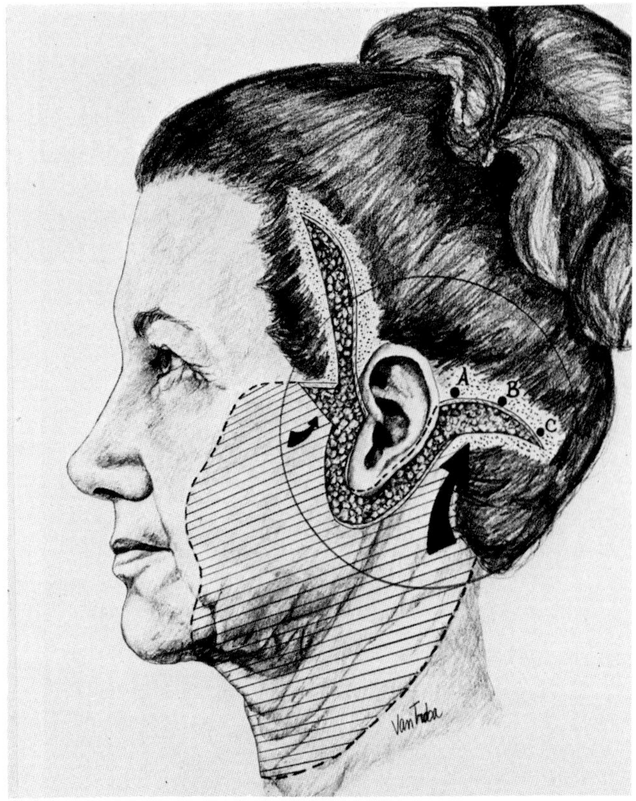

Figure 3.

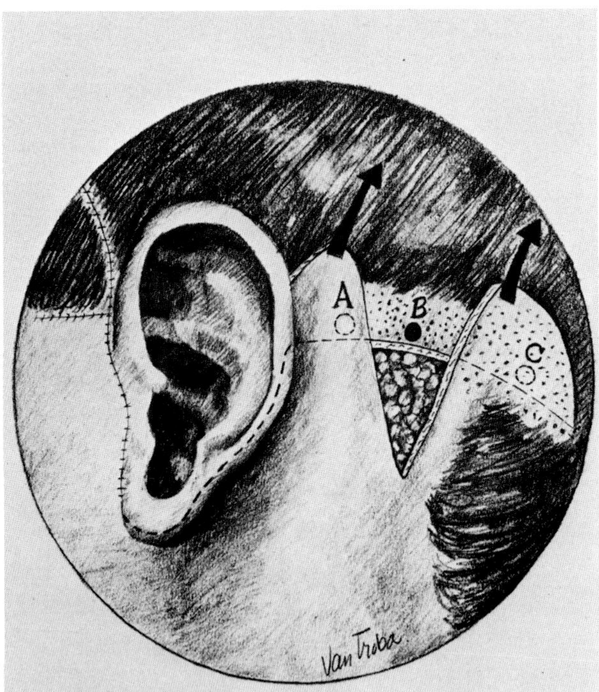

Figure 2.

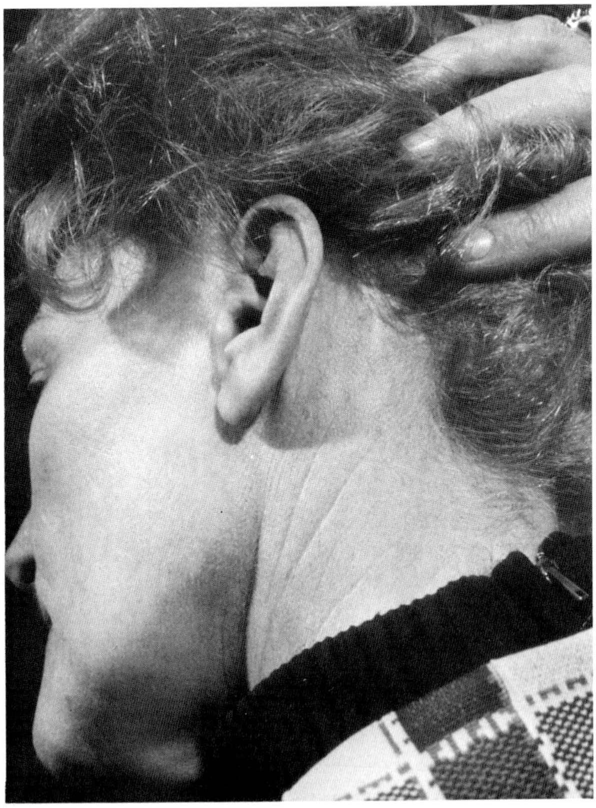

Figure 4.

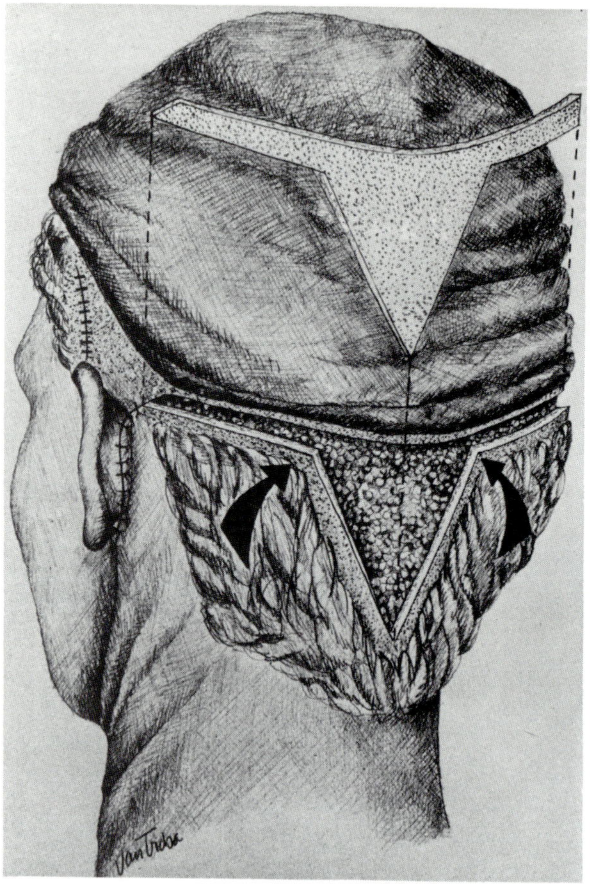

Figure 5.

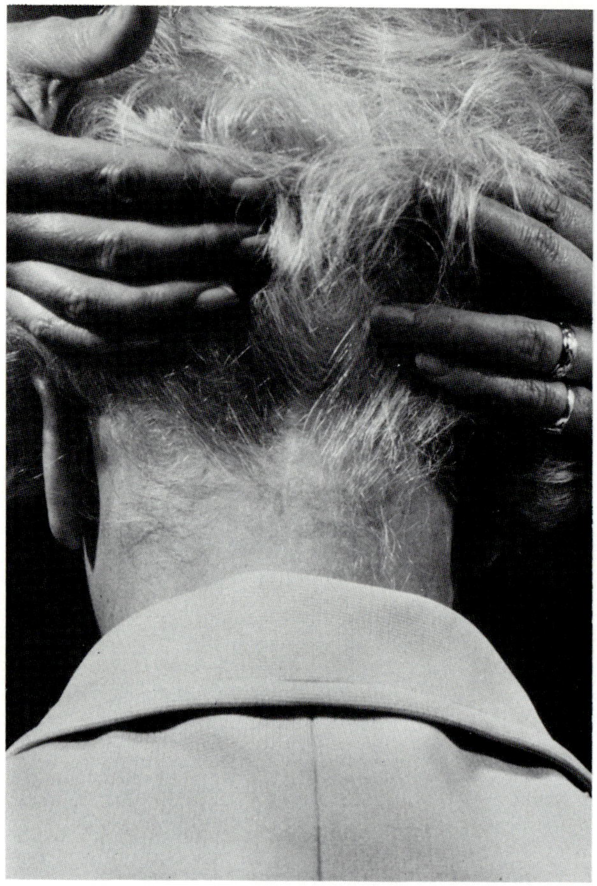

Figure 6.

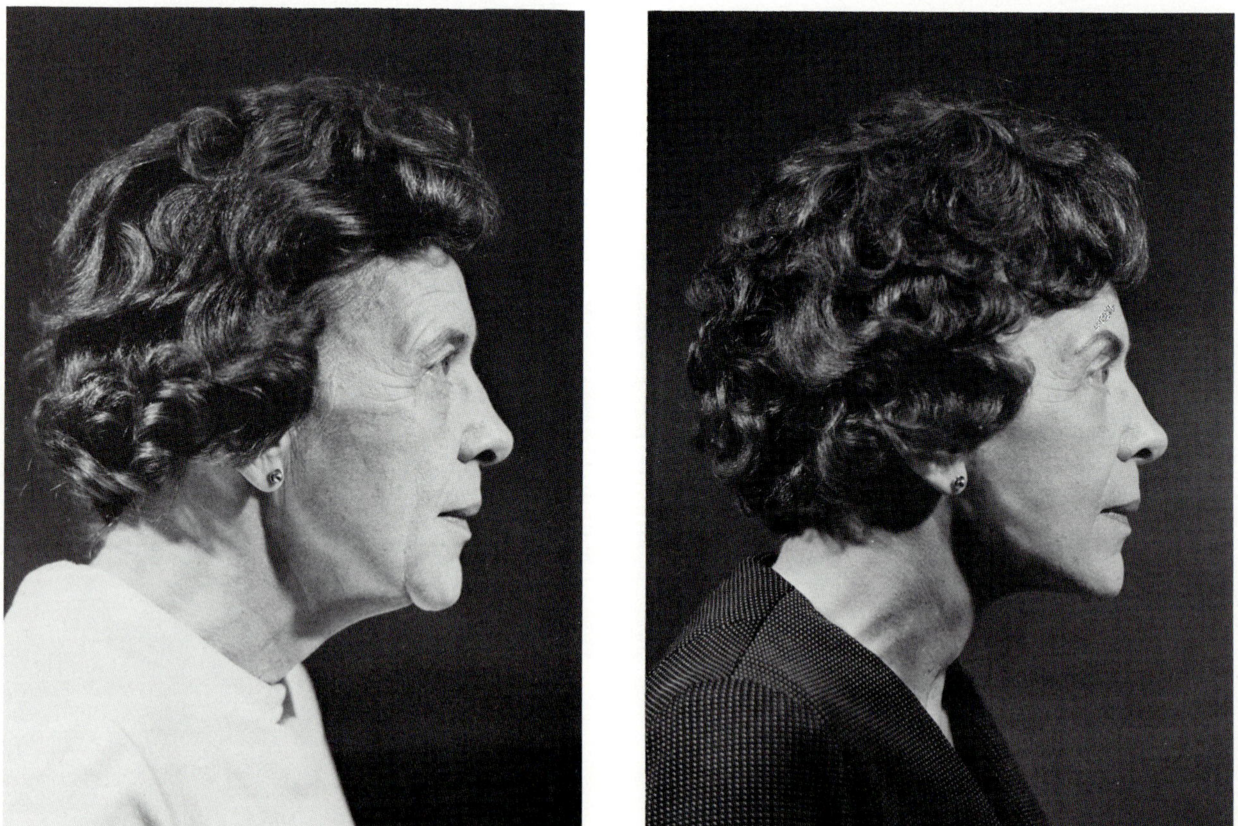

Fig. 7. See legend on facing page.

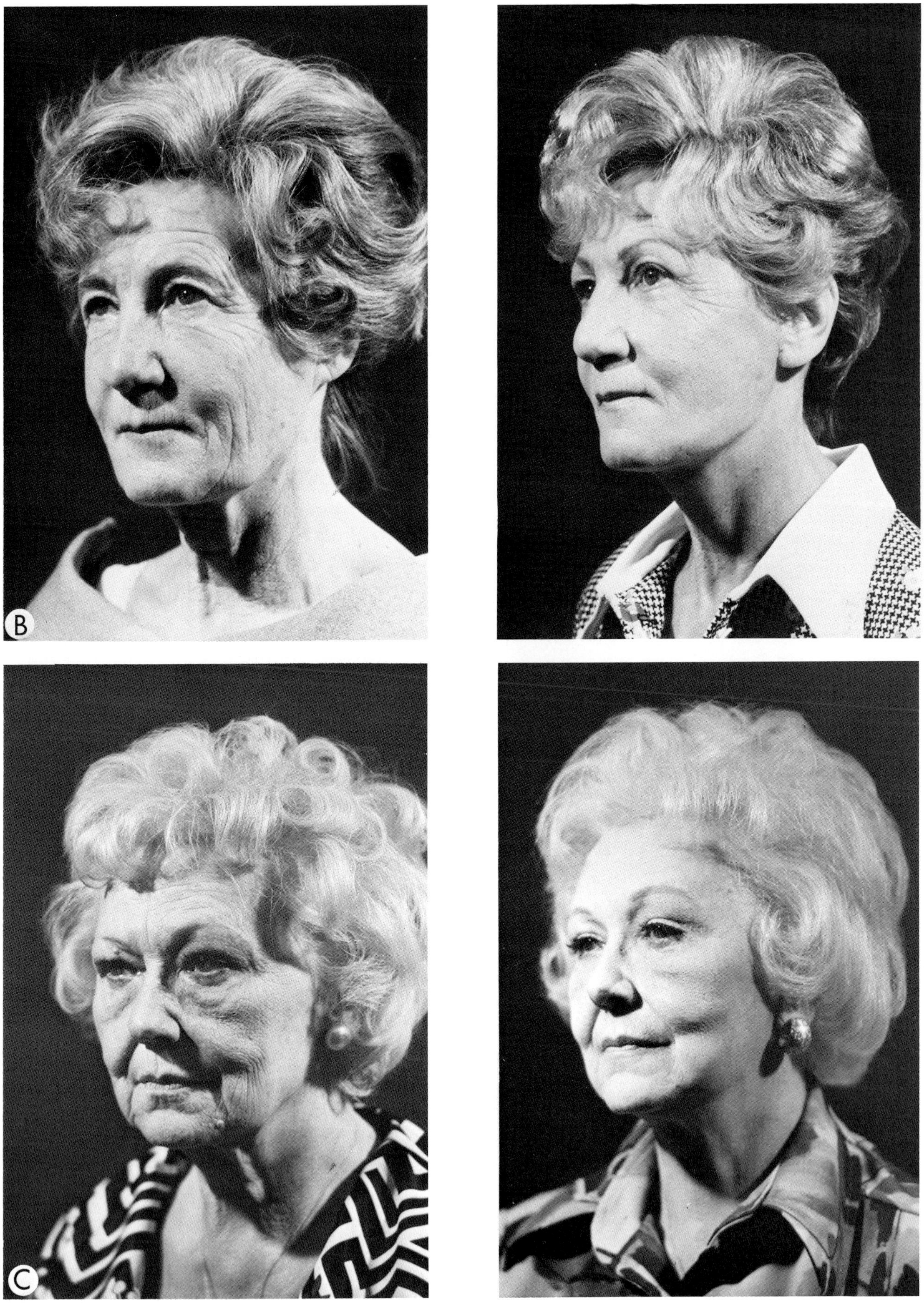

Fig.7. Post operative results using extended posterior dissection to correct anterior cervical redundancy.

of the lower flap must be moved to an extended posterior position (Fig. 3, Point C) and tacked in position (Fig. 4). When Position C is selected, the extended posterior dissection is indicated to completely smooth the posterior aspects of the neck flap and to give adequate lateral cervical symmetry.

Extended Posterior Dissection

The patient is placed in the supported sitting position and the posterior rhytidectomy incision from either side is joined in the midline posteriorly. It is important to direct the posterior rhytidectomy incision toward the inferior aspect of the external occipital protuberance in patients where posterior positioning the face lift flap is contemplated. Thus, if an extended posterior dissection is selected, the union of the right and left posterior rhytidectomy incisions can be completed with a smooth flowing circumferential incision line. The dissection is now begun at the nape of the neck and extends inferiorly into the base of the hairline completely freeing the base of the flap. The dissection than extends laterally completely joining the anterior cheek-neck pocket flap with the posterior nape of the neck dissection. The posterior redundancy is treated by excision of a winged wedge (Fig. 5) of posterior cervical tissue. Simultaneous advancement, elevation and medial rotation of the two posterior cervical flaps results in a T-shaped closure that adequately pulls the cervical tissues into proper alignment. This incision is adequately camouflaged by growth of adjoining cervical hair (Fig. 6).

Additional Flap Adjustments

The hairbearing incisions are closed with interrupted suture and the autostaple suture device. The ear lobe is now freed by making a short anterior and inferior incision. It is important that this incision be conservative in length so that the flap acts as a hammock support to the inferior aspect of the auricular cartilage. This slight upward tension prevents inferior migration of the lobular scar during the later stages of healing. Trimming the preauricular tissues must be precise to allow adequate approximation of flap to the auricular area. It is best to avoid tension when suturing the preauricular flap. The postauricular incision is closed using a nylon pull out suture.

Posterior Operative Care

The patient is examined the morning following surgery. The entire dressing is removed. Incisions are carefully checked for hematoma and signs of early infection. The wet dressing is then reapplied. The patient is dismissed from the hospital 24 hr following surgery. On the fourth day following surgery the dressing is removed in the office. Suture removal is done at intermittent intervals during the 10-day period following the operative procedure. Discoloration and ecchymosis are common following surgery and usually recede over a two to three week period of time. The patient is socially presentable with cosmetic cover two to three weeks following the procedure. Postoperative photography is deferred for two to three months following corrective surgery to allow for adequate diminution of the postoperative swelling and to accurately document the long term aesthetic result (Fig. 7).

Surgical correction of the aging face requires thoughtful analysis of presenting pathology. Vector forces created by posterior and superior pull of the face lift flap must be carefully applied to achieve the maximum aesthetic result. The surgeon should be prepared to utilize all stages of flap adjustment to create a satisfying aesthetic result.

References

1. Bettman AG: Plastic and cosmetic surgery of the face. Northwest Med 19:205, 1920
2. Passot R: Chirurgie Esthetique Pure (Technique et Resultats). Doin et Cie, Paris, 1931
3. Joseph J: Plastic operation on protruding cheek. Deutsche med Wchnschr 47:287, 1921
4. Lexer E: Die Gesamte Wieder Herstellungschirurgie. JA Barth, Leipzig, Vols 1 and 2, 1931
5. Noel A: La Chirurgie Esthetique, Son Role Social. Masson et Cie, Paris, 1926
6. Aufricht G: Surgery for excess skin of the face and neck. Trans Interna Soc Plast Surgeons, Second Congress. E and S Livingstone, Ltd; Edinburgh and London, 1960
7. Pitanguy I, Ramos H, Garcia LC: Philosophy technique and complication of rhytidectomies. Rev Brasil Cir 62:277, 1972
8. Stark RB: Hoeber Medical Division, Harper & Row, New York, 1962
9. Anderson J: Surgical treatment of periorbital aging. Plastic and Reconstructive Surgery of the Face and Neck. Pro-

ceedings of the First International Symposium, Vol 1, Aesthetic Surgery, p 73
10. Conley J: Face-lift operation. Springfield, Ill, Charles C Thomas, Co, 1968
11. Rees TD, Guy CL: Patient selection and Technique in blepharoplasty and rhytidoplasty. Surgical Clinics of North America, April, 1971
12. Gonzales-Ulloa M, Stevens FE: Sectional rhytidectomy. Plastic and Reconstructive Surgery of the Face and Neck. Proceedings of the First International Symposium, Vol 1, Aesthetic Surgery, p 29
13. Webster RC: Eyebrow position in selection of procedure for rehabilitating the aging face. Plastic and Reconstructive Surgery of the Face and Neck. Proceedings of the First International Symposium, Vol 1, Aesthetic Surgery, p 23
14. Edergton MT, Webb WL Jr, Slaughter R, Meyer E: Surgical results and psychosocial changes following rhytidectomy: an evaluation of facelifting. Plast Reconstr Surg 33:503, 1964
15. Castanares S: Forehead wrinkles, glabellar frowns and ptosis of the eyebrows. Plast Reconst Surg 34:406, 1964
16. Johnson JB: The problem of the aging face. Plast Reconstr Surg 15:117, 1955
17. Pangman JW, Wallace RM: Cosmetic surgery of the face and neck. Plast Reconstr Surg 40:551, 1967
18. Millard RD, Pigott RW: Submandibular lipectomy. Plast Reconstr Surg 27:544, 1968
19. Rees TD, Lee YC, Coburn RJ: Expanding hematoma after rhytidectomy. Plast Reconstr Surg 51:150, 1973

Nuances in Face Lift Surgery

Walter E. Berman and Charles M. Monell, Beverly Hills, Calif.

Introduction

A wishful hope was captured by Shakespeare in a few lines from a sonnet:

> Devouring time . . . O, carve not
> with thy hours my love's fair
> brow,
> nor draw no lines there with
> thine antique pen.

Yet, inevitably, the lines are drawn, and the brows are carved. We turn them to thoughts of rejuvenation. The word itself derives from a late latin word meaning "to make young again." Although this is obviously impossible, we like to think of cosmetic surgery as a type of facial rejuvenation, which at least is a delaying action against the ravages of time. In our youth-oriented society, physical appearance can be the doorway to personal success. The social and economic advantages of a pleasing physical appearance are obvious, and are openly discussed today without the false modesty so common in the past.

Our goal is a happy patient after surgery, and a surgeon pleased and proud of his work. Our quest is for maximum results with a minimum of hazard. We feel that a careful preoperative evaluation of the patient's physical appearance and emotional health are the keys to success. The discussions should also concern the possibility of scar formation and a realistic approach to the subject of complete healing. A preoperative approach that is realistic and honest will avoid future misunderstanding and disappointment.

Many of the complications of facial plastic surgery are iatrogenic, and therefore preventable. Untoward effects may follow a surgeon's well intentioned attempt to overextend the surgical procedure in the hope of achieving a supermaximal result. Although perfection is a logical goal, in facial plastic surgery attempts to reach this goal must at times be tempered by conservatism. A summary of what can and what cannot be done with safety and some techniques in handling unfavorable results are the subjects of this discussion.

The patient and the surgeon must agree in advance that there will be variations in tissue healing between individuals. A well-prepared preoperative patient, who has a good rapport with his surgeon, is the best form of malpractice insurance.

The manner in which the patient is prepared before surgery will strongly influence his attitude after surgery. Total honesty and frankness, even pessimism when indicated, are the best approaches to educating the potential patient.

The material presented in this discussion is based on our series of approximately 500 facelift operations and 1000 blepharoplasties. Some of the more recent literature and current texts have also been reviewed.

The Preoperative Examination

Our patients are usually seen two or three times well in advance of surgery so that all points of the interview and the examination will be reviewed in detail with adequate time available. As the doctrine of "informed consent" becomes the law of the land, it is all the more important that the doctor and his staff take care to make all problem areas evident to the patient. In the history and physical examination the vital organ systems are surveyed.

Pertinent Points in the Preoperative Examination

1. Vital organ survey: Contact a doctor who knows the patient, preferably the family physician. Obtain an electrocardiogram and chest films.
2. Evaluate skin healing: Basic tissue healing, such as the knuckles that are often subjected to minor traumas.
3. Question regarding bleeding tendencies.
4. Question regarding medications and toxic reactions. Is there excessive use of aspirin?
5. Psychological evaluation: Obtain a clearance if the patient has been treated by a therapist in addition to one's own psychological clearance. Question the patient to discover what he expects to derive from the surgery.
6. The patient should be seen a few days before surgery to reassure him, to answer any questions, and to obtain a final evaluation of heart, lungs, blood pressure, and so forth.
7. Test visual acuity with Snellen charts prior to any surgery involving eyelids. Evaluate visual fields if indicated.

Rationale

Several techniques of face lifting have been advocated over the years. Incisions have been placed in various patterns, areas, creases, and folds with varied degree of success. But the one important requirement in any worthwhile face lift is extensive undermining. The "minilift," in which only a fold of skin is excised without undermining will accomplish nothing. To achieve and sustain a serviceable lifting procedure it is mandatory to create a sufficiently dissected area so that a skin flap can be repositioned and held in a new location. Skin tension along the line of simple excision will not hold a lift. A layer of fibrosis must be laid down between the skin and the deeper layers of the dissected tissues. This layer of fibrous scar helps hold the skin flaps to the deeper tissues in the newly established relationship. We consider this fibrous layer to be important in slowing down the relaxation process, for it replaces in function the elastic fibers of the skin, which disappears with age. This is as important as the actual excision of excess skin during the procedure. The amount of undermining is proportional to the degree of success.

Pathogenesis of Wrinkling

Understanding why wrinkles appear can be most helpful. A professor once said, "if you know the diagnosis, you know the prognosis. You will know what can, and more importantly, what cannot be done." A young adult has taut skin, solid bones, firm muscle, and a certain amount of fat for contour. With age, there is atrophy of fat pads. There is loss of the teeth and absorption of the alveolus. The ligaments relax, the muscles shrink, the skin has stretched, and time and gravity take their toll. It is easy to understand why we end up with too much skin to cover our shrinking frame. A description of an aging Falstaff makes it all too plain, "have you not a moist eye? A dry hand? A yellow cheek? A white beard? A decreasing leg? An increasing belly? Is not your voice broken? Your wind short? Your chin double? Your wit single? And every part about you blasted with antiquity?" Not a very pleasant picture, and one we hope to partially correct with proper surgery.

INCISIONS AND UNDERMINING

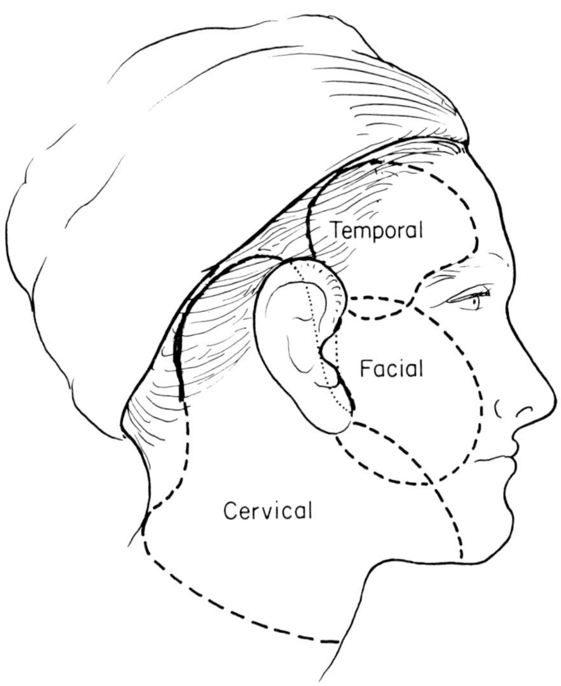

Figure 1.

Regional Face Lift

We divide the face lift operation into three areas or regions: The temporal, facial, and cervical (see Fig. 1). Some patients may need surgery in one, two, or all three of these regions to achieve the maximal results. The degree of relaxation in any one area will determine the amount of undermining needed before the excess skin is excised.

The temporal, or upper third, incision is hidden in the hair bearing area. It extends from the top of the ear, curving superiorly, and about 4 cm behind the patient's temporal hair line. The skin is elevated from the incision forward on the superficial (not the deep) temporal fascia. Just below the level of the hair follicles, which should not be visible on the undersurface of the flap. The dissection is above the temporal vessels. In the nonhair bearing portion of the forehead flap, the dissection is very superficial to avoid branches of the facial nerve. This superficial dissection may extend as far as the brow if necessary. In this manner a "browlift" can be accomplished via the temporal incision without producing the obvious scars seen with the usual brow incisions.

The middle third, or facial, incision extends from the top of the auricle, down to the lobule, and then up the back of the auricle. However, in the region of the tragus, the incision is carried behind the tragus, into the ear canal. This requires more care than the usual incision in the preauricular crease, but the result is well worth the trouble. There will be no visible scar in the tragal area, and this is of cosmetic importance to many patients. The skin flap over the tragus must be thinned to achieve a natural tragus postoperatively. The incisions of the lower third, the cervical incisions, extend along the back of the auricle, about 1.5 cm from the auriculomastoidal crease to the top of the auricle. At this point it will be only a few centimeters away from the bottom of the temporal incision. From this point it extends down the neck along the edge of the thicker hair bearing skin. The length of the incision varies according to the needs of the patient. Most incisions end at about the level where the hair of the neck begins to thin.

These incisions help eliminate the usual preauricular and postauricular tell-tale scars of face lift surgery (see Fig. 2). The incisions and permanent tension sutures we have discussed are not a panacea, but they have markedly decreased the obvious signs of face lift surgery.

We have a head holder that is used primarily for face lifts, enabling bilateral surgery. Our technique is to complete the eyelid flaps. I will then perform the face lift on one side, while my associate sutures the eyelid surgery. Secondarily, while my associate is suturing the first operative side of the lift, the flaps of the second side are being developed. The operating table is quite high and we are seated. Besides the obvious time saver, the patient's head is not moved during the entire surgery or dressing. The latter point causes less postoperative throat irritation when an endotracheal tube is used, and may even keep the anesthetist quite happy. Here these aluminum parts disassemble and can be autoclaved as a relatively small unit. This photograph shows how we can raise, lower, go forwards or backwards, all of which can be particularly important when an endotracheal tube is not elected.

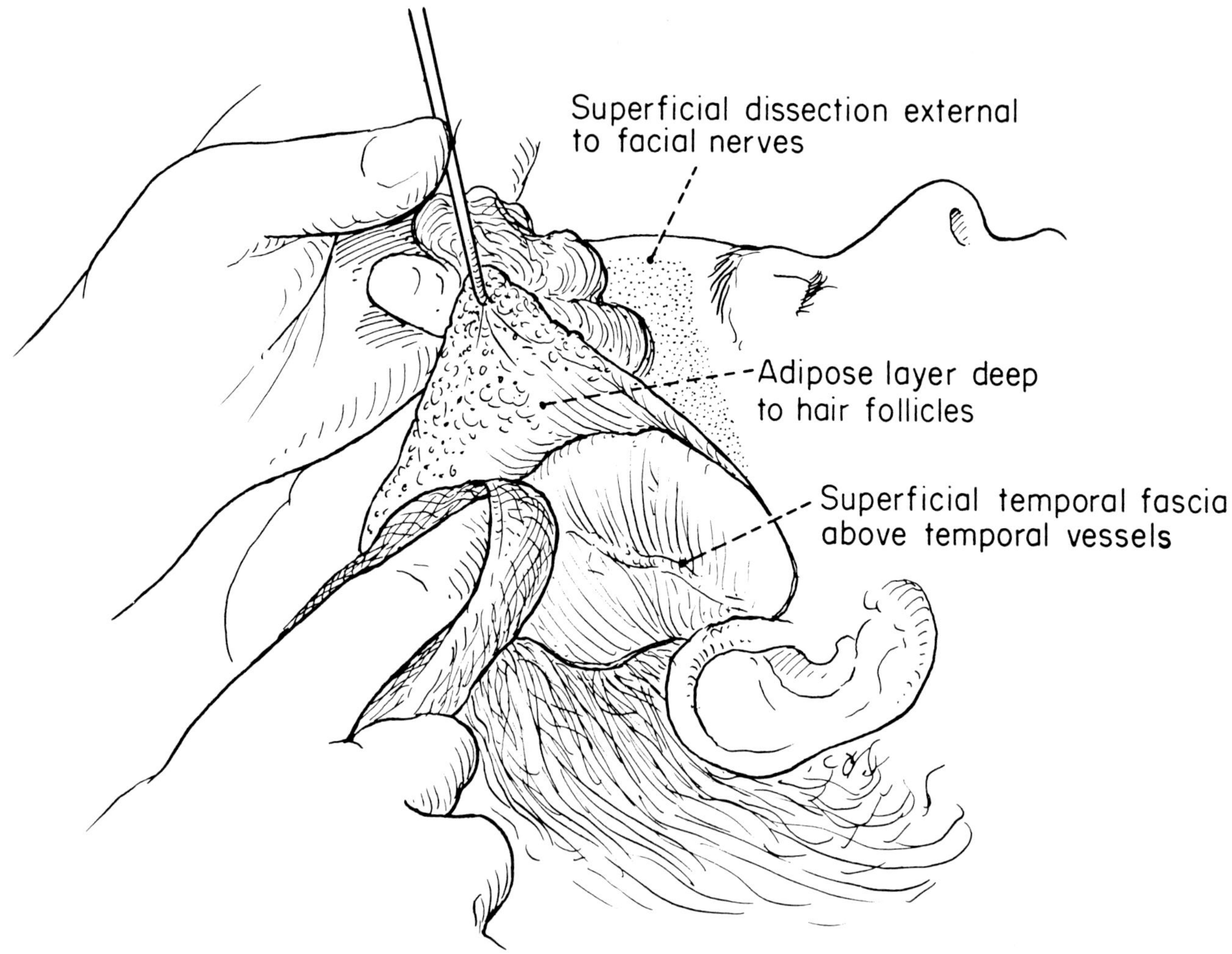

Figure 2.

We inject the entire area to be dissected with one-half percent solution of xylocaine with 1 to 200,000 adrenalin per ounce. Approximately 30–40 cc for each side of the face will be used. We have found it most helpful, particularly when doing a lift with eyelid surgery, to inject one side of the face. Do the lids and then 15 min before the second side of the face is done, inject to allow adequate vasoconstriction before the facial surgery is done. This is the position that will be maintained throughout the surgical procedure. If, at any time, rotation of the patient is desired, the table is rotated.

The temporal portion of hair is tied forwards with Selvedge gauze. Methylene blue is used to demarcate the future incisions. You will note that no shaving is done. We have done this for many years and have not noticed any morbidity from this technique. The temporal and preauricular incisions are completed at this time. The dissection of the posttragal flap and adjacent tissues are done with a fine forceps and a small Stevens scissors. I have found this technique preferable in this area, to sharp dissection. The mid-facial or buccal area dissection can then be carried forward with a long double edge dissecting scissors, utilizing a superficial plane through the nasolabial folds. With gauze packs in place in the midfacial dissection, we then go superiorly, and take care of the temporal dissection as previously described in the diagrammatic picture. Here, we can see the plane of the temporal vessels inferiorly, while the hair follicles are in the dissected flap, held in a distal position.

The seventh nerve is most superficial as it courses over the zygoma. This is probably the most frequent site of nerve injury during the face-lifting procedure. Creation of superficial skin flaps over the zygoma, as well as using absorbable ties on bleeding vessels, rather than cautery or permanent sutures will also be a good safeguard.

The cervical dissection is dependent on the needs of the particular patient. It may vary from meeting in the midline, going inferiorly to the clavicle and extending posteriorly until the incisions almost meet; or a much more minor procedure.

The dissection has now been completed. Hemostasis is obtained, and the flaps elevated at about 45° to be tacked to their new positions.

Tacking Sutures (Fig. 3)

The first tacking suture is at a level just above the superior and anterior portion of the auricle. This is held with a Brown Adson forceps and pulled posteriorly. Remember that the undissected tissues posterior to the incisions also have some give. The two meet with some tension. A splitting incision is done and our first tacking suture placed.

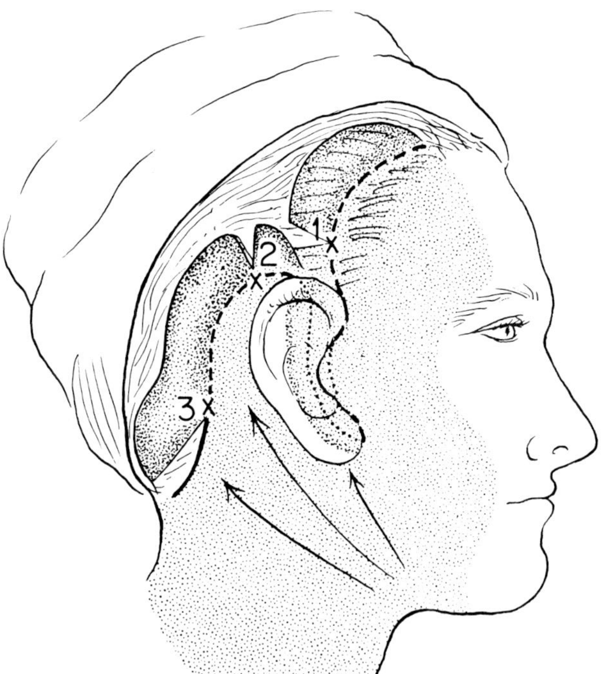

Figure 3.

A similar procedure is carried out in the superior postauricular area. This flap is then placed with the second tacking suture. The first and second tacking sutures are the major forces or vectors of pull in a 45° upward and backwards direction. The third tacking point is approximately at the level of the inferior auricle but is at the posterior incision, or the incision of the cervical hairbearing line.

Second and Third Tacking Sutures

I like to use a Brown Adson forceps, grasping this elevated flap and measuring until it approximates the point of the incision at the hairbearing area and marking with a scalpel. The flap is the incised from this point inferiorly until it meets the end of the inferior portion of the original cervical incision.

For purposes of clarification, this diagram shows the three tacking sutures we have used to reposition our flaps. One, just above the auricle anteriorly. Two, at the top of the postauricular incision behind the ear. Three, the point of the stab incision in the middle of the posteriocervical flap. Our butterfly flap is at least descriptive, if not out and out pure surgical license. This is related to the flap created in the cervical dissection. The upper portion of the flap, or left wing when standing behind the patient, is related to the excessive post auricular tissue. The lower is formed by measuring the redundant skin from the posterior neck incision. This forms a right wing. The possibilities of dog ears are eliminated by this technique.

Three tacking sutures are in place, showing the redundant skin in the temporal, preauricular, and cervical areas to be removed.

All but the pretragal flaps are trimmed. This flap is left in place without any excisions, at this point, so that when the suturing is complete elsewhere, this will be done last. This will enable us to have the least amount of pull on this flap without causing any postoperative pulling and possible distortion of the postoperative tragus.

Trimming has now been completed, except for untrimmed tragal flap.

This is grasped with a curved kelly, extended with minimal tension, and marked with methylene blue for the flap incision. This will, of course, fit into the prior incision of the external portion of the ear canal behind the tragus. At the same time, the flap is thinned with a small scissors practically leaving a full skin thickness without subcutaneous tissue for adherence on the tragal cartilage. Suturing is now complete. No drains are used. After many years of to drain or not to drain, in our experience it seems that no benefit is derived from the use of drains.

The submental fat pad may be a problem. We can connect the dissected cervical planes from each side and still be left with an undesirable submental bulge. This may be related to the actual muscular contour; but most frequently the cause is excessive fatty tissue in this particular area. We have found that through a small incision, over the point of maximal bulge in a horizontal direction, the submental fat pad can be separated from the overlying skin. By use of a cup biting forceps sizable amounts of fatty tissue may be removed. These are removed in many small pieces. The fibrosis from this procedure also helps hold this dependant area in a better position after surgery.

Fine Lines

There are many modalities of treatment. Particularly with the fine points of facial surgery. Various chemical peels, injections of synthetic materials, which is not approved by the food and drug administration at this time, superficial irritants which are usually of short lived duration and merely have an effect through the swelling they cause. Youth pills, which are quite problematical and certainly unproven. Fifth—plastic surgery.

I like treating fine lines of the face that are not related to loose tissues with dermabrasion. Perioral lines are a tell tale sign of mother nature's relentless effort to age people. Whether superficial lines are improved with the aid of a dermabraider or skin peeling is not important. I feel that there is better control, as to depth, with a dermabraider than with a peeling mixture. There are fine results from both techniques. This may be carried out in other sections of the face; but I would not suggest this where simultaneous undermining of the same tissue had taken place.

Cleaning and Dressing

The drape is then removed from the head area. Any prep solution, dried blood, etc., is then removed with sterile water by the use of a water basin underneath the patient's head, and using abdominal laps to cleanse off any extraneous material.

The postoperative dressing may sound routine or even mundane but can eliminate any problems. The application of a firm, comfortable nonconstricting dressing that applies even pressure to the entire operative area is most desirable. Telfa and cortisporin ointment are applied over the incisions. Three layers of roller cotton are then placed under the chin and dissected flaps. These are held in place with a 6 in. bias dressing. The direction is under the chin, over the vertex and secondarily from the forehead around and under the occiput. Never use a roller type dressing around the neck. This type of described dressing holds up the chin for an even better airway exchange.

We use a thin foam rubber whiplash type collar, that we give to the patient on the fourth postoperative day. This is the same time that the eyelid sutures are also removed. This collar is done as a reminder not to stretch the incisional areas by turning for a similar period of 6–8 weeks as a definitive time of histological healing of tissues. This has been particularly useful with a cervical dissection. Logically, with less stretching of a scar, we may expect a thinner scar.

Special Problems (Fig. 4)

Scars

No matter how carefully the work is done, a certain amount of scar formation is inevitable. Most are not a problem, but some are objectionable:

1. Thickened, keloid-like, either vascular, fibrotic, of some combination of the two.
2. Broad and flat; these may be consequences of the first type.
3. Changes in pigmentation: Hyperpigmentation or hypopigmentation.

The first two groups appear to be related primarily to postoperative tension on the line of the incisions during the first two months.

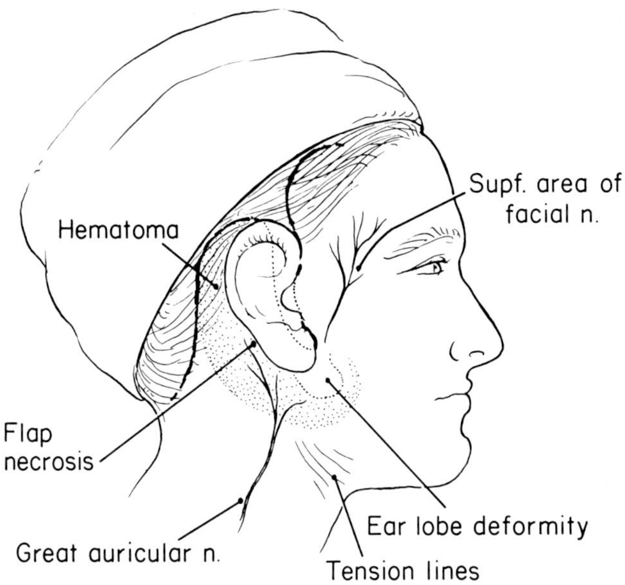

Figure 4.

Undermining also decreases the tension on the lines of incision so that the scars do not stretch unduly in the postoperative period. Inverted buried 4-0 clear nylon sutures are also used in the subcutaneous tissue along the incision to help prevent stretching of the scar. We consider there to be a critical period of two months, for healing of the skin edges. Some of the buried nylon sutures may be extruded after many months. However, they are important during the first critical weeks. During this early healing period we also partially immobilize the neck with a soft 2 in. foam rubber whiplash collar to prevent excessive turning of the head and neck and stretching of the cervical incisions.

The red vascularized scars respond well to local infiltration with steroids. Multiple injections of the small particle (10 mg per ml) corticosteroid at weekly or biweekly intervals have been helpful in controlling this problem. A spring loaded instrument is available that will inject 0.1 ml as a jet directly into the tissue. Surgical tampering with these scars prior to their maturation usually leads to poor results. After full healing has taken place and there is some relaxation of the tissue, it may be possible to excise this type of scar and resuture without tension.

If necessity dictates that surgical removal be done before the scar has matured, immediate postoperative irradiation is used. Delaying the start of radiation for only a few days appears to have an adverse effect.

Pigment Changes

Pigmentary changes are expected primarily in the more heavily pigmented skins. These are indeed a challenge. Preoperative warnings and even trial incisions can be of value. We have not been happy with the results of tattooing the hypopigmentary changes. The pigment from the tattoo always seems to change in time, and the skin tones alter with other variables, such as exposure to sun. A cosmetic skin dye that lasts a few days has been the most acceptable but is not a permanent answer.

Hematoma Formation

The fragile nature of face lift flaps makes a hematoma a most serious complication. The facial skin flaps must be thin and the extensive undermining necessary further impairs the circulation. It is only the abundant blood supply of the face and neck that maintains the viability of this skin. A hematoma, causing pressure and impairment of the circulation, can be a major disaster.

It is strongly recommended that at the time of surgery all visible bleeding vessels be suture ligated, and that cautery be reserved for incision edges and small bleeders. If the blood pressure has been lowered during the procedure to decrease the bleeding, the pressure should be returned to near normal before the flaps are closed and sutured. If the patient complains of postoperative pain or if there is marked firmness of the cheek skin or mucosal surfaces, immediate inspection of the flaps is indicated. A major hematoma requires a return to the operating room, general anesthesia, release of the flaps, irrigation, control of bleeding points, and resuturing. A smaller hematoma in the postauricular area or near the angle of the mandible may be treated by inserting a sterile number 30 catheter through the cervical incision to remove the clots. This conservative approach should be used only when all signs of active bleeding have ceased. Insertion of a 1/4 in. penrose drain for 24 hr and reapplication of a firm pressure dressing are also indicated. A small hematoma near an incision line should be drained by inserting a small straight forceps through the line of incision to evacuate the clot. At this time the skin flaps are fairly insensitive and a local anesthetic is not required.

Occasionally there is evidence of a hematoma after a few days. The pathogenesis appears to be related to a deep muscle hematoma that required a few days to become evident. Aspiration with an 18 gauge needle can be accomplished. This type of hematoma often requires multiple aspirations at one to two day intervals as liquefication progresses. A bimanual technique with one finger in the oral cavity and the other on the cheek is helpful in confirming the presence of a deep hematoma.

To Drain or Not to Drain

Several years ago we stopped the routine use of suction drains under the flaps. The pressure dressing permitted only local drainage anyway. On one occasion a large hematoma resulted when a perforated suction catheter drain was removed after 48 hours.

Even after the use of meticulous hemostasis, pressure dressings and preoperative clotting studies, a hematoma may occur at times. Probably the most common cause is a marked blood pressure elevation, which is usually noted in the recovery room. An uneven pressure dressing may also permit collections of serum and blood clot. A firm uniform pressure applied over thick cotton padding is preferred to a constricting uneven dressing.

All bandages are removed the next morning for inspection of the skin. A light cotton padded dressing is reapplied, leaving the ears uncovered for comfort.

Skin Necrosis

Skin necrosis most often occurs after hematoma formation. It may also be noted if there is undue tension on a flap, excessive pressure from dressings, or lack of a proper blood supply. If the etiology is obvious and treatment provided, such as evacuation of a hematoma, the course of action is easily apparent. Often the situation is not simple, and judicious treatment of both the skin and the patient will be needed. Above all, one must explain what is happening to the patient and offer reassurance that all possible is being done, particularly if secondary repair may be necessary. Telling the patient that the condition will rectify itself may be far from the truth and also create the nidus for litigation.

If cyanotic changes are present, it may be helpful to decrease the local metabolic level with ice packs. If there is marginal circulation, the decreased metabolism may afford time for the development of an adequate blood supply. However, the flap fails to blanch with digital pressure, there is little likelihood that the skin will survive.

If skin loss appears inevitable, spontaneous demarcation and conservative superficial debridement yield the best result. While waiting for demarcation to occur, the skin is covered with cortisporin and bacitracin ointments twice daily. If a large area of necrosis has occurred, it has been helpful to administer antistaphylococcal medications systemically. Postauricular skin is probably the most easily necrosed because of the thinness of the flap and the scant circulation. However, the amount of spontaneous repair has often been remarkable. Recovery may be prolonged and the patient may be anxious for more vigorous treatment.

Asking the patient to wait for a more opportune time for repair may be more difficult. I feel that patient acceptance is closely related to the rapport created prior to the surgery. Tincture of time and gentle debridement require the least amount of surgical repair and insure an optimal result.

Infection

A serious infection is most unlikely in this procedure unless there has been a marked impairment of the blood supply to a skin flap. We do not shave the hair preoperatively. The hair is combed and parted along the incision lines and held in place by ties or by soft soap. The face and exposed areas are given the usual skin preparation in the operating room. To date, we have had no problems with infection. If infection should occur, the most likely organism will be a Staphylococcus, but cultures should be taken and treated accordingly.

Hair Loss

Hair loss is rarely a complication and results when the temporal flap is very thin with an actual loss of the hair follicles, or it may result from the application of too much tension or pressure to the hair bearing skin. Prophylaxis is the best treatment. If an area of marked alopecia forms, spontaneous recovery may occur during the first six months. Any persisting bald areas can be treated with hair transplants, using a punch technique.

Facial Nerve Injury

Injury to a branch of the facial nerve should be rare or, preferably, occur not at all. It is a reminder that one has dissected in the wrong plane, in the wrong place. The most vulnerable nerve is the zygomatico-temporal branch where it courses over the zygomatic arch. If dissection is done in this area, extreme caution must be taken to remain very superficial. Bleeding points should be tied, not cauterized. Occasional injury to mandibular branches has occurred. Most often these are not main branches and spontaneous recovery will occur. The nerve most commonly injured is the great auricular. If the fibers of the sternocleidomastoid muscle are not visualized during the dissection, the nerve will not be injured. Anesthesia of the inferior half of the auricle connotes damage.

Elevation of the facial flaps usually produces temporary anesthesia of the facial area supplied by the trigeminal nerve. This numbness subsides spontaneously as the postoperative edema decreases.

Other nerve injuries have been reported, such as that of the spinal accessory and the lesser occipital nerves.

Use of a curved dissecting scissors under the flaps with the points toward the skin is helpful in keeping the surgeon from going into the deeper dangerous planes. The presence of adipose tissue below the skin flap should be a most reassuring sight.

Pain

Pain is a highly subjective matter. Most of our postoperative patients require no pain medication. Occasionally a patient complains of severe pain for prolonged periods of time. If the pain is generalized, I would tend to discount the veracity of the complaint on a physical basis. If the pain is localized, there may be a secondary neuroma or neuritis during the healing phase. Appropriate excision of the neuroma and the use of nerve blocks for the neuritis would then be in order. In our series of cases I have seen one neuroma and only transitory neuritis.

Ear Lobe Deformity

The so-called "devil's ear," or inferiorly pulled auricle, results from excess traction. The points of tension, when the face lift flaps are repositioned, must be temporal, postauricular, and cervical, almost forming a hammock for the lobule of the auricle, without causing downward traction of the ear lobe.

Chronic Edema

Localized areas of hard swelling may persist for many months. Aspiration is invariably not productive. The etiology appears to be a localized area of lymphedema, which persists until the lymph vessels have formed new anastomoses. Other lumps may result from localized fat necrosis or be secondary to the trauma of cauterization, suture ligation, or dissection. Our treatment has been local injection of corticosteroids with massage. Even without active treatment, these problem areas gradually resolve. We have not seen any permanent problems resulting from these minor irregularities.

Secondary Surgery

A secondary benefit of face lift surgery is the development of a fibrotic scar layer between the skin and the muscles. This not only helps to hold the skin over the muscles but tends to slow the process of facial relaxation, referred to as aging. With this thought in mind it appears rational to assume that a secondary lift should have an even more beneficial result than a primary operation. This has been well borne out in our experience. When a complete primary lift is done, we have found that about a ten year period passes before a second lift is indicated. The results of a secondary procedure last an even greater length of time. These times depend upon differences in skin and the aesthetic demands of the patient.

The dicta for secondary face lift procedures are the same as for primary procedures. The planes of dissection may be readily available or extremely fibrotic. The tissues usually have less elasticity but hold their new positions to a better degree. We have often been able to move a noticeable preauricular incision to a less noticeable posttragal position. The inferior postauricular scar may also likewise be raised higher up onto the auricle, eliminating this obvious line. If the first procedure was a minimal dissection, the secondary procedure will almost be the same as that in an adequate primary dissection. We have not noticed a lesser degree of flap viability, although theoretically one could expect this possibility. A secondary procedure is often ideal for a regional upper, mid, or lower third, rather than performing a complete face lift.

While on the subject of photography, our standards committee are trying to have everybody take their photographs under similar conditions. These photographs are at right angles and straight forward and the lighting is similar in all views. We also think it is important that the post operative photographs not be taken until all swelling is gone. In face lifts and eyelid surgery, six months is usually alright. With a nose, particularly with heavy skin, a year may be too early.

As for sutures, running locked are used predominantly with interrupted as necessary; 5-0 for the anterior part of the auricle, including the ear canal. We remove the preauriculars in one week.

We have been pleased with stainless steel staples for the hair bearing areas. The staples evert the skin edges and eliminate the possibility of suture, or "cross hatch" markings. The staples are removed at 10, 14, or even 21 days.

Summary

If there is a face lift philosophy, I feel it can be summed up thusly. A patient who is well prepared prior to the surgery will receive an inside as well as an outside lift.

References

1. Berman WE, Monell CM: Complications in blepharoplasties and face lift operations. *Otolaryngol Clin N Amer* 7: No. 1, February 1974
2. Conley J: Face-lift operation, Springfield, Illinois, Charles C. Thomas, 1968
3. Goldwyn RM: The unfavorable result in plastic surgery. Boston, Little, Brown Co, 1972
4. Rees TD, Wood-Smith, D: Cosmetic Facial Surgery, Philadelphia, W.B. Saunders Company, 1972
5. Gonzalez-Ulloa M: The ethiology of the progressive changes observed in facial senility. 7th International Congress of Gerontology Vienna/Austria, June 26–July 2, 1966.

Facial Analysis in Patient Evaluation for Physiologic and Cosmetic Surgery*

Carl N. Patterson and Donald G. Powell, Durham, N.C.

Introduction

The purpose of this paper is to present some anatomic and artistic relationships that must be known, appreciated, and used by the reconstructive facial surgeon. In order to construct a well balanced face, the surgeon must adhere to certain principles of proportion, symmetry, and balance. Beauty can be achieved only by adherence to these principles. Various standards of proportion have been formulated and charted by Michaelangelo, Leonardo da Vinci, Albrecht, Schadow and others. While these criteria cannot be rigorously followed, they are valuable in that they express a relationship from which there cannot be a great deviation without transgression on the laws of harmony.

* Presented at the Meeting of the Souther Section of the American Laryngological, Rhinological and Otological Society, Inc., Williamsburg, Va., January 11, 1974.

A facial operation involves a great responsibility on the part of the surgeon. He must take apart irregular or deformed tissue and remodel it to render it acceptable to the patient, relatives, friends, and the most severe critic, the surgeon himself. No standard norm can be slavishly followed; however, one can establish a fictional norm for each individual on the basis of the deformity encountered. Such a norm is desirable since criteria of ideal forms are by no means universally accepted. For example, the facial proportions which are acceptable and pleasing to one ethnic group would not satisfy the concepts of another. Judgment will be necessary in the applications of rules to prevent all individuals to be cast in the same mold.

Since standards of beauty differ from race to race, this discussion will be confined to the Caucasian.

History

History shows us that standards of beauty have changed through the ages; but it has been said that the prime requisites of civilization are intellectual energy, freedom of the mind, and a sense of beauty. Paintings and sculptures from ancient civilizations show an appreciation of beauty, and the tendency to enhance beauty through adornment. Ancient Egypt of 2000 B.C. is represented by the classic beauty of Queen Nefertiti. Artifacts from Minoan civilization of 1800 B.C. show that their women curled their hair elaborately and applied heavy lip rouge and eye shadow. The most dramatic legends of the early Greeks are based on the kidnapping of a beautiful woman, with the subsequent ruin of the City of Troy, for the sake of the beautiful Helen. Greek statuary of the Golden Age provides many examples of the classic "Greek profile." In the First Century A.D., another Egyptian beauty appears, Cleopatra, whose legendary beauty captivated her Roman conquerors, and who was known to have spent hours at her toilette applying cosmetics to enhance her beauty. Women of Rome at the time of the Caesars adorned themselves with various facial cosmetics, including eye liners and eye shadows.

From the drawings, paintings and sketches of the immortal Leonardo da Vinci, we get a concept of the almost perfect type of beauty that was obtained by strict adherence to the rules of balance and proportion.

The French court women of the 17th and 18th centuries were tremendously beauty conscious, and spent a great part of their days in arranging elaborate wigs, adding rouge, powder and beauty spots. Josephine, wife of Napoleon, in the early 19th century, was not a classic beauty, but she had the ability to give the illusion of beauty.

A woman whose beauty was said to have transcended changing standards in the early 19th century was the famous Lola Montez. Daguerrotypes taken at the time show her to be far less lovely to our eyes than her reputation would lead us to believe, but to those who saw her, she appeared ravishing.

A real American beauty of the late 1800s was Jennie Jerome, the young New Yorker who married Randolph Churchill, of England, and was the mother of Sir Winston Churchill. It is said that, at a party, she was invariably the most beautiful woman in the room, and very often conversation hushed at her entrance.

The beauty ideal of the early 20th century was the "Gibson Girl," the creation of artist Charles Dana Gibson. His drawings are a composite of the beauties of that time, with round, wide-eyed feminine features, and the full hair styles of the day.

In 1921, in Atlantic City, the first "Miss America" was crowned. Each year that succeeded this first, a young lady was selected who represented not only the concept of beauty for that year, but other characteristics which made her a true "Miss America." In today's concept of beauty, movies and television have played dominant roles in establishing the criteria of what is attractive and beautiful; however, in my opinion, few can surpass the classic face of Garbo.

Strictly speaking, one must differentiate between beauty *per se* and self adornment. Adornment and beautification are well recognized features of man from the dawn of civilization. In the primitive people this consisted of mutilation by scarring and distortion. Designs were cut or burned into the skin of the face, arms, chest, back or legs to provide distinction. Perforations were made in the ears, nose and lips to hold various pieces of adornment. Parts of the body were molded into various forms and designs to conform to certain requirements of beauty of the times. Who performed this esthetic surgery at that time? The medicine man—have things really changed much today?

Our lives and thoughts today are much related to physical appearance. People want to fall within the dimensions of normal. Crossed eyes, hair lips, lop ears, grotesque noses and "Andy Gump" chins are now corrected universally.

Our society would like to halt the hands of the clock of Father Time. We know we can't even slow it down, but by rearrangement of tissue, an individual can be made more youthful in appearance. This can play a great role in the person's self esteem and self image. This kind of surgery is now being done, not only for purely esthetic but also for economic reasons, as the older citizen many times is desirous of remaining in the employment market; hence, baggy eyes, saggy jowls, flabby wattles, deepening wrinkles, and drooping noses need to be corrected. It is not only for medicine to add years to our lives but to add life to our years.

With this general background, I will deal with some specifics regarding facial analysis. The proper form and dimensions of the part to be reconstructed can be determined by the comparison of the deformed part with some standard. As previously stated, obviously no single standard is applicable to all cases. The deformed part must be related to the parts surrounding it and reconstructed to blend into a harmonious picture. The aim of reconstruction is not to obtain perfect symmetry but merely to bring an abnormality within the realm of normalcy for the specific individual. The greatest enemy to excellence is perfection.

General Considerations

Even though the surgeon is taught not to operate by the protractor he would do well to utilize the instruments of artistic measurement to comprehend better the anatomic relationships of structures requiring his reshaping skill. As the artist adheres to certain rules of construction in the systematic rendering of a portrait, so can the reconstructive facial surgeon utilize the same fundamental tenets of drawing in the actual reshaping of the human countenance.

The ancient Greeks established the norm for the proportions of the human figure as precisely seven and one half head lengths long.

The neck is one-half the head length, from the point of the chin to the hollow at the supra-sternal notch (Fig. 1).

The hand is three-fourths of a head in length or the distance from the point of the chin to the hairline. Placed on a parallel axis with the nose it covers half the face (Fig. 2). As a perpendicular axis with the nose (Fig. 3) it covers one-fourth the face length, or the distance from the base of the nose to the point of the chin. The hand plays an important role for the portrait artist in establishing facial proportion.

Generally speaking, the head, as seen in an anterior-posterior view, is oval shaped, with the width of the head two-thirds of its length. From the side, two such ovals superimpose one over the other: one on its side, the other upright.

The cranial mass is two times as large as the facial mass. From an anterior-posterior projection, a horizontal line through the upper eyelids divides the face and head into two equal parts (Fig. 4). The face is divided into three equal segments by horizontal lines (Fig. 5) from the hairline to the glabella, from the glabella to the columellar-labial angle, from the columellar-labial angle to the chin. Ideally, the face should be divided into equal thirds.

Da Vinci described a method of analyzing the face from a lateral view (Fig. 6). Using the ear canal as the center of a circle, ideally the forehead, tip of the nose, and chin should touch the margins of the circle.

Specific Considerations

A general impression of the configuration of the face can be obtained by observing the head. You may note a brachycephalic (a short-wide head), a dolichocephalic (a long-narrow head) and a mesocephalic (a middle-sized head). Each principal component part of the face plays a role in the general configuration. The size, the location, the angulation, and the symmetry of each of the specific parts is most important in facial harmony. Each part will be considered in some detail.

Ears

The physical anatomy of the external ear is not so important from an esthetic or artistic point of view as its size, position, and angulation. The ear

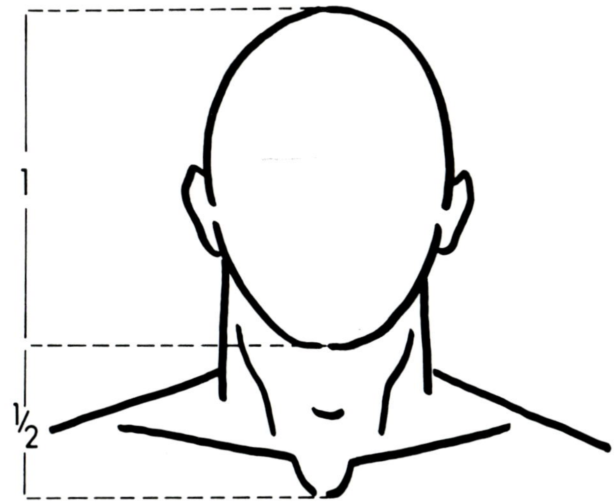

Fig. 1. The neck is one-half the head length, from the point of the chin to the hollow at the suprasternal notch.

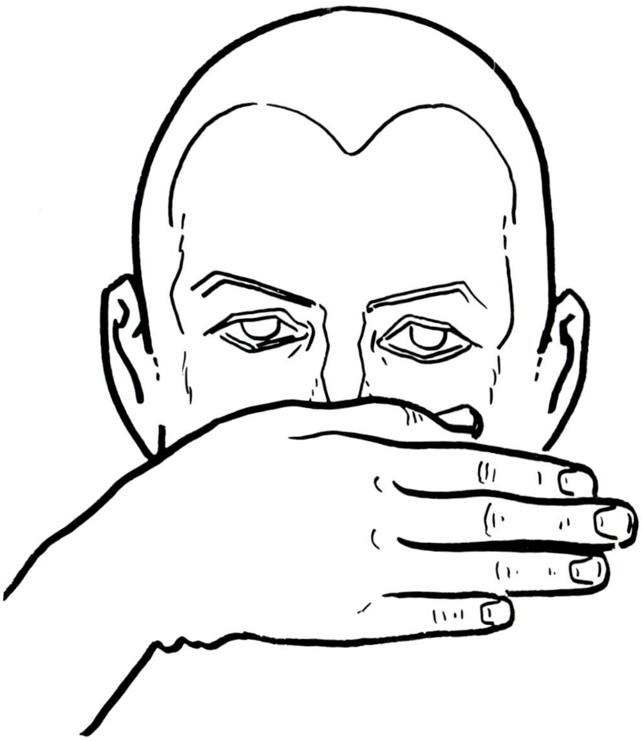

Fig. 3. Hand covers one-fourth the face length.

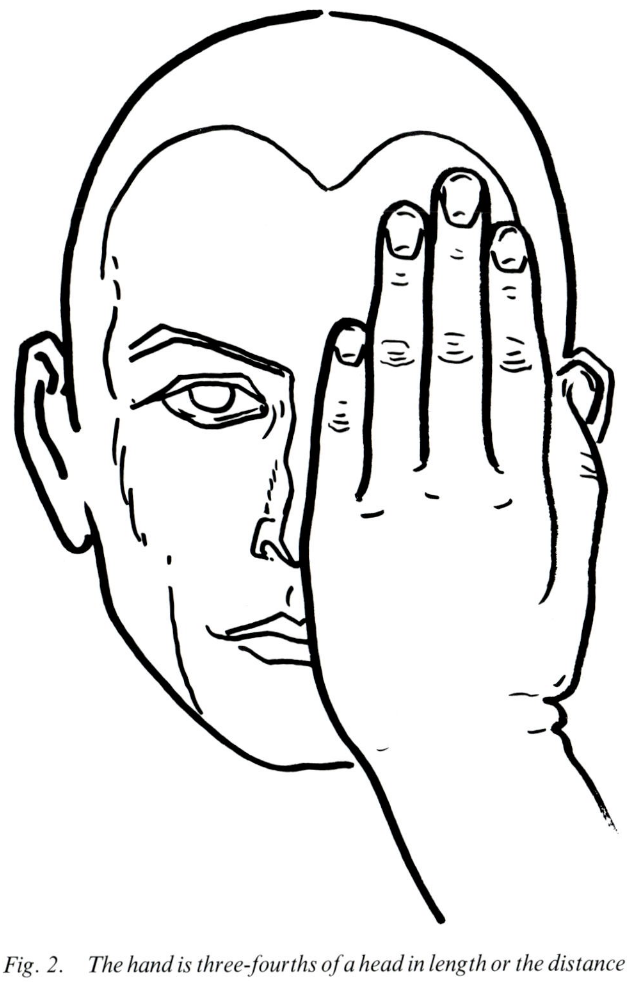

Fig. 2. The hand is three-fourths of a head in length or the distance from the point of the chin to the hairline.

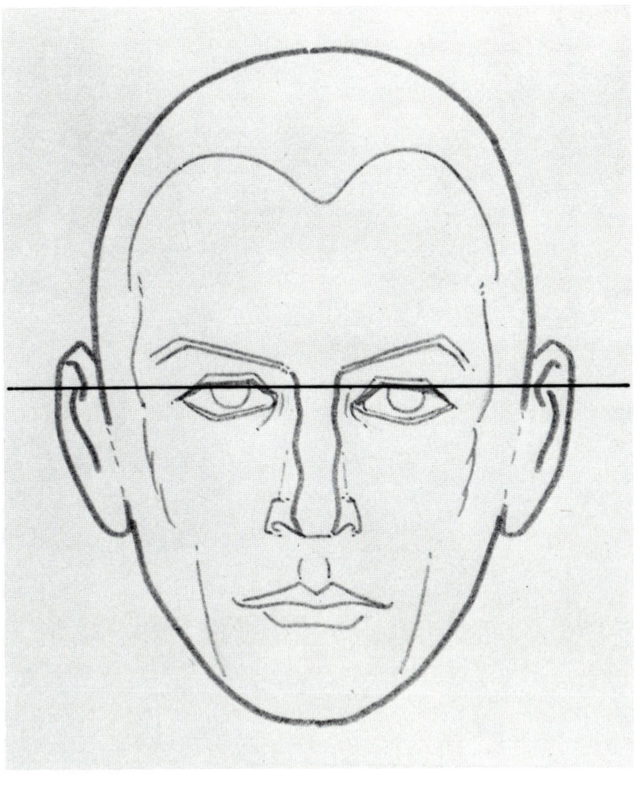

Fig. 4. Horizontal line through the upper eyelids divides the face and head into two equal parts.

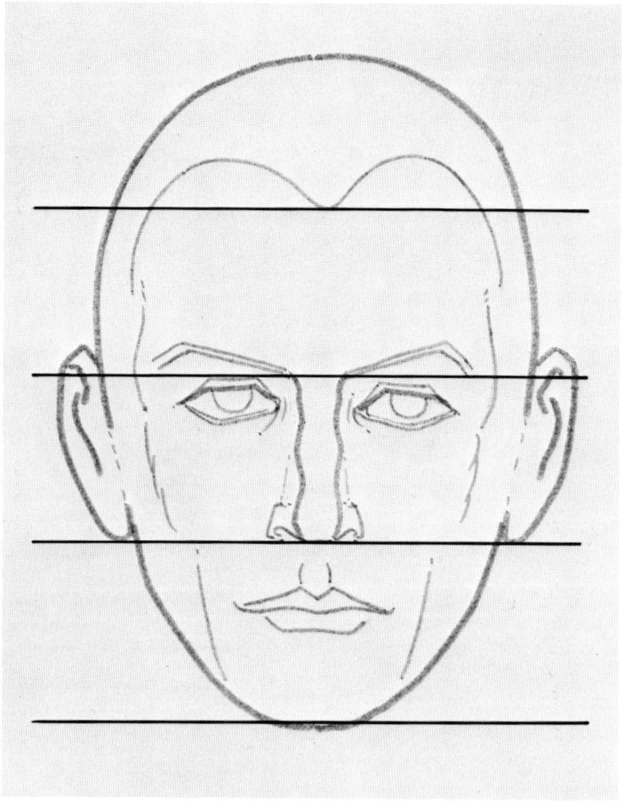

Fig. 5. The face is divided into three equal parts.

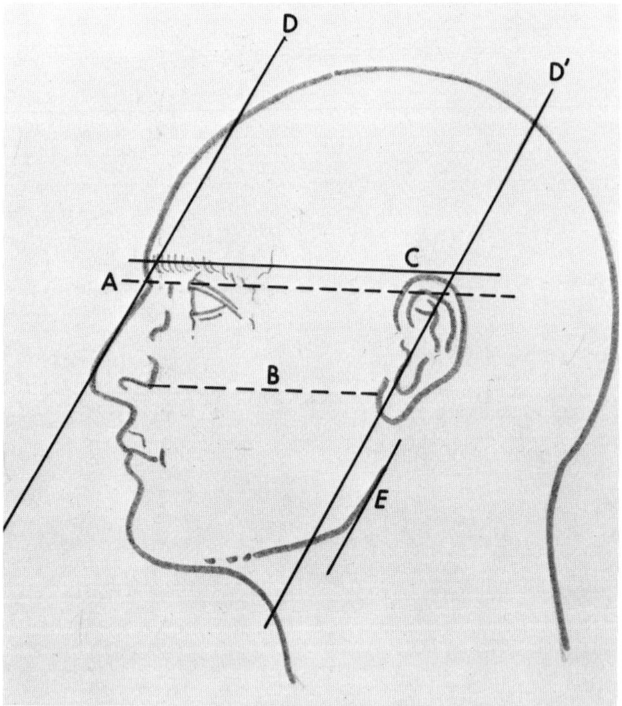

Fig. 7. The ear canal is located on a horizontal line halfway between the outer canthus of the eye and the alar facial junction, and halfway between the back of the skull and the frontal facial plane.

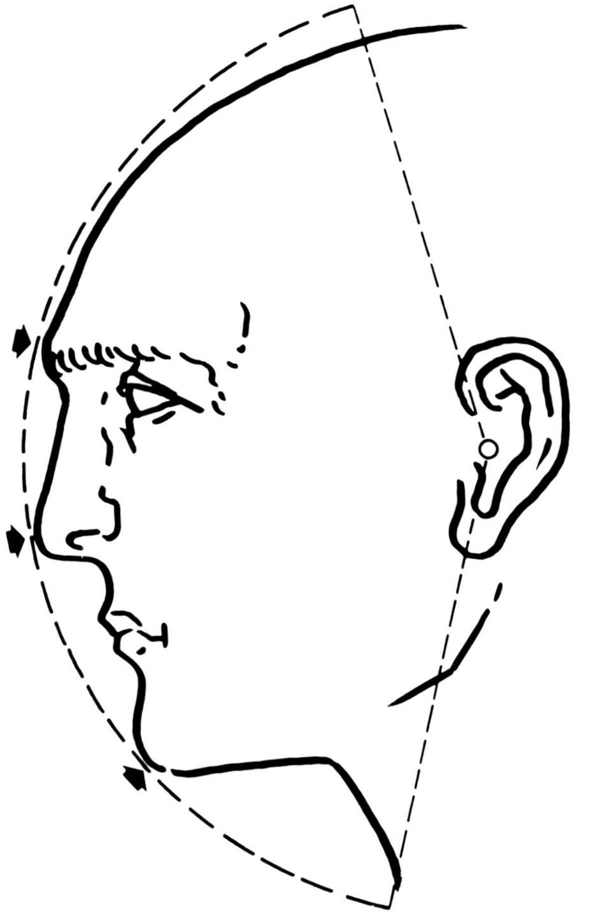

Fig. 6. DaVinci described a method of analyzing the face from a lateral view.

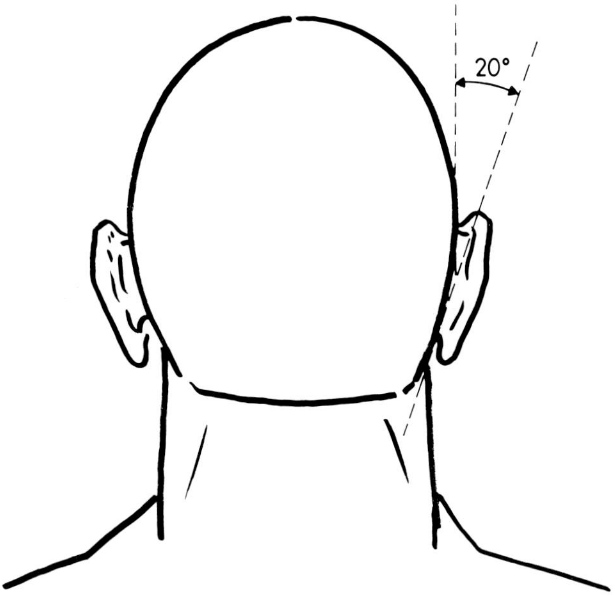

Fig. 8. The ear protrudes from the skull posteriorly at an angle of 20°.

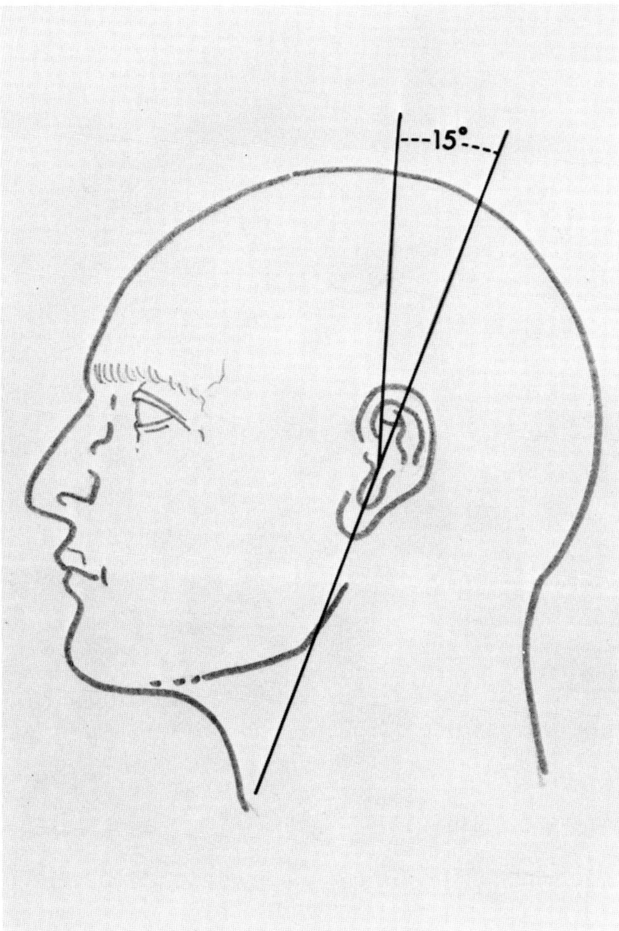

Fig. 9. The long axis of the ear is rotated backward about 15° from the vertical line.

canal is located on a horizontal line halfway between the outer canthus of the eye and the alar facial junction, and halfway between the back of the skull and the frontal facial plane (Fig. 7). The superior point of attachment of the ear to the head is just above the upper lid. The inferior point of attachment of the ear to the head is just above the upper lid. The inferior point of attachment of the ear lobe is in line with the alar facial junction. The helix rises away from the head on line with the eyebrows. The width of the ear is one-half the length.

The long axis of the ear (the highest point of the helix to the anterior attachment of the lobule) is parallel to the long axis of the nasal dorsum. A line joining the anterior attachment of the helix and the lobule is continued along the ramus of the mandible. The ear protrudes from the skull posteriorly at an angle of 20° (Fig. 8) and the long axis of the ear is rotated backward about 15° from the vertical line (Fig. 9).

Eyes

The eyes along with the nose and lips form the principal focal points of facial beauty, expression, and animation. Attesting to this fact is the multiplicity of eye make up cosmetics that have been present through the ages and today. The eyes are situated at the junction of the upper and middle thirds of the face. They are globes lying in a protective bony cave. They are covered by two lids which appear as visors to the eyes (Fig. 10). The upper lid is larger and more fully curved. It is much more active and movable than the lower lid. The eyelids form an irregular parallelogram. The high point of the upper lid is at the junction of the medial and middle thirds; the low point of the lower is at the junction of the medial and lateral thirds. The upper lid has an upward slant parallel with the vermillion border of the upper lip (Fig. 11). The eyes are separated by the root of the nose one eye width

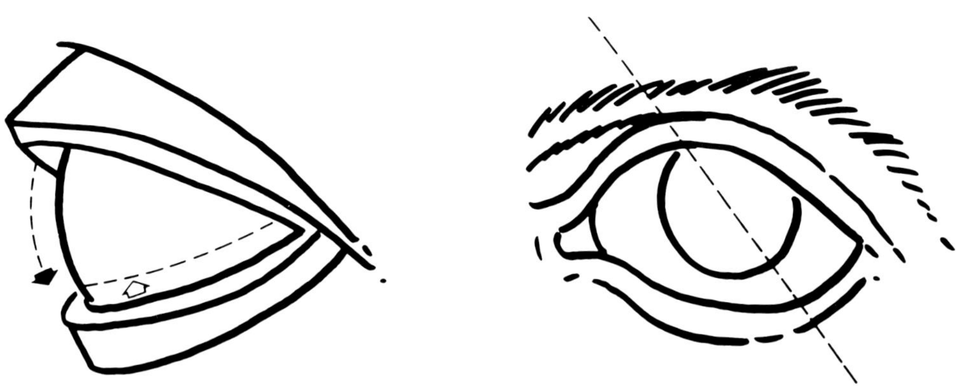

Fig. 10. The eyes are covered by two lids which appear as visors to the eyes.

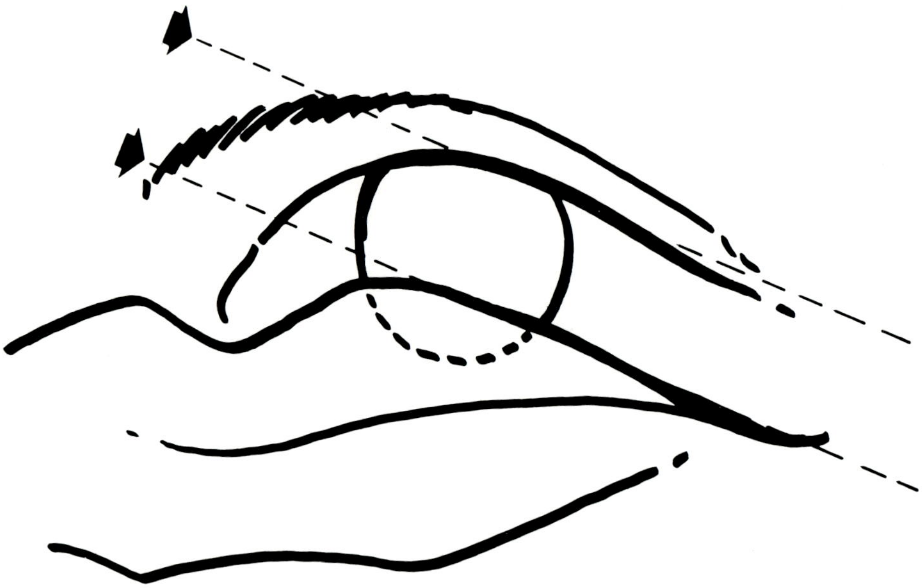

Fig. 11. The upper lid has an upward slant parallel with the vermillion border of the upper lip.

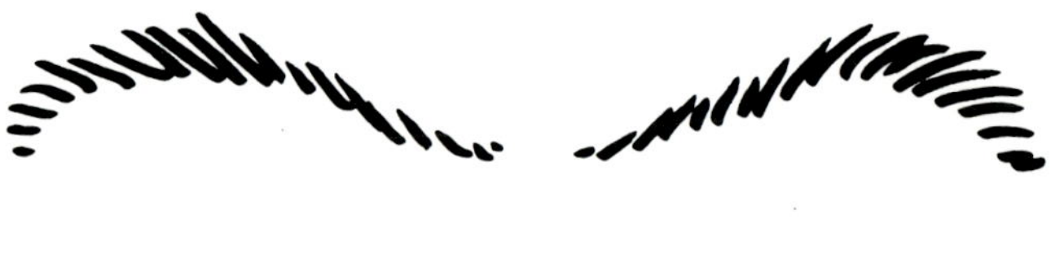

Fig. 12. The eyebrows vary in shape and position.

apart. The eyebrows vary in position and shape (Fig. 12). Normally they are located on the upper orbital rim.

Mouth and Lips

The lips, like the eyes, are important structures for expression and animation. They are located in the lower third of the face (Fig. 13). In the straight forward gaze the outer borders of the upper lips are in line with the medial border of the iris. The distance from the base of the nose to the lower border of the upper lip forms one-third of the lower third of the face; from this point to the chin makes up the lower two-thirds. The vermillion border of the lower lip is midway between the base of the nose and the chin (Fig. 14). The vermillion border of the upper lip is parallel with the margins of the upper eyelid. The upper lip is wider and overhangs the lower lip (Fig. 15). It is shaped like a flattened M. The groove of the M thrusts forward like the prow of a ship. Since the upper lip covers the greater dental arch it is somewhat more arched and wider than the lower.

The lower lip is more delicate and in some portions, particularly toward the corners, may have no visible contour. The lower lip resembles a flattened W, just opposite to its counterpart. The lower lip is recessed about 20° in relation to the upper lip. Both lips have thinly edged margins which outline

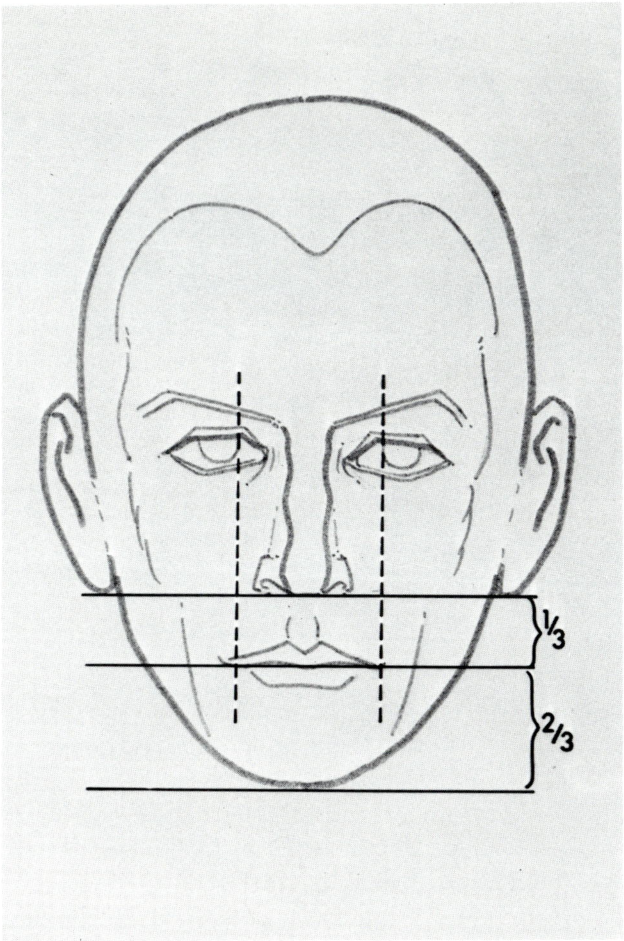

Fig. 13. The lips are important structures for expression and animation. They are located in the lower third of the face.

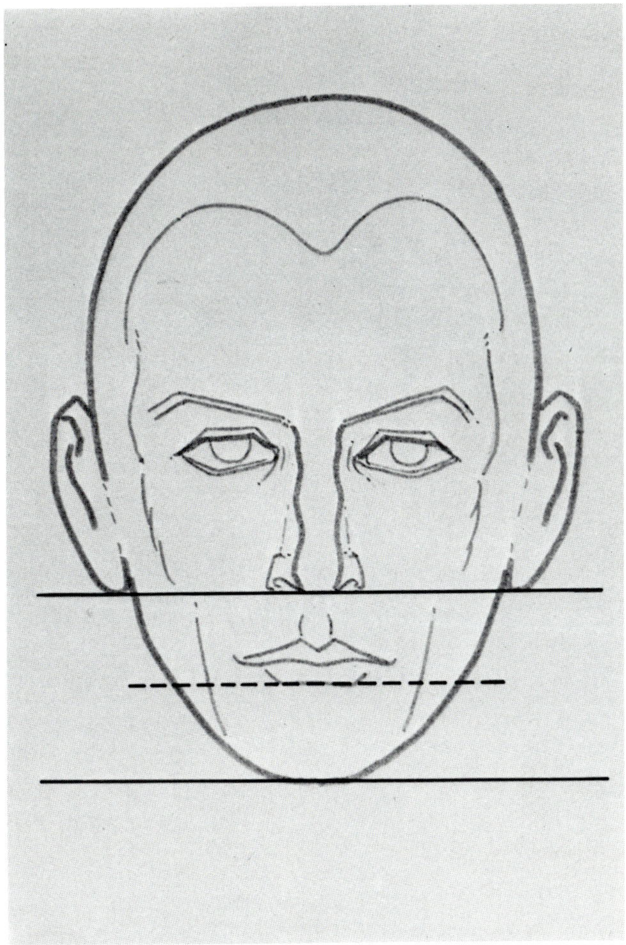

Fig. 14. The vermillion border of the lower lip is midway between the base of the nose and the chin.

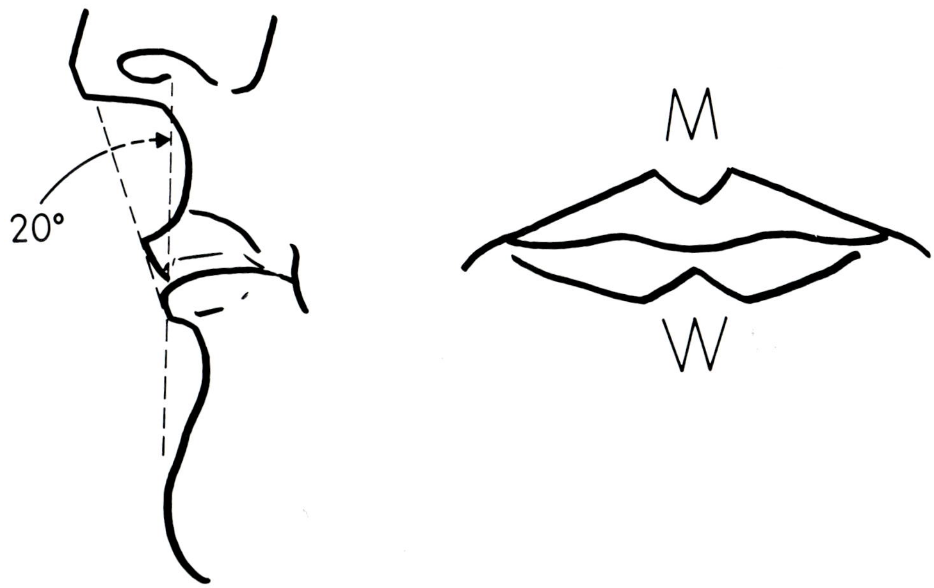

Fig. 15. The upper lip is wider and overhangs the lower lip.

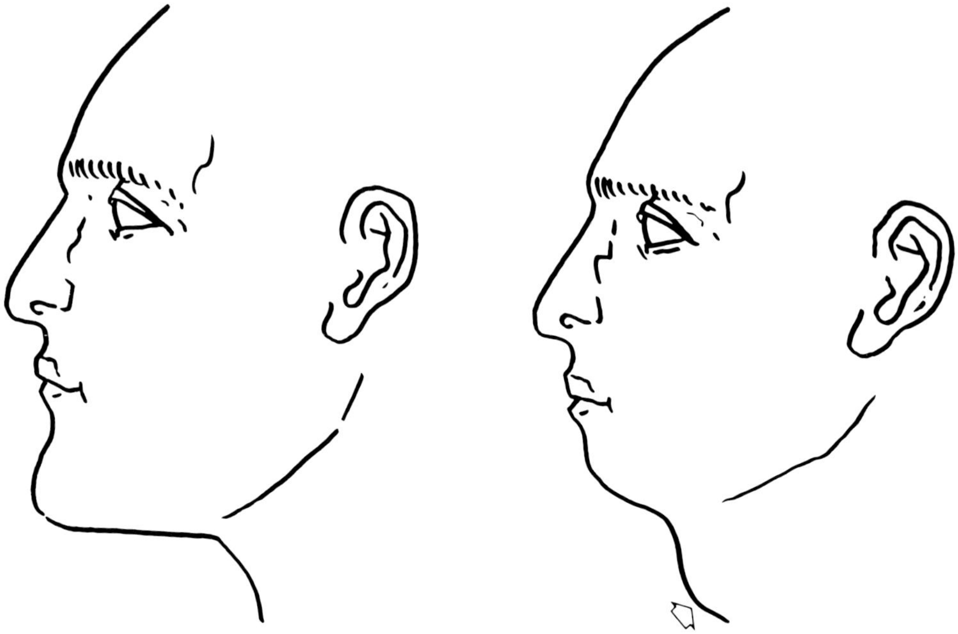

Fig. 16. All facial features are identical except for the chin and the hyoid.

their shapes. The lower lip is more active and mobile than the upper lip.

Chin and Neck

The strength of the face is proportioned to the chin's degree of prominence in relation to the neck. The "Andy Gump" or birdlike weakness of the chin may be due to mere lack of projection of the mandible, but more often is due to this plus the anterior and low position of the hyoid bone. That this relationship is so important is demonstrated in the artist's drawing where all facial features are identical except for the chin and the hyoid (Fig. 16).

Nose

The nose is the principal focal point of the face. It lies in the center of the middle third of the face. Vertical lines drawn through the intercanthus of each eye and perpendicular to these horizontal lines designate the symmetry, length, and width of the nose (Fig. 17). The nasal bones and the nasal processes of the frontal bones make up the upper two-fifths; the upper lateral cartilages, septum, and lower lateral cartilages make up the lower three-fifths (Fig. 18). The nose is one eye length wide at the naso-labial junction (Fig. 19). The angle of projection of the nose from the face is 30° to 36° (Fig. 20). The columellar-labial angle varies from 90° in men to 95° to 110° in women (Fig. 21). In profile, 2 to 3 mm of the columella show below the rim of the alar. The nostrils are oval in shape and are obliquely directed toward the tip (Fig. 22). From the basal view, the nose should be roughly triangular in shape with a rounded apex. Its width at the apex of the nostril should be three-fourths of the width of the nose at the alar-facial junction.

The application of these principles can be illustrated in the following demonstrative cases:

Case Reports

Case 1.

Using the criteria of Da Vinci's circle, this patient does not have the correct proportions. He has a large bony and cartilaginous nose, a retracted columella, downward rotation of the lobule plus a receding chin (Fig. 23). By correcting his nose and chin his features fall within the proportions of normalcy. Note the nasal dorsum is parallel to the long axis of the ear (Fig. 24).

Case 2.

In this case the chin-hyoid problem is the more significant (Fig. 25). Her nasal deformity is not so

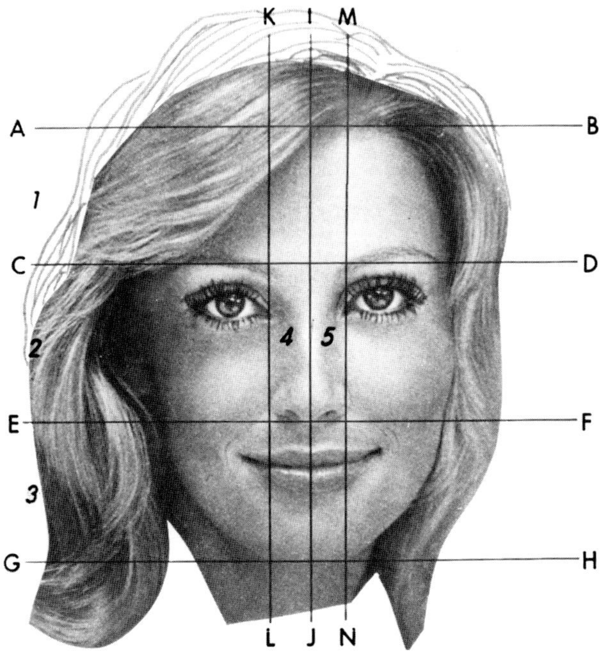

Fig. 17. The symmetry, length, and width of the nose.

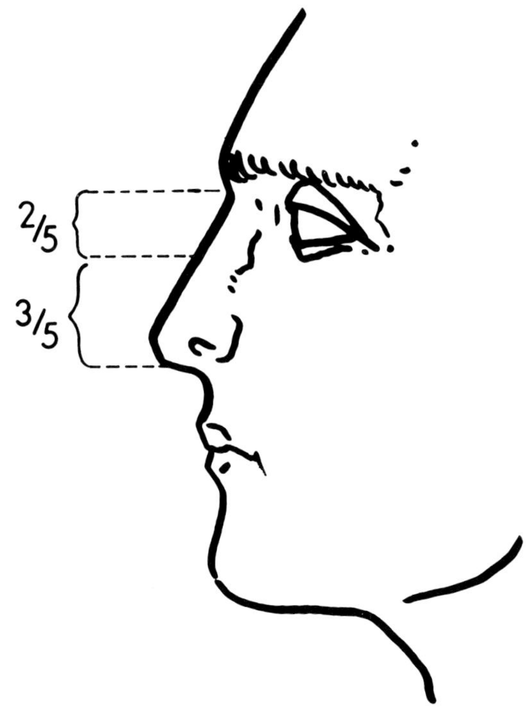

Fig. 18. The angle of projection of the nose (see fig. 20).

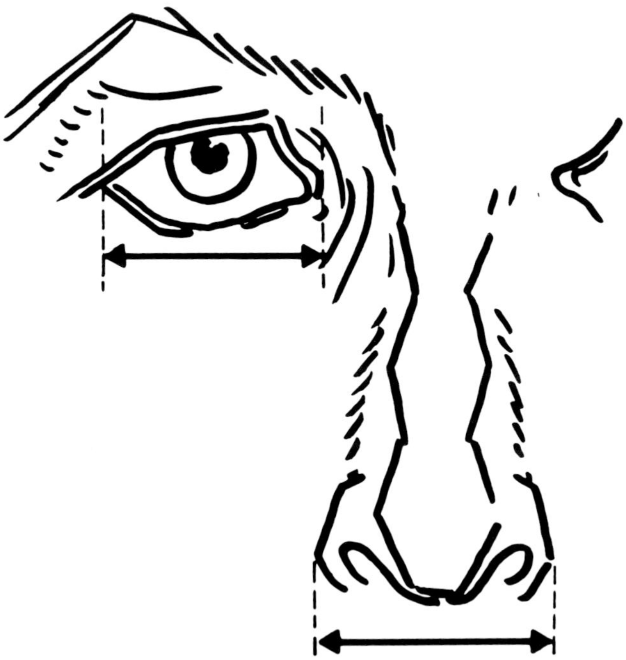

Fig. 19. The nose is one eye length wide at the naso-labial junction.

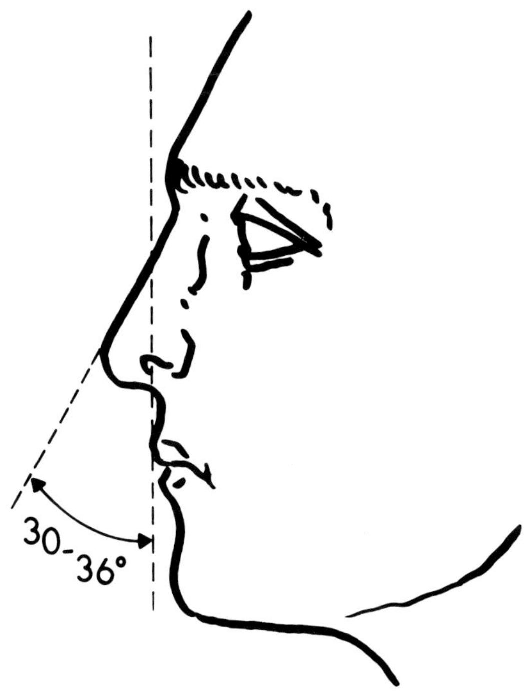

Fig. 20. The angle of projection of the nose from the face is 30° to 36°

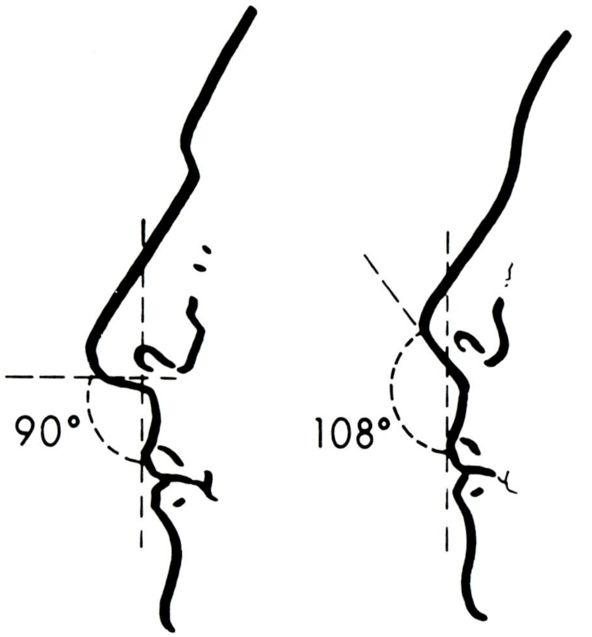

Fig. 21. The columella-labial angle varies from 90° in men to 95° to 110° in women.

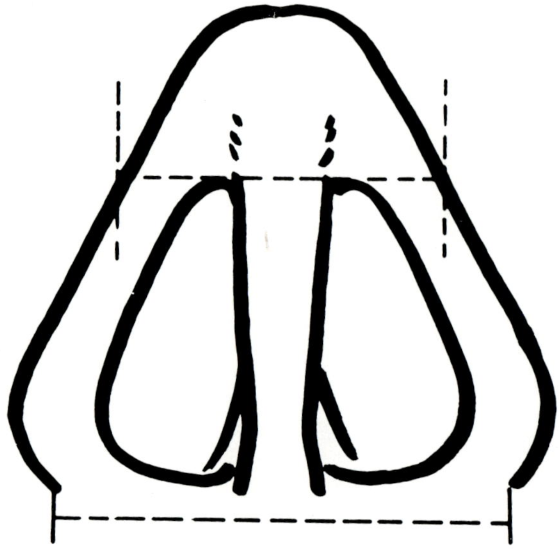

Fig. 22. The nostrils are oval in shape and are obliquely directed toward the tip.

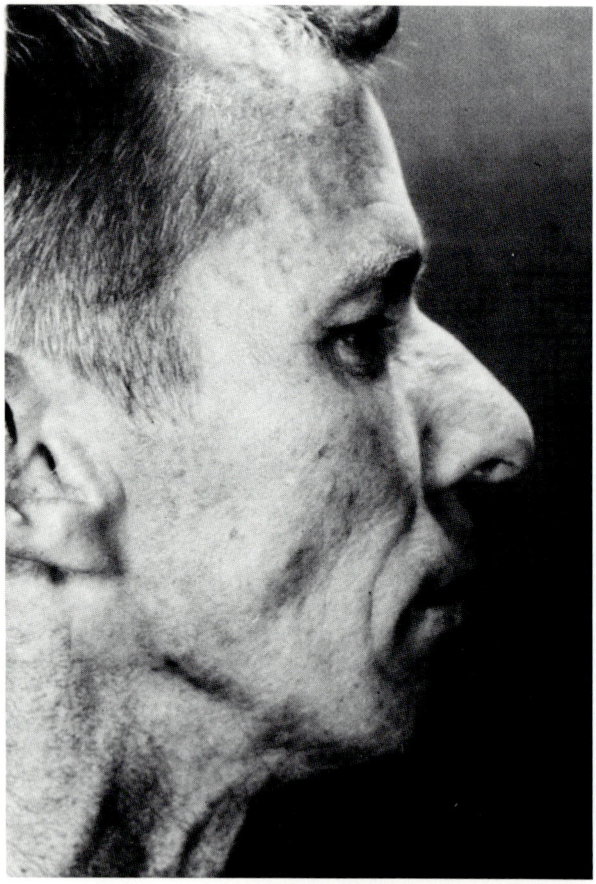

Fig. 23. Preoperative.

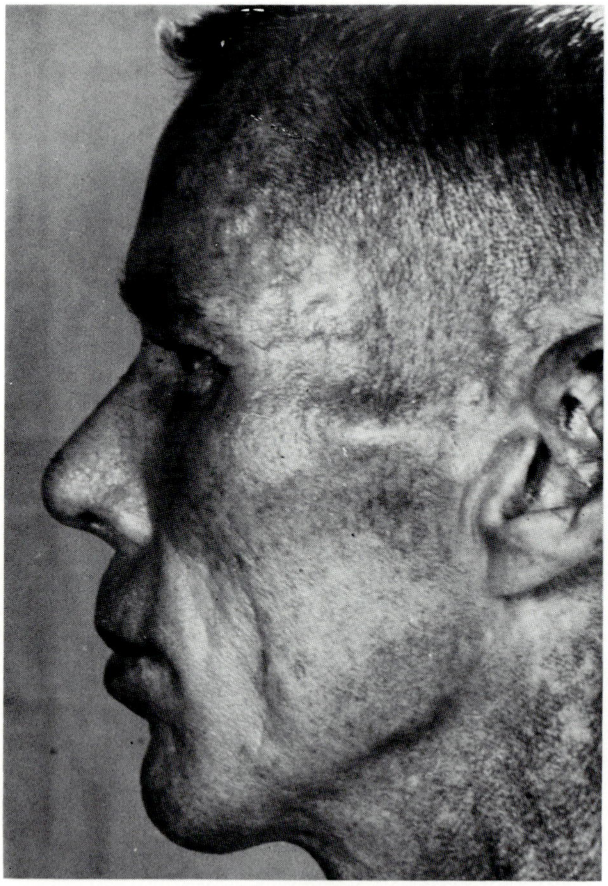

Fig. 24. Postoperative.

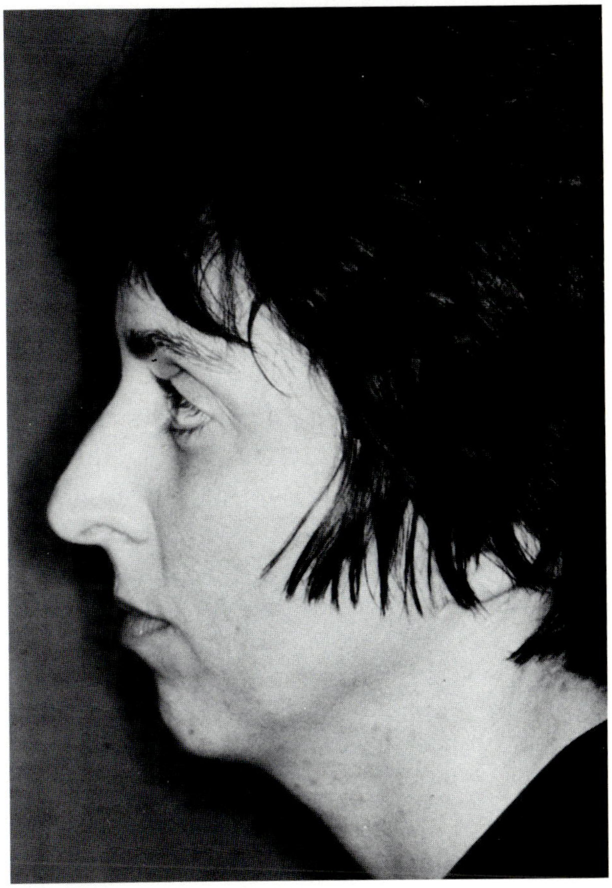

Fig. 25. Preoperative.

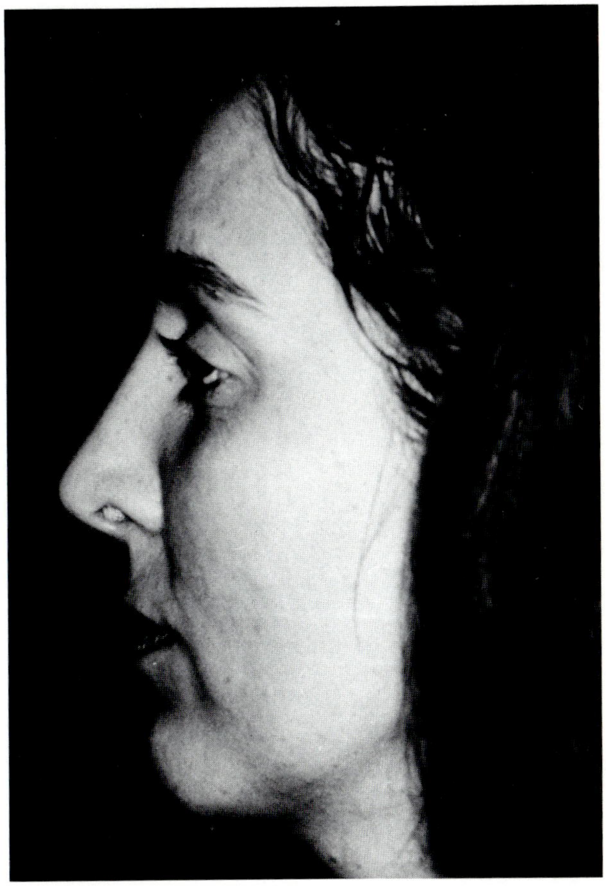

Fig. 26. Postoperative.

marked. With correction of her chin problem, plus rhinoplasty, all her proportions balance (Fig. 26).

Case 3.

A high slanting forehead is accentuated by a "pulled back" hair style (Fig. 27). A moderate nasal deformity, and chin recession plus a satyr-shaped ear completes the picture. Note how these disproportions are significantly exaggerated by her hair styling. Improvement is obtained by rhinoplasty and chin augmentation plus hair styling (Fig. 28). The hair styling decreases the forehead length and covers the ears.

Case 4.

In analyzing this face you find problems in all facial compartments plus outstanding ears (Fig. 29). His hair is not styled to help his physiognomy. The eyes are too far apart. The nose is large, crooked and asymmetrical (Fig. 30). His lips are too small and asymmetrical. The shape of maxilla, lower jaw and chin are not complimentary to upper face.

Most times you cannot easily alter the bony structures, but by altering hair styling, (Fig. 31) and in this case adding a moustache and beard, plus correction of the nose and ears (Fig. 32) this person falls within the realms of normalcy.

Summary

With a knowledge of the size, shape, location and relationship of these important structures, the facial plastic surgeon can reconstruct the deformed part to blend in harmoniously with the other features for that particular individual.

By utilizing the methods of analysis and proportions provided for us by the artist, we can more properly judge and execute the correction of the deformed part.

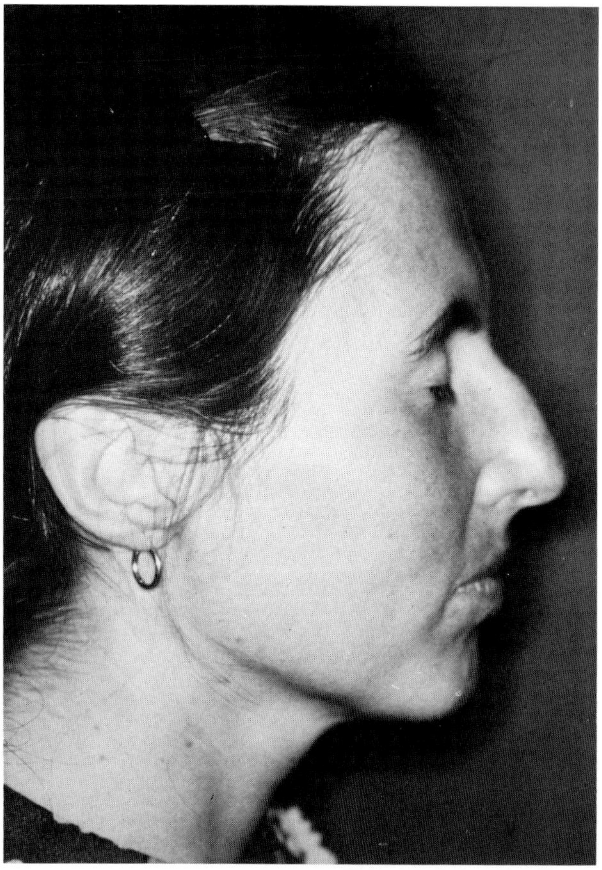

Fig. 27. Preoperative.

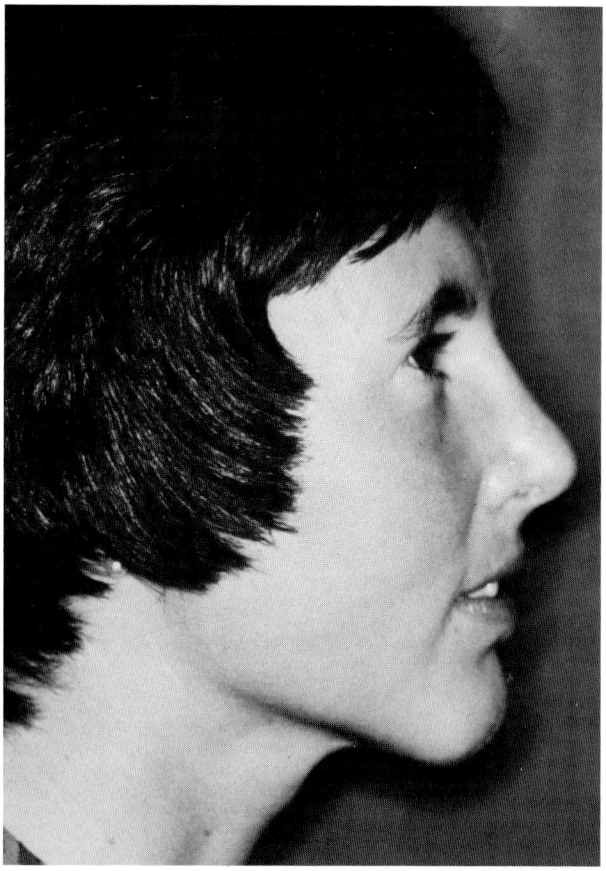

Fig. 28. Postoperative.

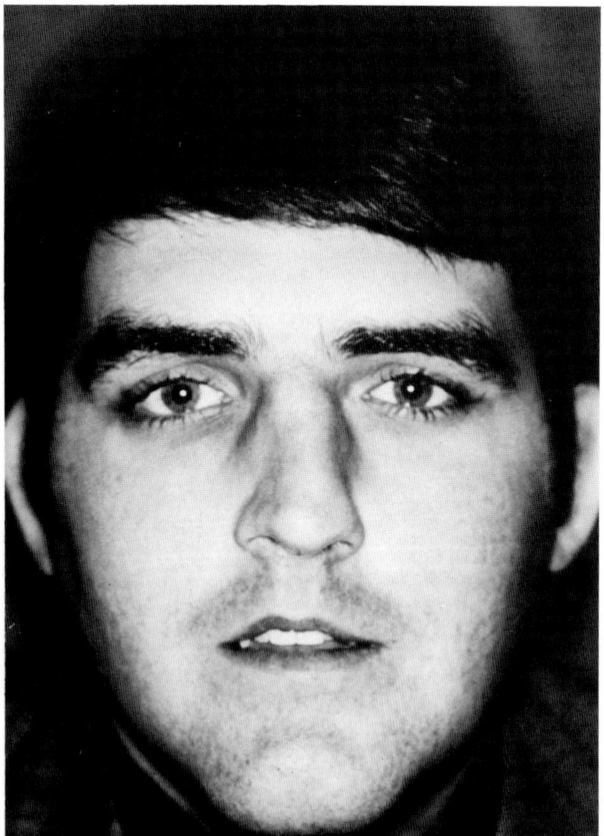

Fig. 29. Preoperative.

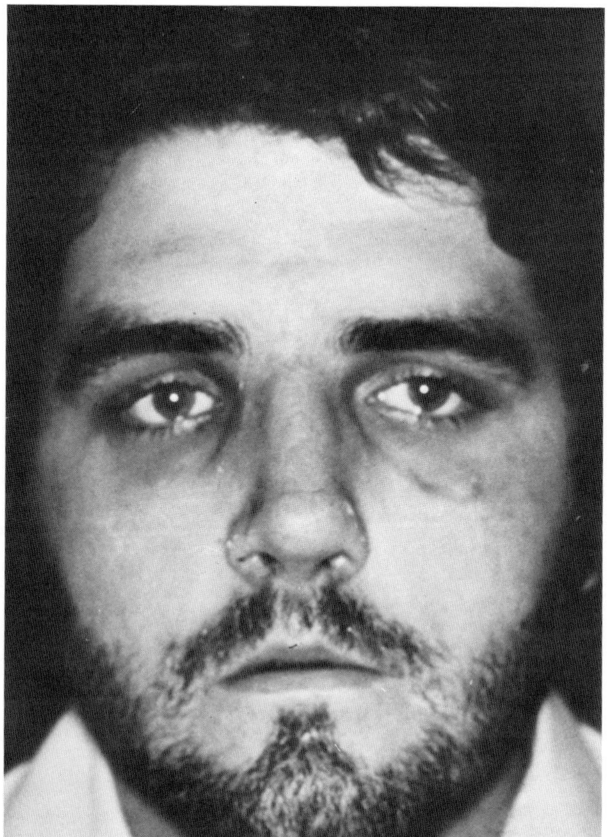

Fig. 30. Postoperative.

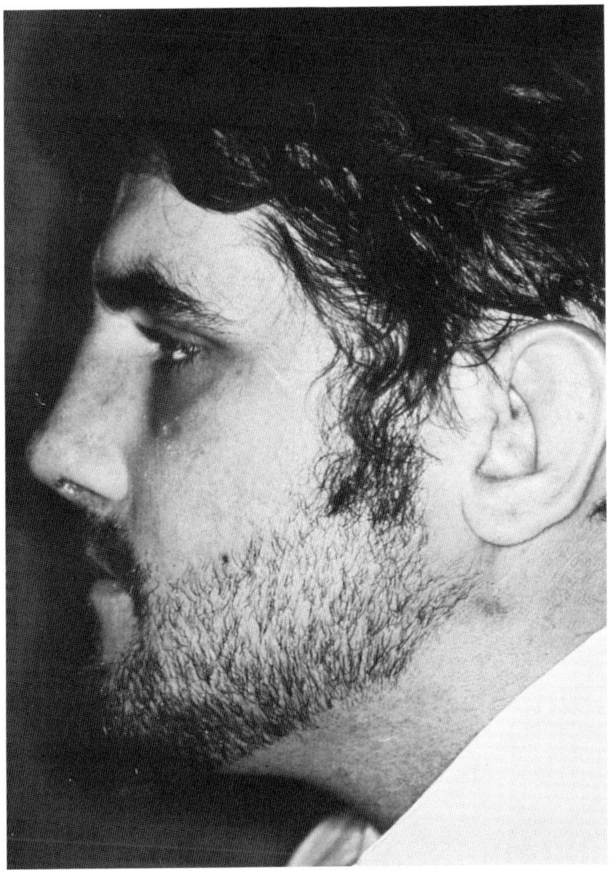

Fig. 31. Preoperative.

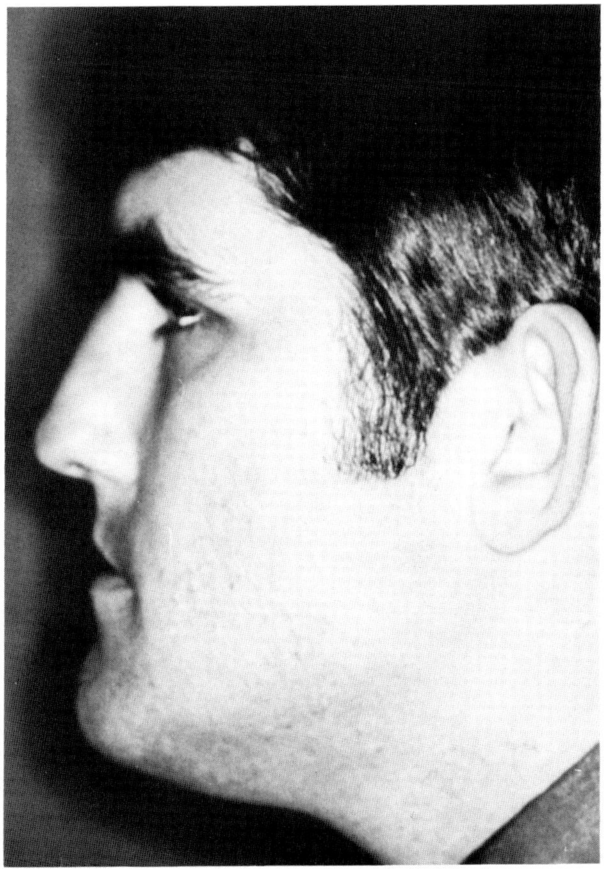

Fig. 32. Postoperative.

Arteriovenous Fistula of the Superficial Temporal Vessels: A Complication of Face Lift

Sidney S. Feuerstein, New York, N.Y.

Fistularization of the superficial temporal artery and vein is an extremely rare occurrence, both after facial injury and surgery. One case will be described following a "mini-facelift" procedure. A search of the literature failed to reveal other such cases following rhytidectomy or meloplasty. The presenting symptoms were unilateral auditory pulsating tinnitus, a localized palpable thrill, a diffuse audible bruit, and intermittent physical fatigue. Surgical excision caused immediate relief of all symptoms and complete rehabilitation of the patient.

War-time injuries of the head and neck region have been described as the principle etiology of

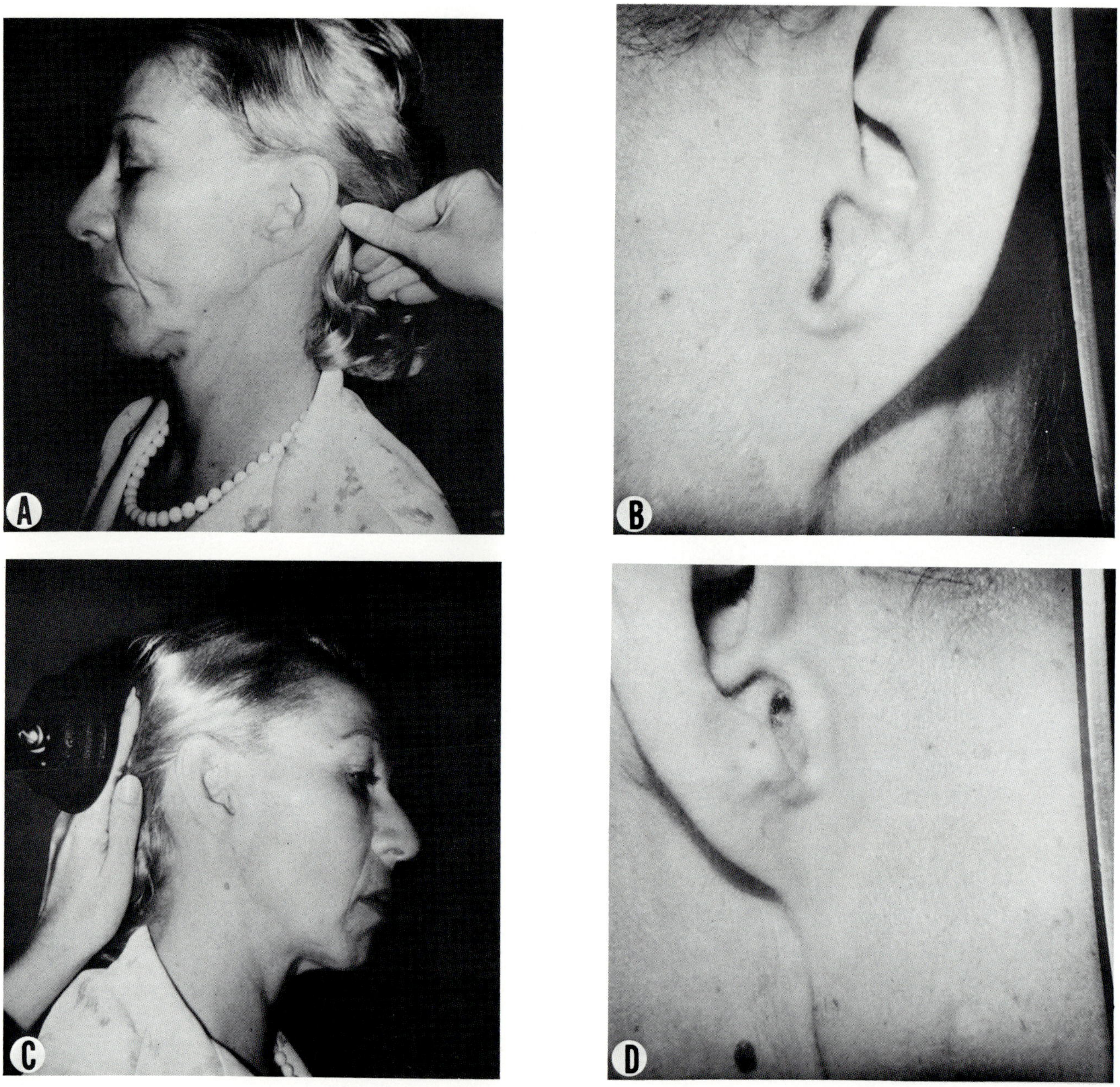

Fig. 1. (A) Left lateral view of face showing widened preauricular scar. (B) Close up of left ear. (C) Right lateral view. (D) Closeup of right ear.

vascular trauma of the cervical and facial arteries and veins. However, iatrogenic injury to these vessels causing aneurysm or fistularization is extremely rare. There has been no case reported of an arteriovenous fistula following a face lift procedure. It behooves us, therefore, to be aware of the potential incidence of arteriovenous fistula especially in the management of the distal branches of the external carotid artery.

One case of arteriovenous fistula involving the superficial artery and vein following a "mini-face lift" procedure will be presented. Both the local and systemic symptoms will be described.

Report of a Case

A fifty year old Caucasian female was first examined in August 1973, with a presenting complaint of "buzzing" in the left ear. In addition, she stated that she felt chronically fatigued. There was no hearing loss, headache or vertigo. She had been examined by several internists and ear specialists during the preceding 24 months and no definitive diagnosis was offered. Politizerizations of the eustachian tube had also been performed without improvement. Careful questioning into her past history revealed that she had only had one surgical procedure performed in her life time, namely, a minor "facelift" operation performed in a doctor's office just 36 months previously. About six months subsequent to this operation the patient noted the onset of "buzzing" in the left ear which became constant and not relieved by tranquilizer medication, sedatives, or vasodilators. The noise had a "whoosing" pulsating character.

Physical examination revealed the following findings. There were widened depigmented scars anterior to both ears extending from the crus helicis superiorally to the lower most attachment of the lobules bilaterally. The scars measured about 5 mm in width (Fig. 1 A–D). The scars were well healed with no evidence of inflammation. Examination of the tympanic membranes and nasopharynx was normal. There were no palpable cervical lymph nodes. A quantitative audiometric examination revealed normal responses to all frequencies. Careful palpation of the face revealed a distinct "thrill" over the left zygomatic arch lateral to the outer canthus of the left eye. Auscultation with a stethoscope over this region and for a radius of 6 cm revealed a loud systolic as well as dystolic bruit synchronous with the radial pulse. The patient was admitted to The Mount Sinai Hospital in New York City on Sept. 4, 1973, where a left percutaneous carotid angiogram was performed under local anesthesia. Hypaque Meglumine* was the contrast material used. Immediate filling of the anterior and posterior branches of the superficial temporal vein on the left side was noted (Fig. 2 A–D) confirming the clinical diagnosis of an arterior-venous fistularization of the superficial temporal artery and vein. Accordingly, the left cheek flap was elevated exposing the superficial temporal artery and vein and indeed a fistulous tract was noted between the

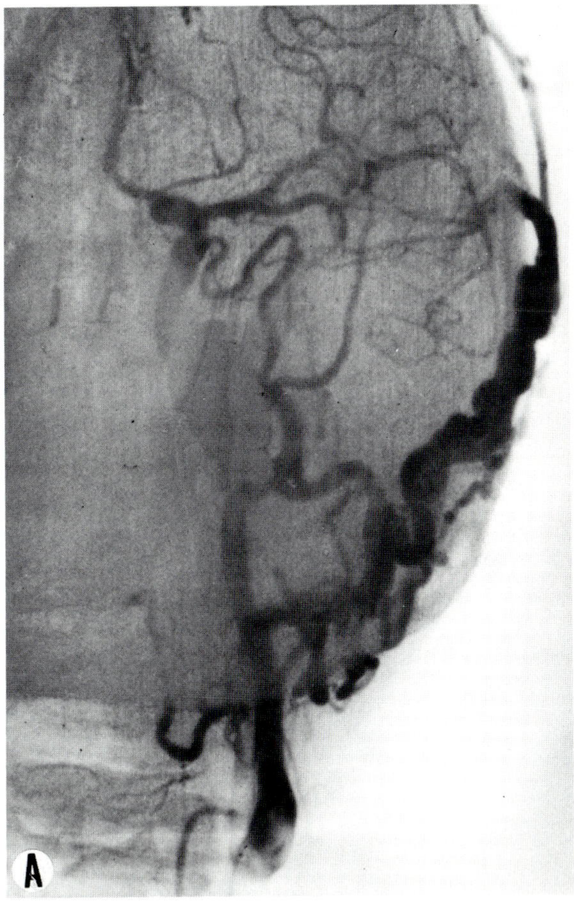

Fig. 2. (A) P-A roentgenogram of left carotid angiogram showing immediate filling of superficial temporal vein.

* Hypaque Meglumine 60 percent manufactured by Winthrop Division of Sterling Drugs, NY, NY 10006.

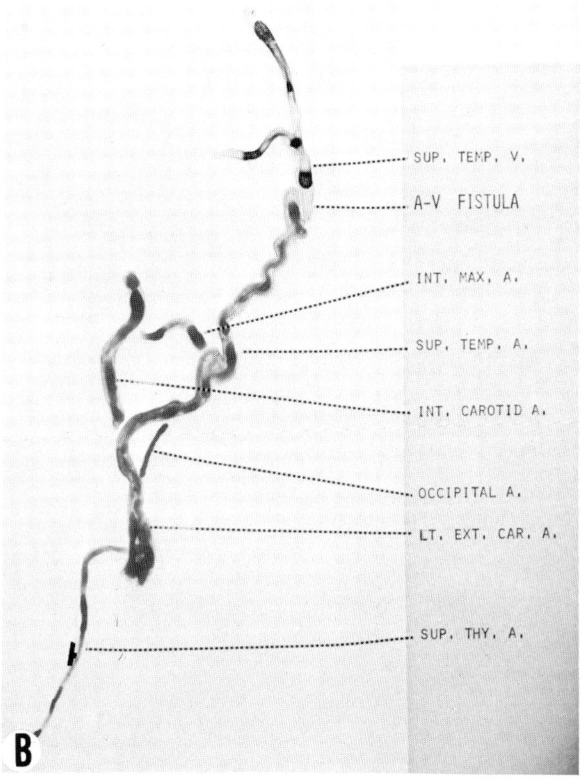

Fig. 2. (B) Diagram identifying arteries and veins seen in angiogram.

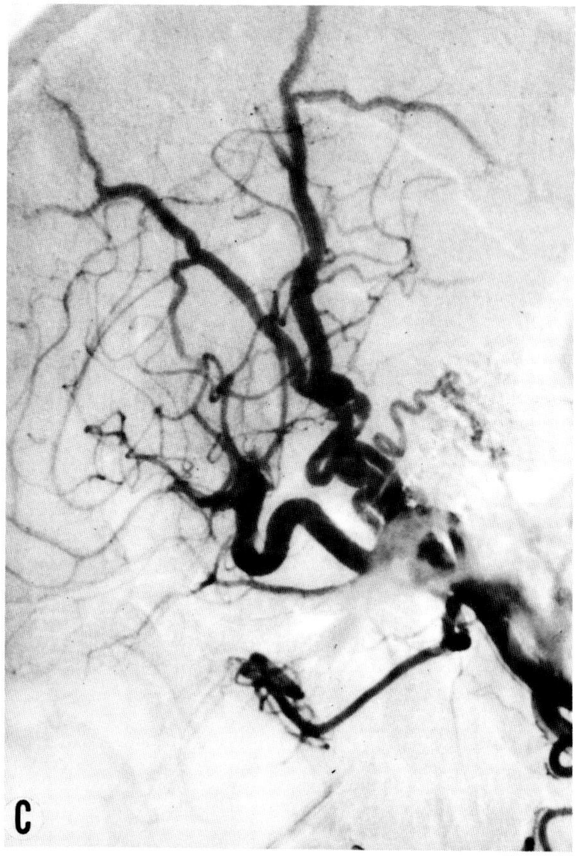

Fig. 2. (C) Lateral skull x-ray with "subtraction" study showing filling of superficial temporal vein at the fistula site.

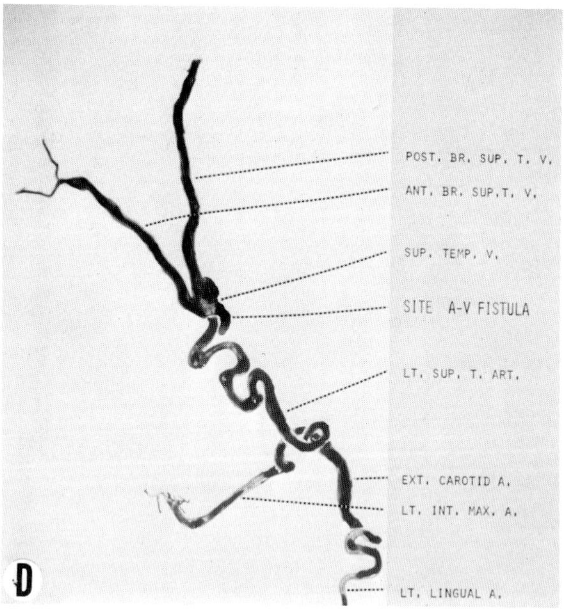

Fig. 2. (D) Diagram identifying arteries and veins on lateral view.

two vessels embedded in a plexus of dilated vessels. All vessels were clamped and ligated and removed after the zygomatic branch of the facial nerve was carefully identified and retracted away from the vessels. Immediately following this surgery the bruit and tinnitus completely disappeared and the patient felt markedly improved. She has remained asymptomatic for the past 18 months.

Discussion

In the case presented one can speculate that perhaps a suture ligature had been introduced into the rather confining depths of a "mini-facelift" wound in an attempt to control unexpected bleeding and the needle probably initiated a small traumatic fistula between the adjacent superficial temporal artery and vein. A small perivascular hemorrhage undoubtedly occurred which subsequently organized and united both vessels creating a fistula.

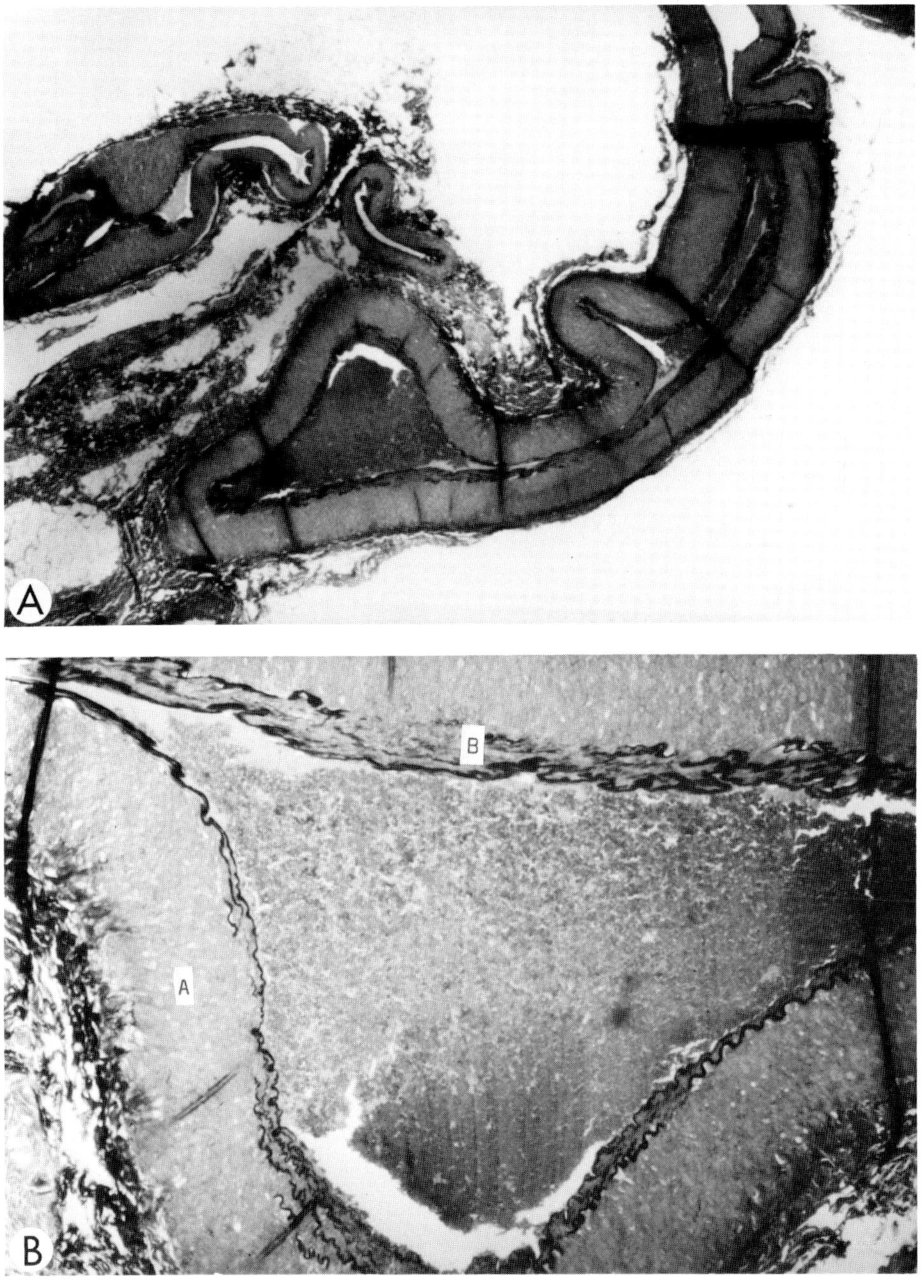

Fig. 3. (A) Histopathological section of superficial temporal artery showing marked dilatation and tortuous elongation. (B) High power of arterial wall showing thickened muscularis (A) and (B) elastic layers.

Thus, it is recommended that a traditional surgical principle of carefully isolating arteries from their venous counterparts before ligation be observed. Upon review of the literature one notes that arteriovenous fistulae may also occur with minimal blunt trauma[1], infection and neoplasm. Following the maturation of the fistula certain generalized hemodynamic changes may occur as follows:

1. Sudden decrease in the peripheral vascular resistance results in a fall in both systolic and dystolic blood pressure.
2. In response, the pulse rate accelerates.
3. Circulating blood volume gradually increases causing secondary cardiac enlargement.
4. Cardiac output increases.

It should be stressed that the physical findings of an arteriovenous fistula are very characteristic as has been stressed by numerous previous authors.[2–5] Probably the earliest description of an arteriovenous fistula was described by William Hunter[6] in 1762, when he reported fistularization of the antecubital vein and artery after a "blood-letting" procedure. A complete reversal of abnormal clinical findings and symptoms following elimination of the fustula was reported in most cases.

Summary

A rare complication of a "mini-facelift" procedure is presented characterized by persistent unilateral tinnitus. The onset of symptoms was noted about 6 months following a "mini-facelift" performed through a limiting preauricular incision without undermining. Chronic moderate fatigue was noted by the patient. Physical examination revealed a loud bruit and a palpable "thrill" over a radius of 6 cm in the preauricular region. External carotid angiography confirmed the diagnosis of an arteriovenous fistula. Uncomplicated surgical excision of the fistula resulted in immediate relief of symptoms and cure of the patient.

Grateful acknowledgment of assistance in the preparation of this manuscript is extended to Dr. Yun Peng Huang of the Neuroradiology department, to Dr. Mamaru Kaneko of the Pathology Department, and to Dr. William Marovitz of the Otolaryngology research laboratories.

References

1. Nunn DB, Harb SK, Jiminez J: Traumatic external carotid—jugular fistula of 33 years' duration. South Med J 67:484–487, 1974
2. Nussbaum M, Lozman H: Traumatic arterio-venous fistula of external carotid artery. NY State J Med 74:2221–2223, 1974
3. Halsted WS: Congenital arterio-venous and lymphatico-venous fistulae. Am J Surg 37:262, 1919
4. Reed MR: Studies on abnormal arterio-venous communications, acquired and congenital. Arch Surg 101:601, 1965
5. Schwartz GF, Rankow RM: Traumatic arterio-venous fistula of the facial artery. Plast Reconstr Surg 40:453, 1967
6. Hunter W: Observations upon a particular species of aneurysm. Med Obs Soc Phys 2:390, 1762 (London)

Cosmetic Repair of the "Marginal Mandibular Lip"

Richard L. Goode, Stanford, Calif.

Injury to the marginal mandibular branch of the facial nerve occurs in a variety of circumstances including parotid surgery, acoustic neuroma surgery, head and neck tumor surgery, cerebrovascular accidents, and skull or facial trauma.

This results in a typical deformity of the lower lip on the involved side consisting of elevation, flattening, inward rotation, and decreased movement. This is due to denervation of the depressor muscles of the ipsilateral lower lip (mentalis, depressor labii inferioris, depressor angularis) plus part of the orbicularis oris muscle. The defect is not apparent when the mouth is closed since the upper lip and/or teeth press down on the elevated lower lip.

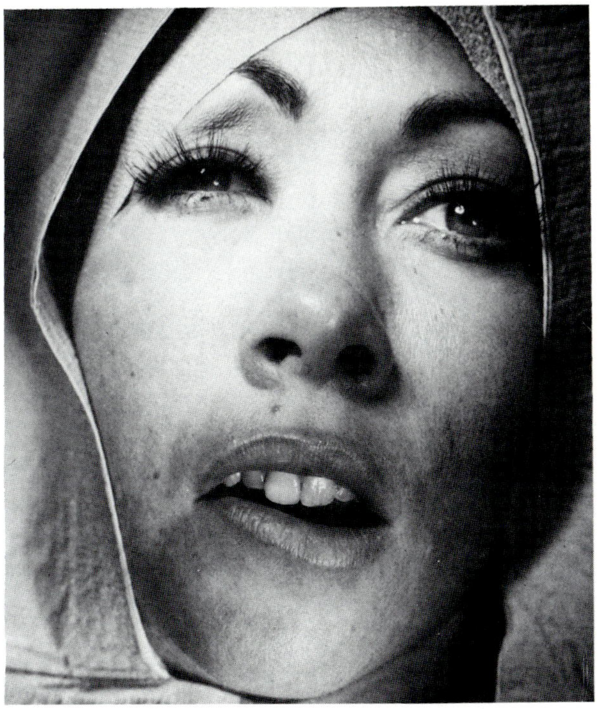

Fig. 1. *The typical "marginal mandibular lip" deformity as analyzed with the mouth half-open. The deformity is aggravated with mouth widening.*

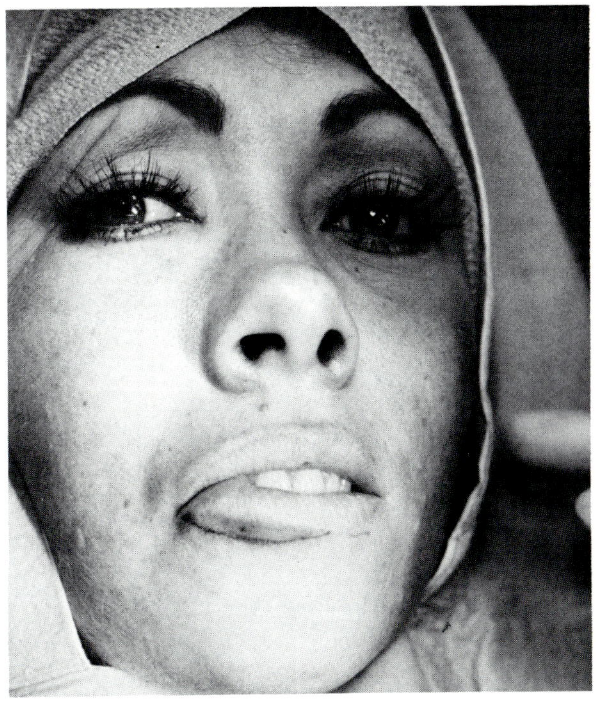

Fig. 2. *The amount of tissue to be resected is outlined. The lower line of the wedge will be the new vermilion border and is drawn to mimic the uninvolved side.*

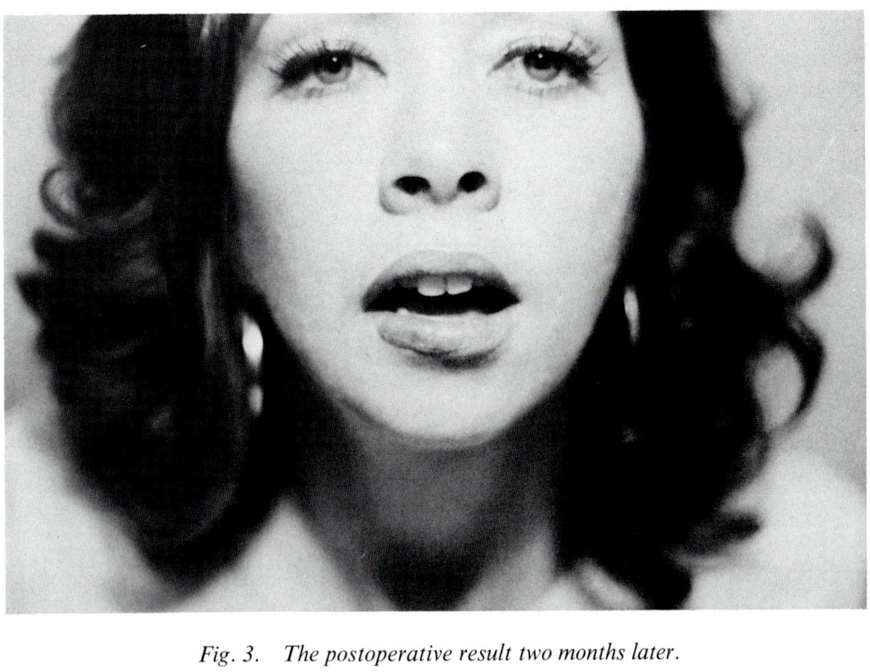

Fig. 3. *The postoperative result two months later.*

As the mouth is opened, the deformity becomes apparent—the wider the mouth is opened, the more the deformity is accentuated. The result is primarily a cosmetic deformity, however, drooling and difficulty with unvoiced speech sounds can occur in some patients.

The need to repair the defect depends on its significance to the patient and the effect of the deformity on the patient's overall facial appearance. For example, the "marginal mandibular lip" deformity as an isolated defect in an attractive young woman after Bell's palsy would be much more significant than the same defect in an elderly man following a cerebrovascular accident.

Technique

Repair of the lip deformity is achieved by removing a horizontal wedge of skin and muscle at the vermilion-skin border on the paralyzed side in order to lower and evert the lip. Part of the orbicularis oris muscle is removed to reduce the elevation while the skin removal provides eversion.

The amount of tissue to be removed is determined with the mouth in half-open position (Figs. 1, 2). The skin incision at the lower aspect of the wedge will be the new vermilion border and should be symmetrical with the normal side. If dentures are worn, they should be in the mouth when the repair is done. The goal is to produce a symmetrical lower lip with the mouth open (Fig. 3). Too much removal of skin and muscle may produce a depressed lip when the mouth is closed with an interlip gap.

If the repair is done as part of total facial paralysis reconstruction, suspension of the oral commissure to the proper position should be performed first. The lower lip wedge is performed later when the exact amount of tissue removal required can be accurately determined. Obviously repair should be delayed until the deformity is known to be permanent.

The procedure is performed under local anesthesia. The deep closure is performed using absorbable 4-0 chromic sutures and the skin closed using 6-0 nylon.

We feel that repair of the "marginal mandibular lip" should be considered in the rehabilitation of patients with facial nerve injuries. The repair is not difficult and produces a more natural appearing lip during speech.

Augmentation Mentoplasty: Comparison of Techniques and Complications

Willard E. Fee, Jr., Stanford, Calif. and
Harold J. Kaplan, Los Angeles, Calif.

Cosmetic facial surgery requires precision preoperative profileplasty in order to obtain optimal results. Since the advent of more acceptable implant materials, the chin has assumed an increasingly important role. Micrognathia, with its usual class II malocclusion, usually requires bilateral mandibular osteotomies for adequate functional and cosmetic rehabilitation. Microgenia, and mild to moderate retrognathia, which may be unrecognized by the patient, respond nicely to a lesser operative procedure—augmentation mentoplasty.

Every esthetic surgeon has adopted and modified a technique of augmentation mentoplasty basically utilizing two different approaches—intraoral or percutaneous. Each approach has a vociferous proponent (Tables 1 and 2), who is, in most cases, a nationally recognized authority.[1–21] Scanty literature has appeared on the complications of each

Table 1. Intraoral Technique Proponents

Name	Material
Millard (1971)[1–4]	Silicone sponge
Converse (1950)[5]	Autogenous bone
Tresley (1972)[6]	Silicone
Newton (1973)[7]	Silicone
Gonzalez-Ulloa (1968)[8]	Silicone sponge
Bell (1969)[9]	Silicone
Pitanguy (1968)[10]	Silicone
Lund (1973)[11]	Silicone

Table 2. Percutaneous Technique Proponents

Parkes	(1973)[12,13]	Silicone sponge
Parkes	(1975—Personal Communication)	Proplast
Safian	(1966)[14]	Silicone
Rish	(1964)[15]	Acrylic
Aufricht	(1958)[16]	Osteocartilaginous hump
Caplan	(1973)[17]	Silicone sponge
Landman	(1972)[18]	Teflon
Penn	(1968)[19]	Kiel Bone
Carlin	(1973)[20]	Silicone
Berman	(1975—Personal Communication)	Silicone
Ashley	(1975—Personal Communication)	Methyl methacrylate
Farrior	(1972)[21]	Silicone sponge

technique, but virtually no reports compare one technique with the other.

Material and Methods

Designed to obtain the highest possible complication rate, this study is a retrospective analysis of 80 augmentation mentoplasties performed by the UCLA Divisions of Head and Neck Surgery and Plastic Surgery and the Stanford University Divisions of Plastic Surgery and Otolaryngology. The majority of cases were performed by senior resident physicians supervised by staff.

A minimum follow-up of 6 weeks was required for inclusion into the study; 8 patients (6 percutaneous and 2 intraoral) were excluded from the analysis because their care was terminated at one month; all, however, were doing well and without apparent complications. The range of follow-up was 6 to 192 weeks with a mean of 34.7 weeks for the 72 analyzed cases.

In addition to method of insertion, other surgical considerations were investigated: supra- or subperiosteal placement of the implant, suturing of the implant to bone or periosteum, type and size of implant, type of sutures used, and the use of antibiotic therapy.

Table 3, modified from Millard,[4] lists the possible complications of augmentation mentoplasty. "Over-projection of chin" is caused by placing too large an implant for the patient, or development of fibroproliferative material about the implant, requiring its removal and/or reduction. "Visual projection" implies that one end of the implant is showing through the skin, secondary to either a too superficial distal end of the receiving pocket, too small a pocket, or ends of the implant not being tapered to proper contour. Subperiosteal resorption, although a well recognized phenomenon,[22,23] was not looked for routinely; thus, no statistics are available for its incidence in this study.

The anatomical approaches have been well described and diagrammed.[4,5,9,10,15,21] The two

Table 3. Complications of Augmentation Mentoplasty

Seroma
Hematoma
Infection
Requiring removal
Not requiring removal
Migration
Requiring removal
Not requiring removal
Asymmetry
Over projection of chin
Visual projections
Extrusion of implant
Mental nerve injury
Subperiosteal resorption

approaches are quite similar, utilizing a sharp incision of skin or mucous membrane and then various amounts of sharp and blunt dissection, creating a pocket just large enough to receive the augmenting material. Most authors agree that there is a greater chance of implant migration if the receiving pocket is made too large.

Migration of the implant inferiorly will often cause a palpable "step-off," or irregularity, but will retain its excellent cosmetic result. Obviously, it can migrate too far inferiorly and require removal. On the contrary, migration superiorly cannot be as readily tolerated by the patient or physician because obliteration of the mentolabial sulcus may occur or the frontal view will show a nonharmonious lateral contour of the chin.

The possibility of obliterating the mentolabial sulcus is slightly greater with the intraoral technique because the implant is more likely to migrate superiorly. However, if the dissection is carried too high via the percutaneous approach, the same situation can occur with superior migration of the implant.

Results

Of the 72 cases analyzed, 20 had complications, with an overall complication rate of 27.7 percent. Table 4 lists the complication rate by the approach used. No significant difference in complication rate can be found between the two approaches. Table 5 shows that 46 percent of the complications occurred more than 6 weeks postoperatively and included 4 migrations, 2 asymmetries, 1 visual projection, 1 extrusion, and 1 pseudo-cyst. This is an important factor when analyzing the results of this study and others. Two patients, who had totally successful results at intraoral and percutaneous placement respectively, developed progressive migration with impending extrusion percutaneously 19 months and 48 months postoperatively respectively. Regarding the onset of complications, however, there does not appear to be any significant difference between the two approaches.

Types of complications can be seen in Table 6. The seromas and hematoma were treated by aspiration and pressure dressing and resolved spontaneously. Three infections were treated with systemic antibiotics and cleared rapidly; interestingly, none required removal. Migration was not only the most common complication encountered, but also the most common requiring removal. One of the percutaneously inserted acrylic implants developed a pseudocyst around it, and eventually migrated. It required removal, and the patient underwent successful reinsertion of a silicone implant. One patient who developed anesthesia along the distribution of both right and left mental nerves resolved spontaneously after several months.

Of the 72 implants, 10, or 13.8 percent, required removal secondary to complications. Stated differently, 50 percent of the procedures which developed complications necessitated removal of the implant. Two additional implants were removed in patients whose operations were considered a total success; one patient became a Kung Fu advocate after his surgery and desired removal to avoid difficulties from a possible blow to his jaw. The other sustained a blow to the chin which caused migration 2 years after a successful procedure—he underwent successful revision. There does not appear to be any significant difference between the two approaches in terms of type of complications, except for the monopoly on asymmetry with the percutaneous approach.

Table 7 shows the results of implant material and complication rate. The large majority of synthetic materials used, versus the very small numbers of autograft material, makes it impossible to make any statement of statistical significance comparing the various materials and complication rates. How-

Table 4. Patient Complication Rate

	Intraoral	Percutaneous
Total number	24	48
Overall complications	6 (25%)	14 (29%)
Complications requiring Implant removal	3 (13%)	7 (15%)

Table 5. Onset of Complication[a]

	Intraoral	Percutaneous
2 weeks	3	7
1 month	2	1
6 weeks	0	1
Greater than 6 weeks	2	8

[a] Total greater than 20 as some cases had more than one complication.

Table 6. Type of Complications[a]

	Intraoral	Percutaneous
Seroma	1	2
Hematoma	0	1
Infection		
Not requiring removal	2	1
Requiring removal	0	0
Migration		
Not requiring removal	1	1
Requiring removal	2	6
Asymmetry	0	4
Overprojection	0	0
Visual projection	0	1
Extrusion of implant	1	1
Mental nerve injury	0	1

[a] Some patients had more than one complication.

Table 7. Implant Material (N) and Complication Rate (%)

	Intraoral	Percutaneous
Silicone	18 (33%)	28 (22%)
Acrylic	1 (0%)	9 (22%)
Bone	4 (0%)	7 (14%)
Cartilage	0 (0%)	2 (0%)
Other		
Heyer Schulte gel-filled prosthesis	1 (0%)	0 (0%)
Dermal graft	0	1 (100%)
Vivacil sponge	0	1 (0%)

ever, there is a suggestion that autograft materials are better tolerated.

Sixteen of the operative reports were not detailed enough to determine whether the implant had or had not been sutured to bone or periosteum. Of the remaining 56 cases, 26 implants were sutured or wired and 30 were not. Seven of those sutured or wired (26.9 percent) developed complications. Eight of those not secured (26.6 percent) developed complications. Five of the sixteen cases (31.2 percent), which did not state the technique, were complicated.

Supraperiosteal or subperiosteal placement of the implant was incompletely evaluated, as only one case had follow-up cephalometric x-rays, and 13 operative reports did not state this method of insertion. Of the remaining cases, 8 of 24 supraperiosteally placed implants (33.3 percent) developed complications. Eight of 35 subperiosteally inserted implants (22.8 percent) developed complications. Four of 13 (30.8 percent) procedures where the implant procedure was not stated, developed complications.

Prophylactic antibiotics were used in 55 cases (76.4 percent). Fifteen of the 55 cases developed complications (27.3 percent). Five of the remaining 17 cases where no antibiotic was used were complicated (29.4 percent). There was no correlation between complication rates and type of suture material used, placement of subcutaneous sutures, size of implant, or whether or not the implant was preformed or formed at the operating room table.

Discussion

Although we deliberately sought to obtain the highest complication rate possible, we were astonished at the high rate of complications which occurred with both techniques and the number of implants which required removal. Most other studies report either no complications or so few complications as to suggest no morbidity. Several factors may contribute to our findings: (1) the design of the study to obtain the highest possible complication rate, (2) performance of the majority of procedures by resident physicians in training, and (3) the lengthy mean follow-up of greater than 34 weeks.

The advantages and disadvantages of each technique are summarized in Table 8. The primary consideration for most surgeons today is operating in the absence of contamination; thus, the presumed higher risk of infection with the intraoral approach has led many to adopt the percutaneous technique. The size of incision limits the rapidity and degree of ease with which larger augmentations can be performed. Having personally performed both techniques with about equal frequency, we agree with the intraoral proponents—that it is technically easier to perform, especially for larger augmentations.

From our analysis of the 72 cases of augmentation mentoplasty, we conclude the following:

1. The procedure has a significant complication rate of 27 percent, and migration was the most common complication. Of the complicated cases, one-half will require removal of the implant, implying a failure rate of 13 percent.
2. Patients need long-term follow-up after augmentation mentoplasty. One half of the complications occur greater than 6 weeks postoperatively and can occur up to 19 months later, or perhaps longer.
3. Securing the implant to bone or periosteum with wire or suture has no advantage in preventing complications.

Table 8. Technical Advantages and Disadvantages

	Advantages	Disadvantages
Intraoral:	No external scar Larger incision if necessary Technically easier Extrusion orally	Contaminated field Migration superiorly Obliteration of mentolabial sulcus
Percutaneous:	Noncontaminated field Migration inferiorly	External scar Smaller incision Extrusion percutaneously

4. Prophylactic antibiotics appear to play no role in preventing complications.
5. This study does not clarify the controversy between supraperiosteal versus subperiosteal placement of the implants.
6. Despite the vociferous proponents of each approach, there is no significant difference in complication rates between the intraoral and percutaneous approaches.

We advocate that esthetic surgeons should know and utilize both techniques, tailored to the patient's needs and the surgeon's skill. Both techniques produce excellent results with equal complications.

Acknowledgments

Our thanks are due to Franklyn I. Ashley, M.D., Walter E. Berman. M.D., and Morey L. Parkes, M.D., of Los Angeles, California, for personal communications regarding this topic.

References

1. Millard DR, Jr: Chin Implants. Plast Reconstr Surg 13:70–74, 1954
2. Millard DR, Jr: Buccal Incision for Chin Implants. South Med J 52:1371–1374, 1959
3. Millard, Jr: Adjuncts in Augmentation Mentoplasty and Corrective Rhinoplasty. Plast Reconstr Surg 36:48–61, 1965
4. Millard DR, Jr: Augmentation Mentoplasty. Surg Clin North Am 51:333–340, 1971
5. Converse JM: Restoration of Facial Contour by Bone Grafts Introduced Through the Oral Cavity. Plast Reconstr Surg 6:295–300, 1950
6. Tresley IJ, Arenberg IK, Polterock J: Augmentation Mentoplasty—Reflections. Laryngoscope 82:2092–2102, 1972
7. Newton RA: Mentoplasty. Can J Otolaryngol 2:235–237, 1973
8. Gonzalez-Ulloa M, Stevens E: The Role of Chin Correction in Profileplasty. Plast Reconstr Surg 41:477–486, 1968
9. Bell WH: Correction of the Contour-Deficient Chin. J Oral Surg 27:110–115, 1969
10. Pitanguy I: Augmentation Mentoplasty. Plast Reconstr Surg 42:460–464, 1968
11. Lund BA, Sather AH: The Chin. Mayo Clin Proc 48:417–425, 1973
12. Parkes ML: Chin Implants with a Newer Plastic Compound. Arch Otolaryngol 75:429–436, 1962
13. Parkes ML: Avoiding Bone Resorption Under Plastic Chin Implants. Arch Otolaryngol 98:100–101, 1973
14. Safian J: Progress in Nasal and Chin Augmentation. Plast Reconstr Surg 37:446–452, 1966
15. Rish BB: Profile-plasty. Laryngoscope 74:144–154, 1964
16. Aufricht G: Combined Plastic Surgery of the Nose and Chin. Am J Surg 95:231–236, 1958
17. Caplan H: Profileplasty. Can J Otolaryngol 2:347–349, 1973
18. Landman MD, Strahan RW, Ward PH: Chin Augmentation with Polytef Paste Injection. Arch Otolaryngol 95:72–75, 1972
19. Penn J: Kiel-Bone Implants to the Chin and Nose. Plast Reconstr Surg 42:303–306, 1968
20. Carlin GA: Personally Fabricated Chin Implants. Plast Reconstr Surg 51:121–128, 1973
21. Farrior RT: Mentoplasty. Ed. by Conley J and Dickinson JT. *Plastic and Reconstructive Surgery of the Face and Neck. Proceedings of the First International Symposium.* Vol 1, pp 291–207, New York, Grune & Stratton, 1972
22. Robinson J: Bone Resorption Under Plastic Chin Implants. Arch Otolaryngol 95:30–32, 1972
23. Jobe R, Iverson R, Vistnes L: Bone Deformation Beneath Alloplastic Implants. Plast Reconstr Surg 51:169–175, 1973

Orbit

Reduction of the Supraorbital Ridges A New Cosmetic Operation?

Jean-Paul Lintilhac, M. D. Paris, France

It has probably occurred, and happened, to some plastic surgeons to reduce a prominent supraorbital ridge be it for asymmetry or abnormal prominence but, to my knowledge, bilateral supraorbital ridge reduction has never been described or considered as a usual cosmetic operation, which it actually should be.

Indications For This Operation

The necessity for this operation first appeared to me by the observation of male transsexuals. Most of these patients have masculine features they want to change into more feminine ones. Once their noses and chins have been reduced, many of them ask that their eyebrows be raised but a skin resection above the eyebrow or a temporal lift does not achieve their goal because they have, in fact, a protruding and thick bony superciliary ridge compared to the thinner and higher feminine ridge.

It seemed to me rather easy to devise an operation for reducing their supraorbital ridge and they accepted it freely and readily as they would accept any operation that makes them look more feminine.

After operating some transsexuals with satisfactory results I realized that many women who have a thicker, low or slanting down lateral part of their supraorbital ridge giving them a "hard" or "sad" look would also benefit by this operation. It was more difficult to convince them to accept this unheard of procedure involving the bone, and only those who had gained confidence by previous aesthetic operations were willing to have it performed. I am convinced that once this procedure gets better known by the public the number of operated cases will increase greatly.

For some men who have a very thick and low supraorbital ridge, giving them a "suspicious" look, the operation might also be useful.

Preoperative Examination

The examination of the candidates for this operation should be thorough and is comprised of:

Inspection. This will determine:

The general shape, the thickness, the protrusion of the supraorbital rim that may be more or less hidden by excess skin or fatty hernias of the eyelid and will be best appreciated by elevating the eyebrow with the finger.

The level of the supraorbital ridge in relation to the eye: low or high, slanting more or less downward in its lateral half.

The level of the eyebrow in relation to the orbital ridge: in young individuals it can be at the same level, above or under it, however there is no doubt that with age the eyebrow has a tendency to fall.

When the eyebrow is low and the supraorbital ridge is also low and prominent, the upper eyelid has generally a normal convex appearance, a marked flexion crease and is usually sagging.

This corresponds to the usual masculine type of supraorbital ridge hypertrophy.

When the eyebrow is high and the supraorbital ridge rather high but prominent and slanting down in its lateral part, the upper eyelid is generally concave and quite hollow under the roof of the orbit. In this case there is usually no flexion crease of the upper eyelid. This hollow eye corresponds more to a feminine type of supraorbital ridge hypertrophy.

The importance of the supraorbital ridge must be compared with other bony structures of the face (nose, chin, cheekbone): it is usually not just mere chance if most patients already had previous nose and chin reductions.

Palpation will allow to appreciate more precisely the shape and contours of the supraorbital ridge. Many men (and transsexuals) have a bony protuberance immediately above the fronto-malar suture.

Roentgenograms, while not absolutely necessary, are interesting in order to study the thickness of the bone, the situation of the supraorbital foramen and the extension of the frontal sinus.

Photographs. Front, $\frac{3}{4}$, and lateral views should be taken routinely.

The examination of existing scars might reveal a tendency to hypertrophy or keloïd formation: in this case the palpebral approach should be preferred.

The usual blood tests and preoperative check-up are prescribed.

Operative Procedure

The operation is usually performed under local anesthesia with 1 percent or 0.5 percent xylocaïne with epinephrine after the usual premedication. Neuroleptanalgesia, or general anesthesia can also be given to apprehensive patients as the use of chisel and mallet is noisy and unpleasant although not painful.

The approach to the bone is different if the eyebrow needs to be raised or if it is already high.

In the first case the supraorbital ridge is approached through a skin excision above the eyebrow: we shall call it the superciliary approach.

In the second case it is approached through an incision (or excision) on the upper eyelid: this is the palpebral approach.

We will describe first the different steps of the operation with a low eyebrow.

Superciliary Approach (Figs. 16, 18, 19)

Skin Excision Above the Eyebrow

The two incisions are marked with Bonney's Blue delimiting the area to be excised.

The upper incision starts from the middle of the eyebrow or somewhat more medially on the vertical passing through the pupil. It describes a regular curve extending 1 or 2 cm outside the eyebrow tail. At its peak it reaches 3 to 6 mm (or more) above the eyebrow according to the degree of elevation needed.

The lower incision follows exactly the upper border of the eyebrow turning up at its extremity to join the upper incision laterally.

The upper and lower incisions should be different in shape although equal in length; the upper being regularly concave whereas the lower should have a double curve.

The incisions using a no. 10 (or 15) blade cut all the way through the skin of which the whole thickness is excised. Some superficial veins and occasionally arteries are electro-coagulated.

Skin Undermining

The skin is then undermined at the lower edge of the excision taking care not to interfere with the hair follicles of the eyebrow. The undermining is initiated with the scalpel and continued with scissors. It should reach the level of the supraorbital ridge.

Incision of the Muscle

Five millimeters above the orbital ridge, as controlled by palpation, the orbicularis muscle is incised following the direction of its fibers from the level of the external canthus to the middle part of the orbit. Both sides of the muscle are retracted using skin hooks or better two prong nasal retractors (which should be blunt because of the vicinity of the eye).

Incision of the Periosteum

After incising through the layer of connective tissue where one generally encounters some blood vessels, the incision is carried through the periosteum down to the bone 5 mm above the lower margin of the supraorbital ridge. This incision should extend from immediately above the external canthal ligament to the midline of the orbit or even a little further according to the shape of the bony ridge but it should avoid the supraorbital foramen and the emergence of the supraorbital nerve.

Elevation of the Periosteum

The periosteum of the lower lip of the incision is raised with a periosteal elevator. A mosquito forceps grasps the periosteal flap as soon as it appears facilitating its elevation. The periosteal elevation should extend from a point between the external canthal ligament (which must not be seen) and the fronto-malar suture (clearly visible once the periosteum is elevated) to past the midline of the orbit.

The lower aspect of the supraorbital ridge (this means toward the roof of the orbit) must also be freed of its periosteum for which I generally use a cleft-palate periosteal elevator. The upper lip of the periosteal incision is also elevated from the prominent part of the bone.

The supraorbital ridge appears then fully exposed in its external half and the surgeon can appreciate its shape, thickness and the aspect of the tubercle often existing in its outer part.

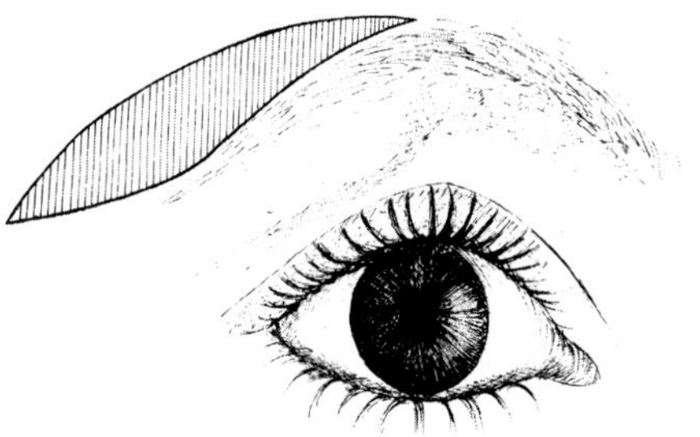

Fig. 1. Skin excision above the eyebrow.

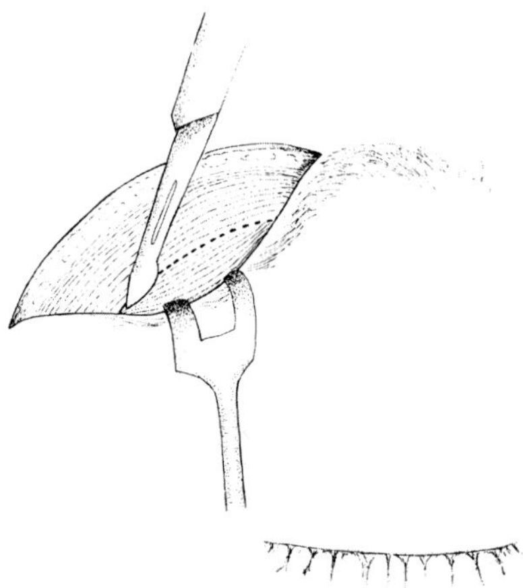

Fig. 2. Incision of the orbicularis muscle after skin undermining.

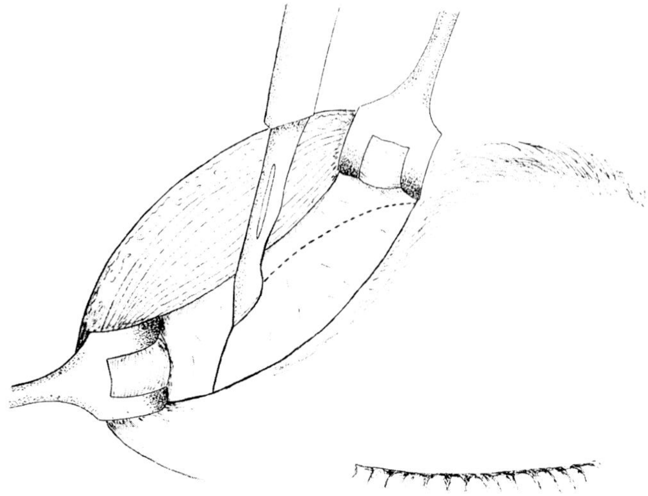

Fig. 3. Incision of the periosteum.

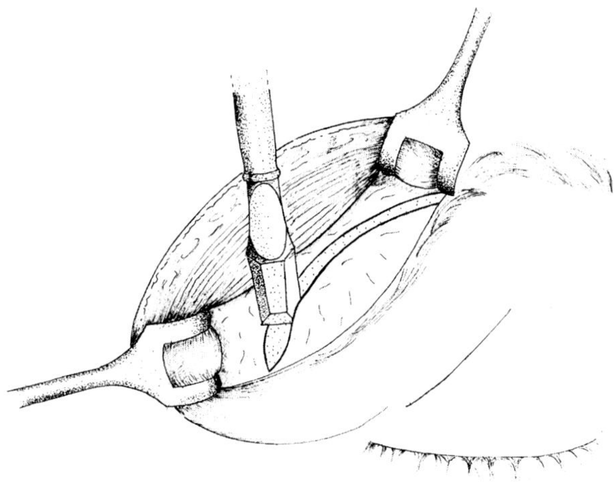

Fig. 4. Elevation of the periosteum on the supraorbital ridge.

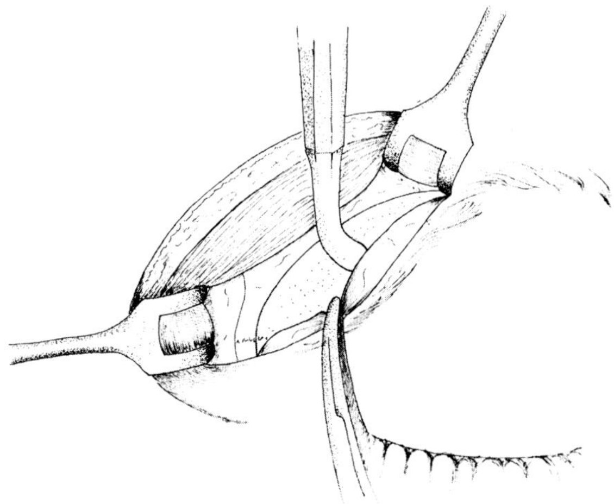

Fig. 5. Elevation of the periosteum under the supraorbital ridge towards the roof of the orbit.

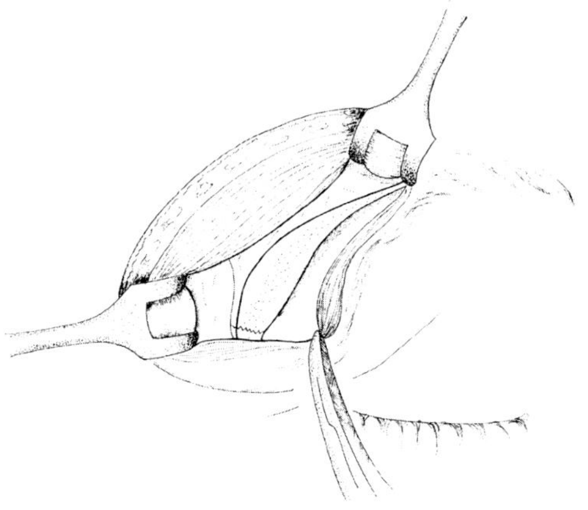

Fig. 6. Exposed hypertrophied supraorbital ridge.

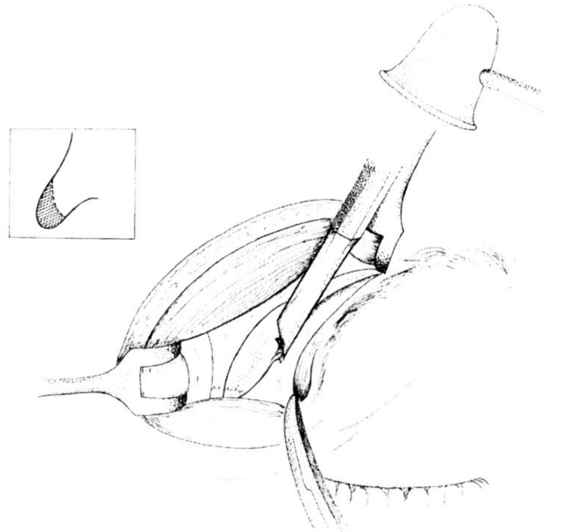

Fig. 7. The supraorbital ridge is resected and reshaped with osteotom and mallet. Insert illustration shows a lateral view of a section of the supraorbital ridge and the way its hanging and protruding part should be resected.

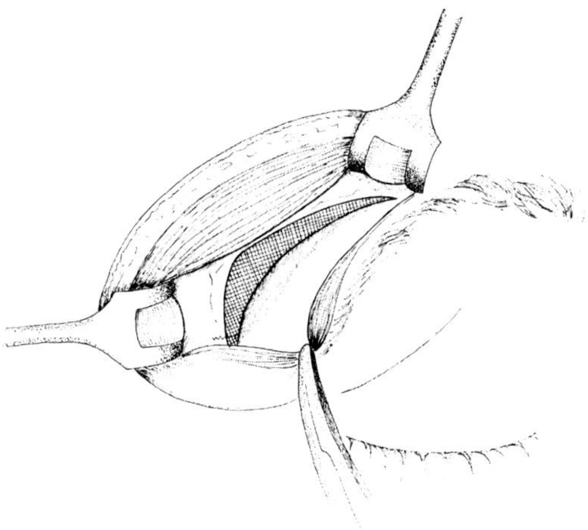

Fig. 8. The checkered area represents the newly cut bone, the periosteum retains its former shape.

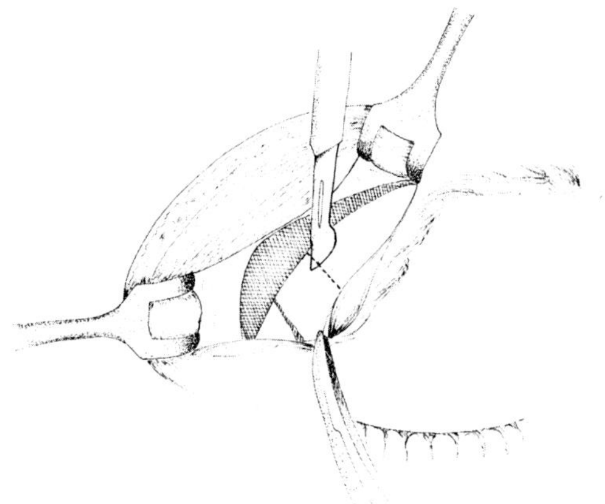

Fig. 9. Incision of the periosteum to allow for its draping on the new bone contour.

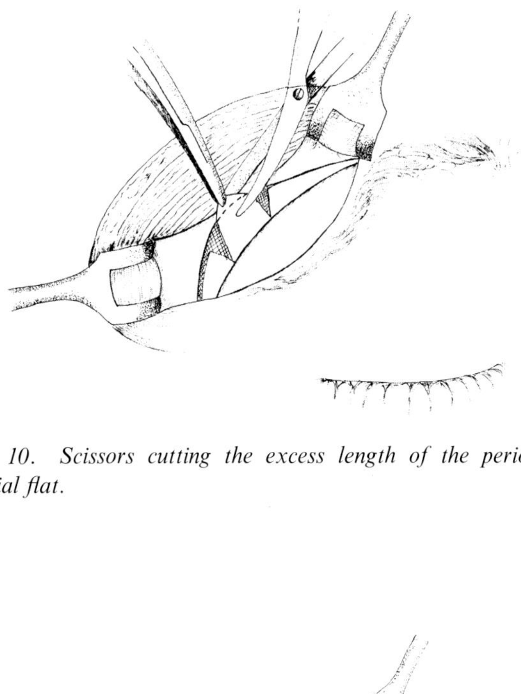

Fig. 10. Scissors cutting the excess length of the periosteal medial flat.

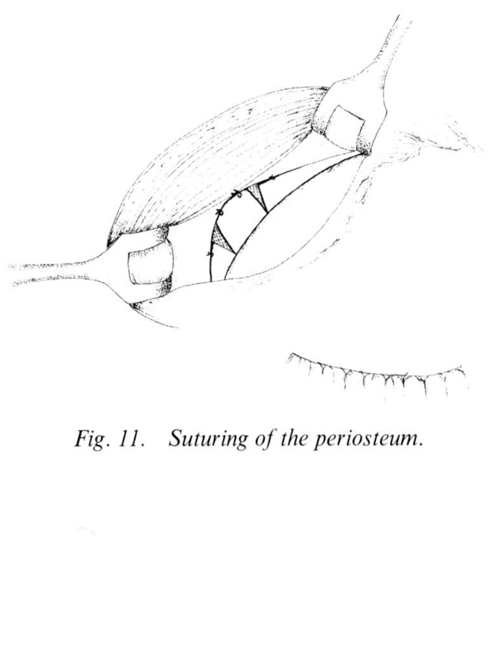

Fig. 11. Suturing of the periosteum.

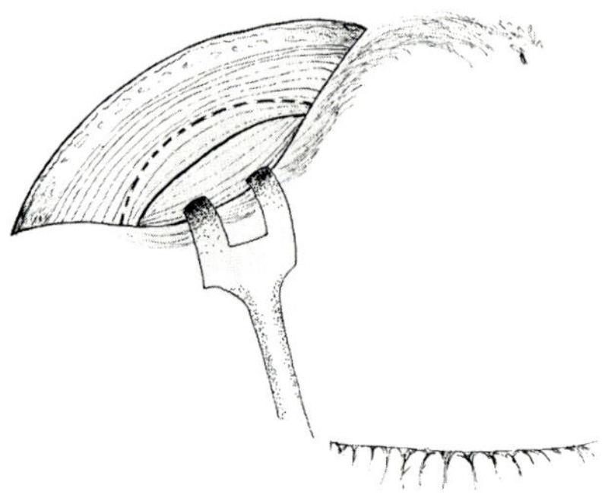

Fig. 12. Excision of a crescent shaped strip of the orbicularis muscle.

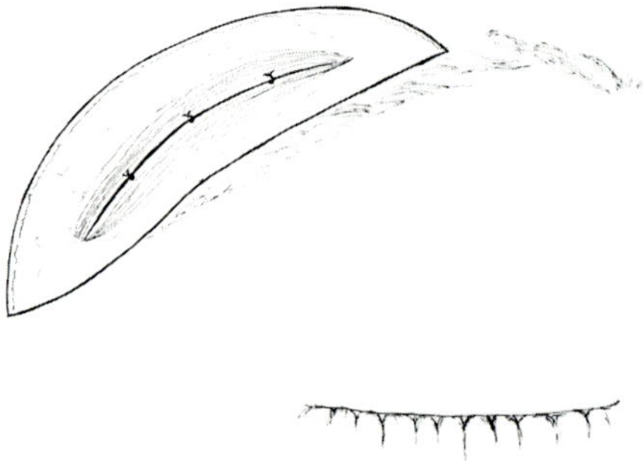

Fig. 13. Suture of the muscle.

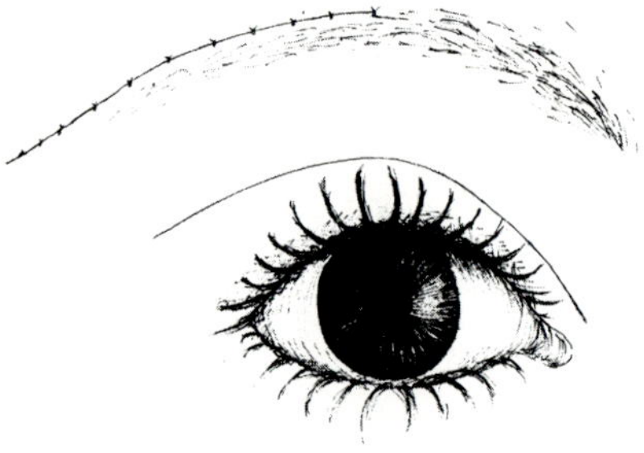

Fig. 14. Skin suture.

Bone Resection and Reshaping of the Supraorbital Ridge

For this purpose I use a fine 8 mm chisel or osteotome and mallet but any other sort of mechanical device could be employed.

The hanging part of the bone is first removed, the orbital ridge is then reshaped so that the lateral upper quadrant of the orbit will take a nice regular curved shape. The bone resection is limited laterally by the external canthal ligament which must absolutely be avoided and medially by the supraorbital foramen. Some of the bone thickness responsible for the forward protrusion of the orbital ridge is also removed so that the bone takes a bevelled shape that will produce a more pleasing supraorbital ridge.

Incision, Draping, and Suturing of the Periosteum

Now comes the most important part in the description of this operation, the only "trick" there is. As can be easily seen by pulling upwards on the mosquito forceps, still holding the periosteum, the latter retains its former shape and will not come into contact with the newly shaped orbital ridge. It stays down like the chord of an arc of a circle. To allow for its coming up and draping over the new bone contour two incisions must be cut with a no. 15 blade in the periosteal flap from its free margin up to the bone and perpendicularly to it. This incision concerns only the periosteum and care must be taken not to open the orbit, letting the orbital fat appear in the incision: in this case the excess fat must be removed and no suture attempted.

By pulling on the mosquito forceps holding the periosteal medial flap the surgeon can check that the periosteum now drapes neatly on the new bone structure. A few millimeters of the medial flap, which is now too long, are cut off and two 3-0 catgut sutures will fix it to the superior lip of the periosteal incision which has been also slightly elevated; one catgut stitch on each lateral flap is sufficient to fix them.

Orbicularis Resection and Suture

A crescent-shaped strip about 3 mm wide is excised with scissors from the upper margin of the incision in the orbicularis muscle. Three 4-0 catgut sutures will approximate the two margins.

Skin Suture

Due to the extensive undermining and to the muscle resection and suture, the skin margins are approximated without tension and sutured with 8-0 silk.

Palpebral Approach (Figs. 17, 20)

When the eyebrow is high or in normal position, the approach will be through the upper eyelid.

If the upper eyelid has no excess skin the palpebral approach will be through a simple incision. The incision follows the normal flexion crease when it exists but extends laterally and upwards for 1 or 2 cm.

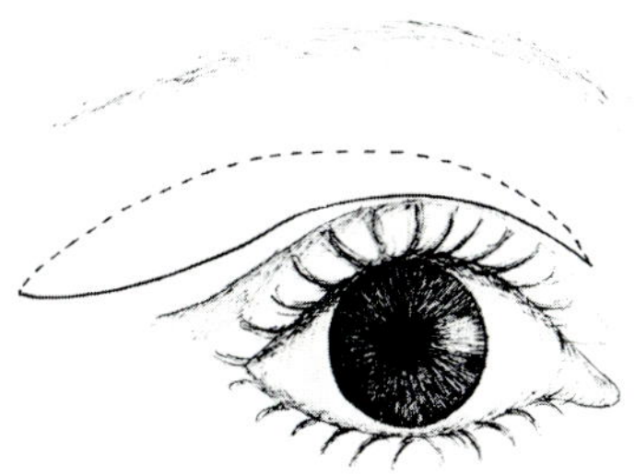

Fig. 15. Simple incision: firm line. Excision: firm + dotted line.

If there is no definite crease, the incision lies in the concavity of the upper eyelid and also extends outwards and upwards across the hypertrophied supraorbital ridge.

If the upper eyelid is wrinkled and sagging with an excess of skin, the palpebral approach will be through a skin excision comparable to that of the usual upper eyelid blepharoplasty extending across the supraorbital ridge.

This excision will expose the orbicularis muscle and the prominent supraorbital ridge.

The following steps: incision of the muscle and of the periosteum, bone resection . . . etc., are similar to those of the superciliary approach.

Postoperative Treatment

A light pressure dressing is applied on the eye for the first night after the operation.

Antibiotics and anti-inflammatory agents are generally given.

The postoperative course is very simple: practically no pain; swelling and ecchymosis of the upper eyelid are usually present for a few days.

Skin sutures are removed after six days in the superciliary approach, after four days on the upper eyelid.

Complications

In seven years I have operated on about 60 cases with no complications whatsoever.

One could probably observe hematomas or injuries of the supraorbital nerve.

Evolution

After 10 to 15 days, edema of the upper eyelid has disappeared but some thickening of the operated tissues will persist for one or two months, so that it will take about three months until the end result is finally obtained.

Results

The cosmetic result of this operation, which is its only goal, is highly satisfactory to both the surgeon and the patient in well selected cases. The scars become practically invisible. The eyebrow is raised when it is necessary and the supraorbital ridge is also made higher and less prominent suppressing the "hard," "suspicious," or the "sad" look.

The only limitation in the result of this operation is at the inner part of the supraorbital ridge when this is specially prominent thus giving a deep-set, sunken eye which cannot be treated in the same way because of the presence of the supraorbital nerve (which could be spared with a little care) and of the frontal sinus which would present more difficult problems.

Summary

The author presents an apparently new cosmetic operation: the reduction of the supraorbital ridge.

Indications are a prominent or hanging supraorbital ridge giving a "hard" or "sad" look.

The approach is through a skin excision above the usually low eyebrow, thus raising it. When the eyebrow is high the approach is through the upper eyelid.

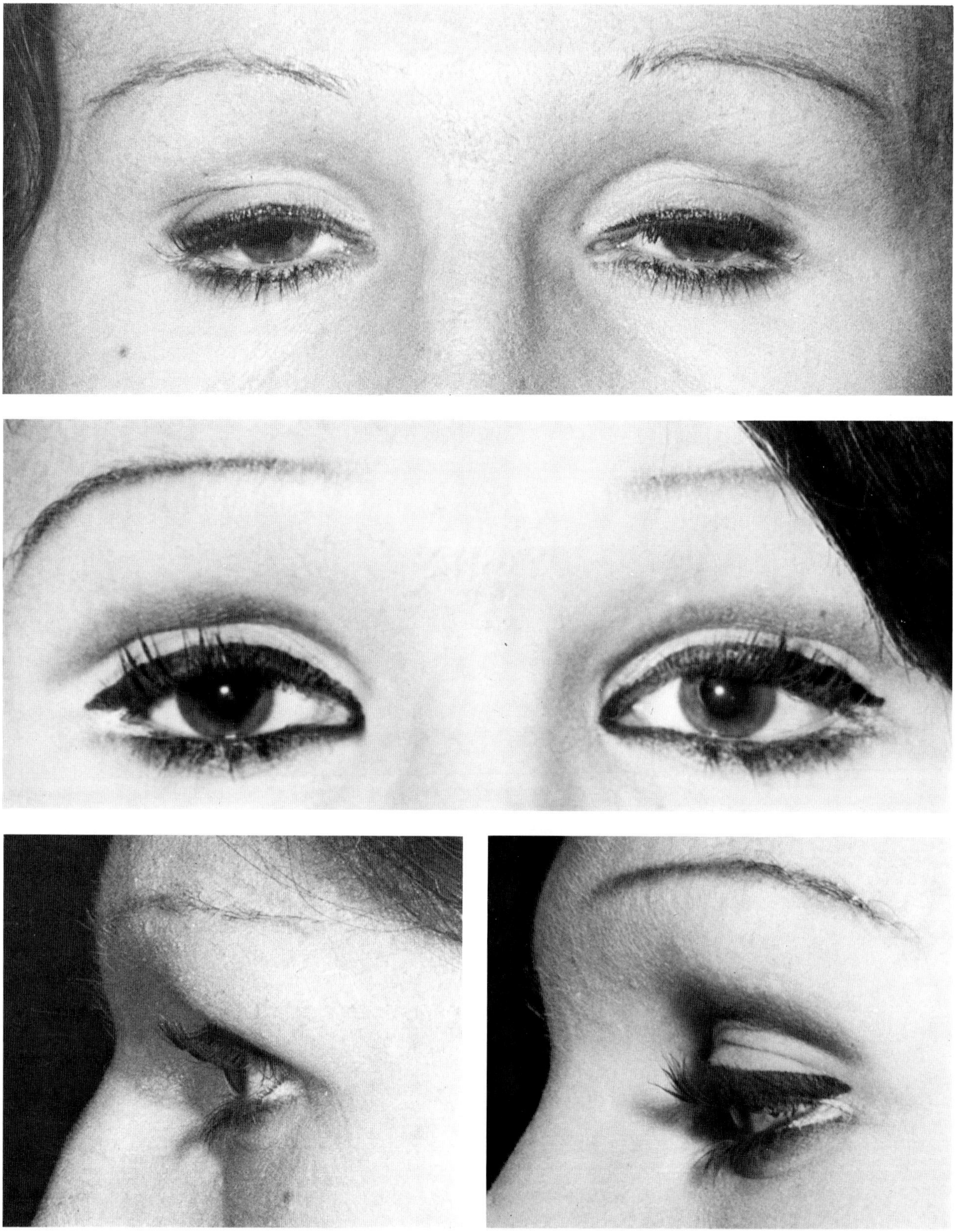

Fig. 16. Transsexual with a low, thick, prominent supraorbital ridge. Superciliary approach.
(Top) Front view before.
(Middle) Front view after.
(Bottom) Lateral view (left) before (right) after.

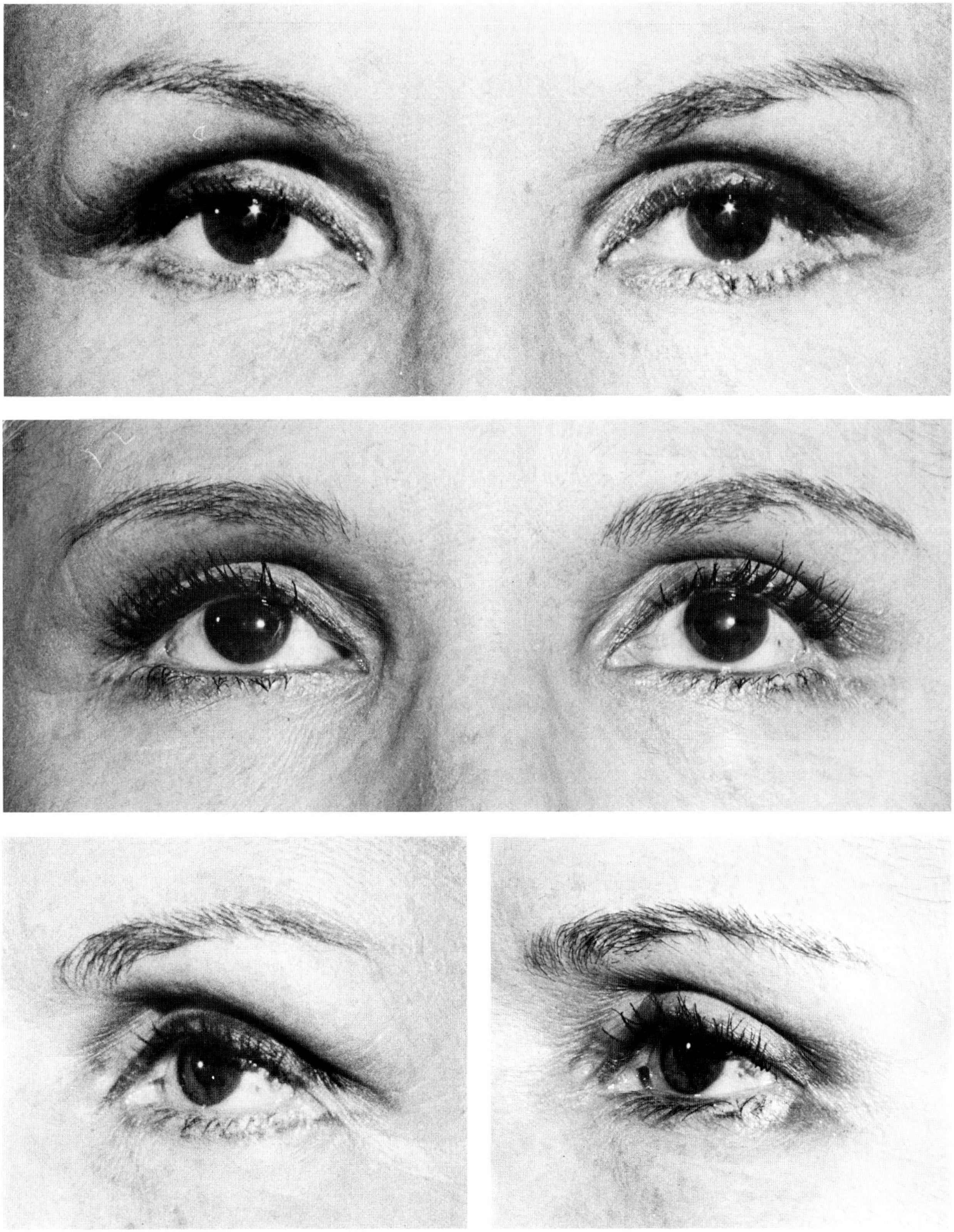

Fig. 17. *Woman with a low, thick supraorbital ridge ("hard, suspicious, look"). Palpebral approach.*
(Top) *Front view before.*
(Middle) *Front view after.*
(Bottom) *3/4 view (left) before (right) after.*

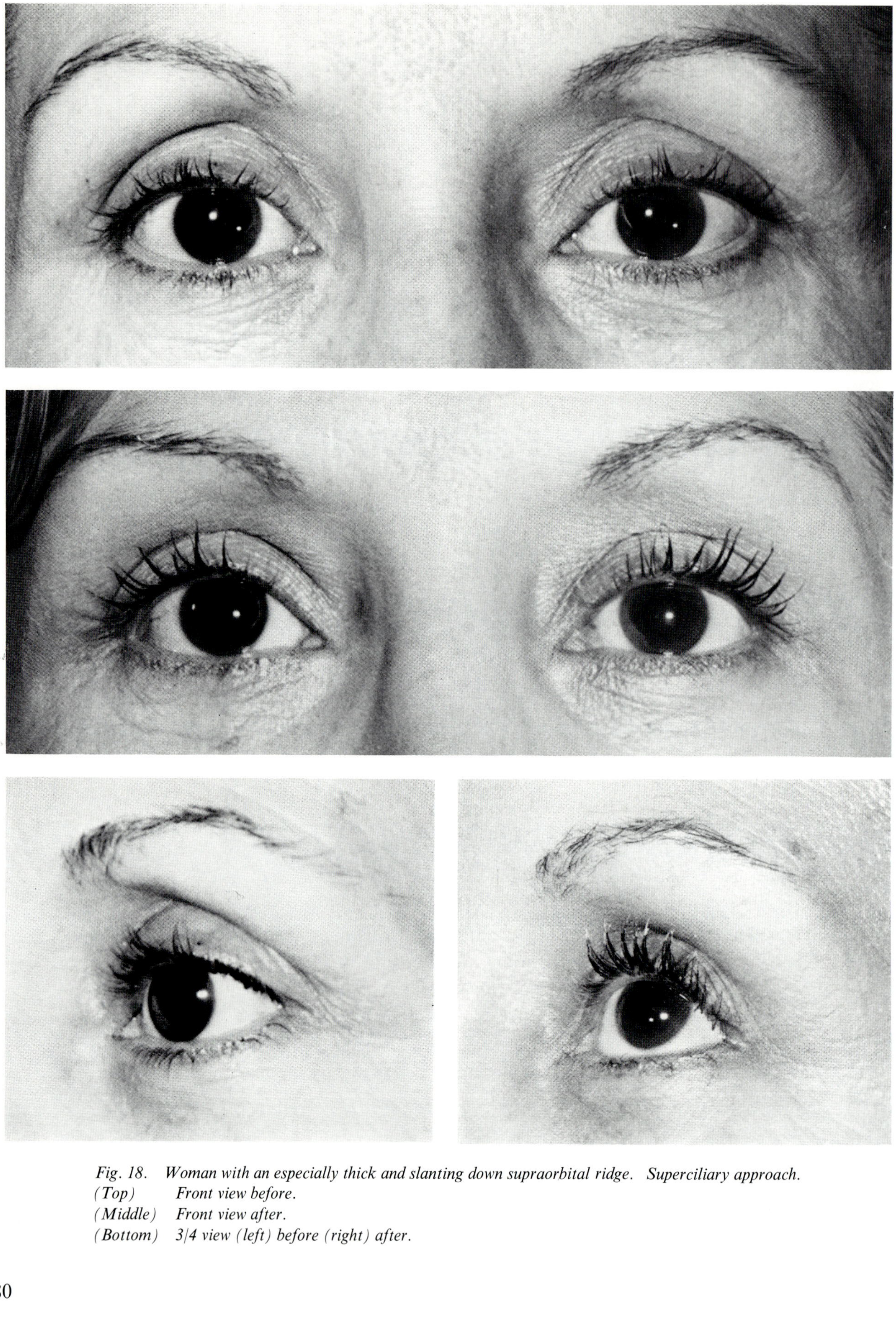

Fig. 18. Woman with an especially thick and slanting down supraorbital ridge. Superciliary approach.
(Top) Front view before.
(Middle) Front view after.
(Bottom) 3/4 view (left) before (right) after.

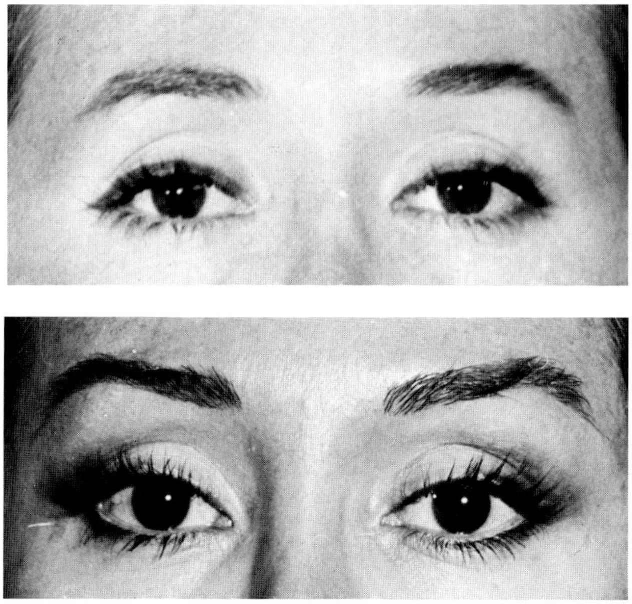

Fig. 19. Woman with a supraorbital ridge slanting slightly downwards whereas the eye slants upwards. The reduction of the supraorbital ridge through a superciliary approach emphasizes the slanting eye and improves the exotic look.
(Top) *Front view before.*
(Bottom) *Front view after.*

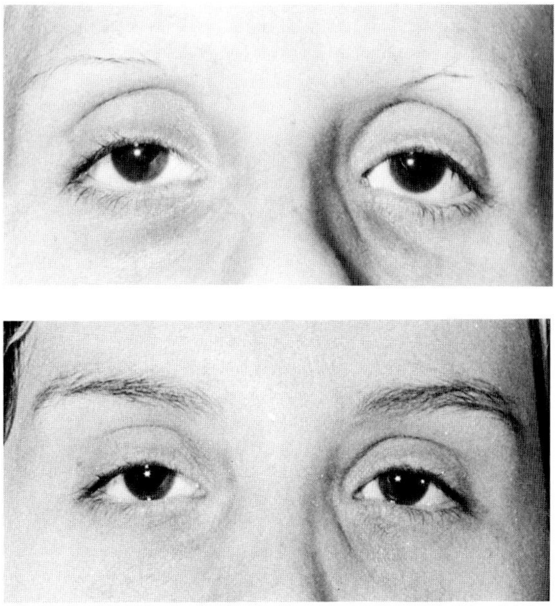

Fig. 20. Woman with a prominent slanting down supraorbital ridge giving her a "sad" look. Palpebral approach.
(Top) *Front view before.*
(Bottom) *Front view after one month.*

After separation of the orbicularis muscle and elevation of the periosteum, the prominent lateral part of the supraorbital ridge is resected with a chisel.

The periosteum must be properly incised and well draped on the new bone structure: *sine qua non* condition of the generally excellent cosmetic result.

Variations in Technique of Blepharoplasty

Jacob S. Aronoff, New York, N.Y.

There exist many choices of technique in blepharoplasty at each step of the operation. This paper attempts to classify these variations with a personal evaluation of each.

Location of Incision

Lower Lid

The standard incision is located 3 to 4 mm below the lid margin. In the older age group with marked chalasis, it might be advisable to increase the margin to 5 or 6 mm to diminish the chance of senile ectropion. Whether to extend the incision beyond the lateral canthus will be discussed under the heading of rotation. If the chalasis is severe and localized at the infraorbital rim, I believe the incision should be localized to the area of pathology, rather than carrying the dissection down from the lid margin area (Fig. 1).

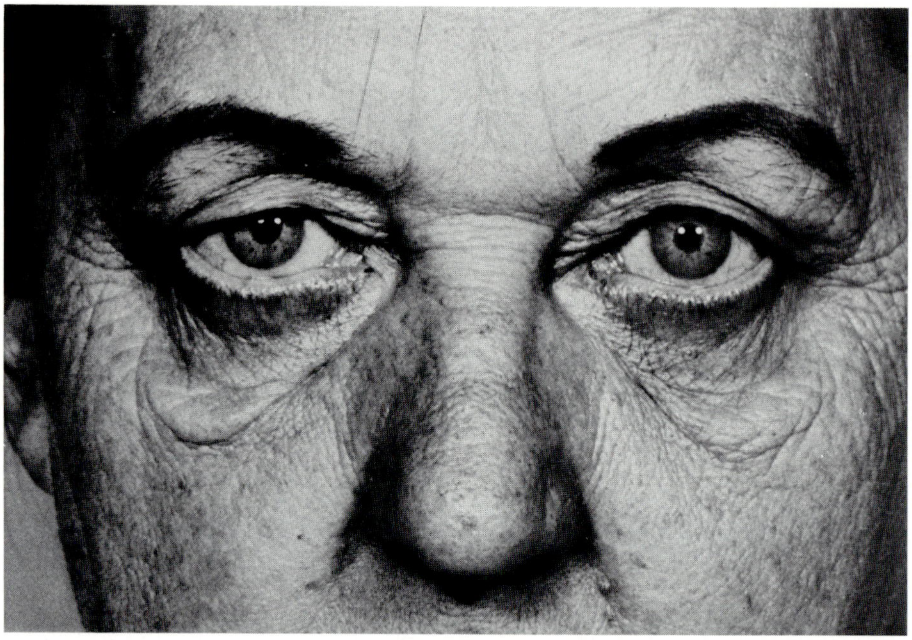

Fig. 1. The lower lid surgery in such a case should be limited to excision of the "bags" at the infraorbital rims.

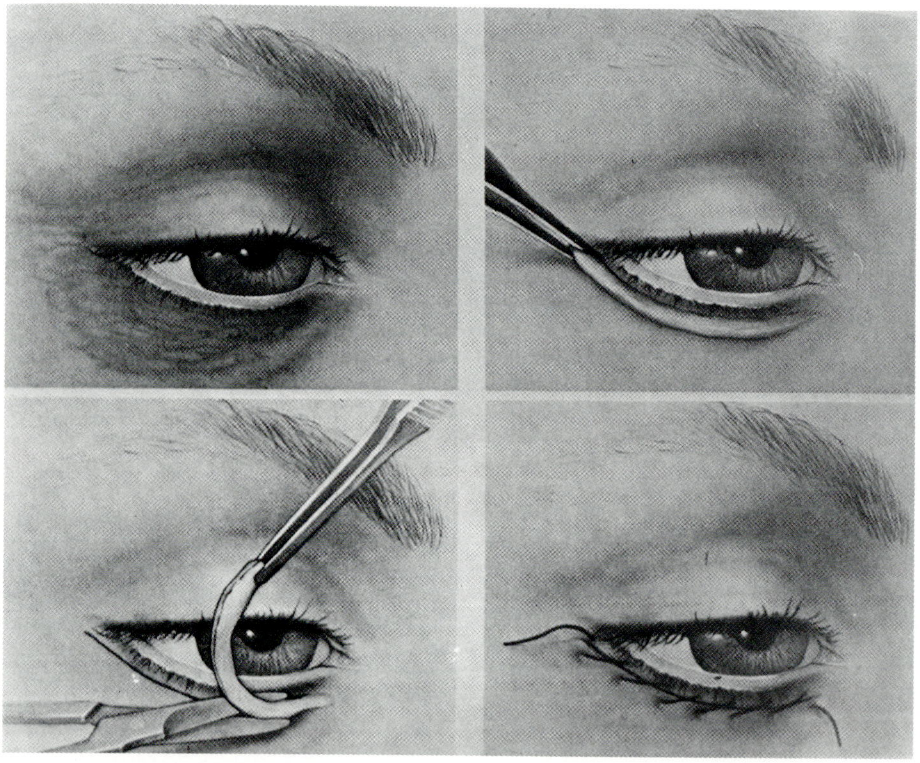

Fig. 2. The excessive skin is pinched into a ridge with the AdsonBrown forceps. The excision is done with straight, sharp scissors (after Parkes, M.).

Superior Lid

The classic crescent shaped incision is made usually with extension beyond the lateral canthus. Mesial extension on to the nasal skin should be avoided. The lower incision is made about 2 mm below the sulcus so as to end up within the sulcus. The upper incision, following the technique of Parkes, is made at the level where the eyelid skin changes its color and texture. This may appear to be radical and does effect a temporary lagophthalmus of 2 to 8 mm. However, it usually prevents the residual fold over the sulcus seen so frequently in blepharoplasty patients. Most of the lagophthalmus disappears in a few days but could persist up to two weeks. The degree of lagophthalmus should be limited in patients with exophthalmos or with deficient tearing revealed by the Schirmer test. It should also be emphasized that no skin is resected over the tarsal plate area.

Technique of Incision

Lower Lid

Here we are confronted by the choice of the knife or scissors on the one hand or the "pinch" technique. I have found the "pinch" technique preferable in patients with minimal to moderate amount of chalasis[1] (Fig. 2). With severe chalasis, I revert to the use of scissors prior to draping the skin. In the "pinch" technique, one can evaluate the ectropion potential after the "pinch" has been effected by the usual tests of having the patient open the mouth and with eyes focused in upward gaze. If these maneuvers do not move the lower lid, the "pinched" skin can be safely removed.

Upper Lid

Incision and excision are made by knife and scissors. The "pinch" technique could be used, but I cannot achieve the same good results as is possible in the lower lid.

Skin versus Skin-Muscle Flap

This problem applies only to lower lid surgery. In the presence of herniated fat, an increasing number of surgeons are finding the skin-muscle flap to be a more direct and less traumatic approach. However, even in the older age group with only chalasis, I see little reason for a skin flap to be separated from relatively atrophic orbicularis muscle. One might chance a wrinkle or two, but the advantage again lies with diminshed reaction and morbidity. Again, where I aim for "100% or more" on the upper lids, one must be more conservative in the lower lids and aim for a "90% result."

Rotation of Flap

This problem is also one confined to the lower lids. The classic technique was to extend the incision beyond the lateral canthus and rotate the lower flap laterally before closure of the wound (Fig. 3). This technique was designed to diminish the chances of ectropion, but I think most plastic

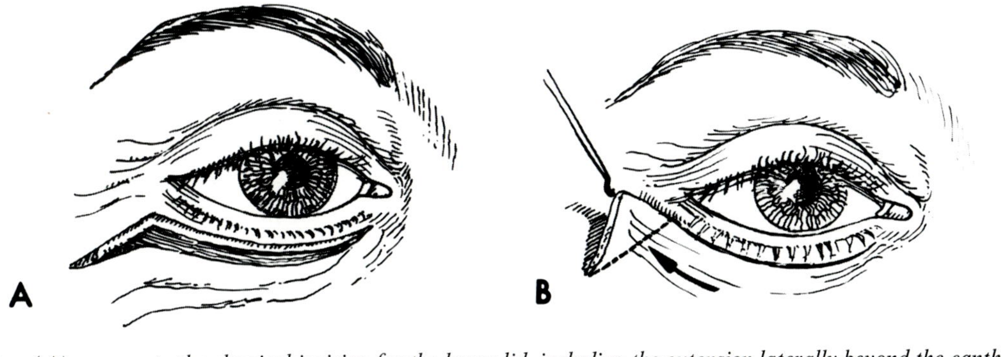

Fig. 3. (A) represents the classical incision for the lower lid, including the extension laterally beyond the canthus. (B) shows the lateral rotation of the inferior flap and the tailoring of the excess skin at the lateral extension (from Rees TD, et al "Cosmetic Facial Surgery").

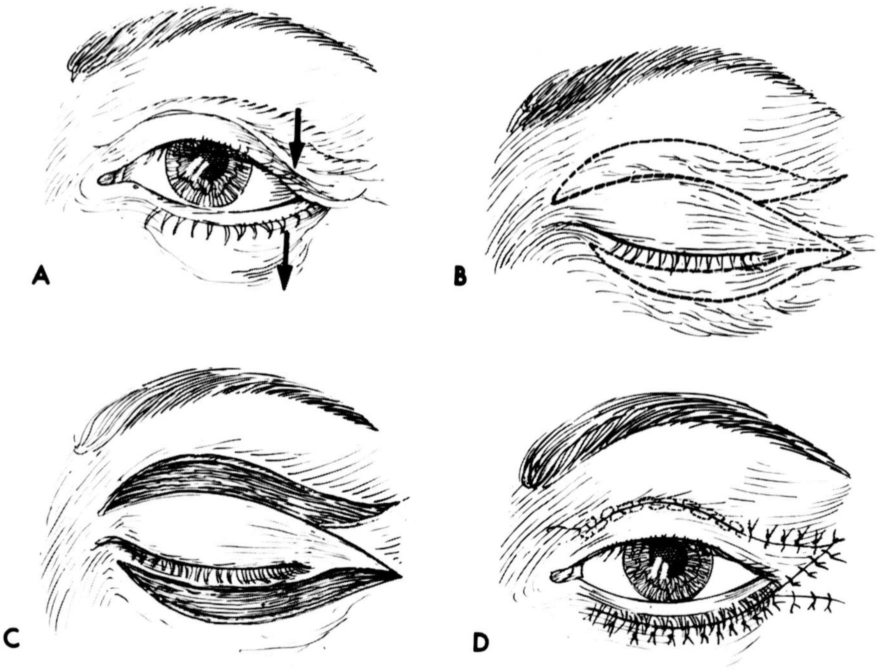

Fig. 4. (B) and (C) represent the outline and excision of the excessive upper and lower eyelid skin, plus the creation of the Z-plasty incision. (D) shows the transposition of the two portions of the Z and the resulting elevation of the lateral canthus (after Lewis, JR Jr).

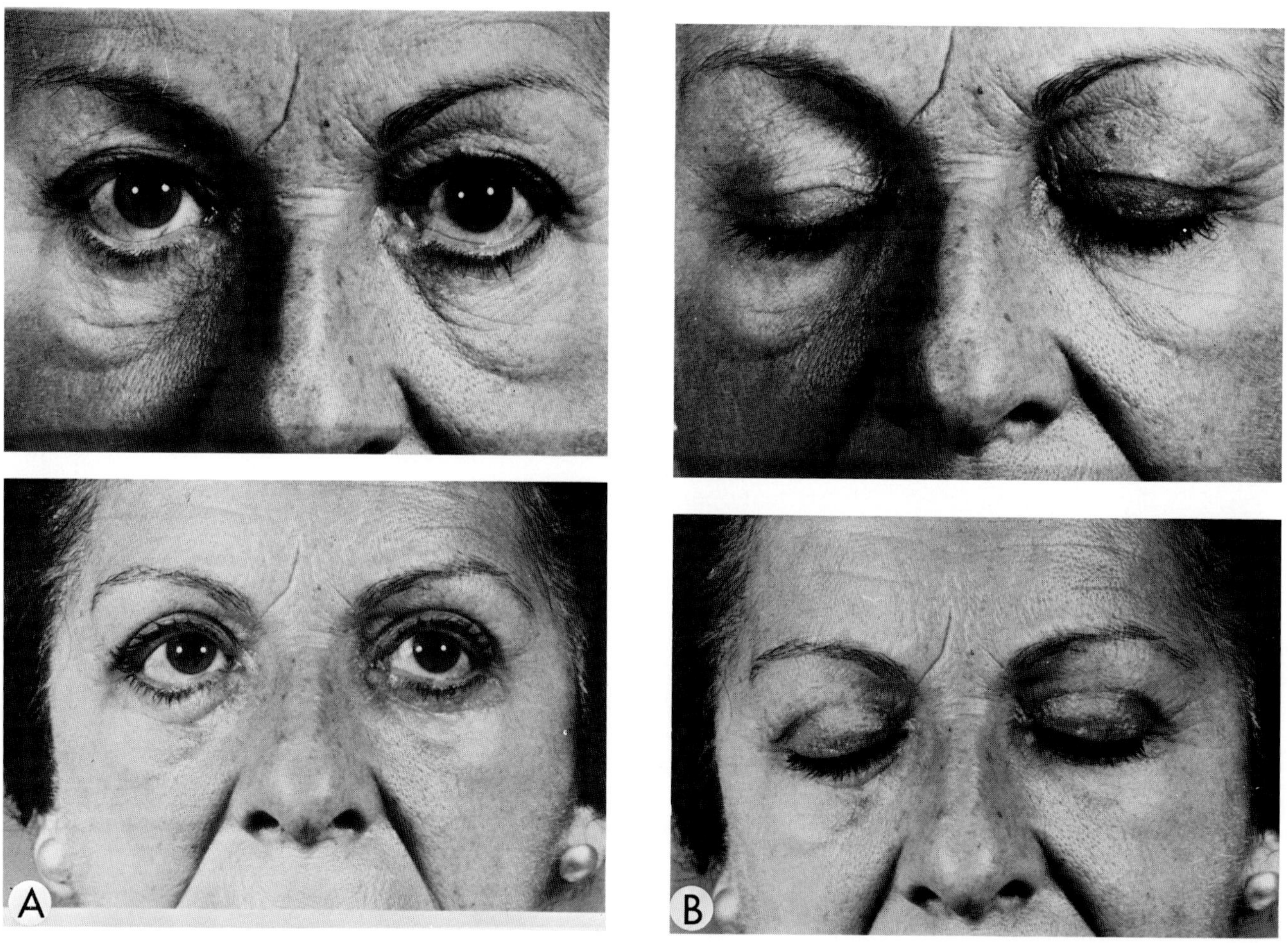

Fig. 5. This patient was concerned chiefly with the folds in the cheeks beneath the infraorbital rims. The problem was complicated by the existence of some ectropion prior to surgery. The incisions were made 7 to 8 mm below the lids. No skin was excised. However, elevation beneath the cheek folds was done after creation of a skin-muscle flap. The postoperative photos were taken six months following surgery.

surgeons have seen enough ectropion with this technique to realize that lateral rotation is not the answer to this problem. Excellent surgeons such as H. Silver[2] and R. Loeb[3] do the lower lids with some mesial rotation. Following the technique of Parkes, Rees,[4] etc., I employ no rotation at all. As the lower skin edge is slightly longer than the upper, a few interrupted sutures are placed at both mesial and lateral canthi and then the intervening space is closed with a minimal "clocking" of the sutures.

Special Situations

Drooping Lateral Canthus

Here Lewis' technique of Z-plasty at the lateral canthus with transposition of the flap would be indicated[5] (Fig. 4).

Chalasis Associated with Cheek Folds

With such pathology, I would advise carrying the elevation beyond the infraorbital rim to all the involved areas. It could be considered a partial meloplasty (Fig. 5).

Most Frequent Technique

After outlining all the above possible variations in technique, I believe it only fair to detail the technique employed in most cases.

Injection

Both lower lids are injected with 1 percent Xylocaine with epinephrine and one unit of hyaluronidase (Wydase) to 10 cc of Xylocaine. The enzyme allows for rapid absorption of the anesthetic and is necessary if one is to use the "pinch" technique. The upper lids are injected heavily with the 1 percent Xylocaine and epinephrine. No enzyme is included as one wants the "stiffening" action of the anesthetic.

Resection of Upper Lid Skin

Each lid is resected immediately after injection. Any hypertrophic orbicularis muscle is also resected at this time. Hemostasis is thoroughly effected with use of electrocoagulating needle.

Lower Lids

The usual approach is by means of the "pinch" technique. Then follows the raising of the skin-muscle flap to expose the herniated fat pads. These fat herniations are removed as required. It should be remembered that, in the older age group, there frequently exists some flattening in the lateral compartment area. Therefore, removal of lateral fat is frequently not needed or, at most, only minimally.

Upper Lids

The fat herniations in the central and mesial compartments are isolated and removed after adequate use of the electrocoagulating needle, especcially in the mesial compartment.

Closure

This should first be completed in the lower lids. The reason is that the upper lid closure may effect lagophthalmos, which simply would expose the eye to the operating room lights and also could interfere with the evaluation of the lower lid results (Figs. 6–8).

The above discussions has been limited to the main techniques used for the upper and lower eyelids. Time does not allow for a discussion of the supra-brow and infra-brow lift procedures. Both of these are important adjuvants to blepharoplasty. In some patients, they may prove to be more important than the surgery performed on the upper lids.

I would close this paper with one word of caution, initially told me by Parkes and often confirmed in my own experience. In the entire field of esthetic surgery, no patient has a higher threshold of satisfaction than the eyelid patient. The wrinkles or "crows feet" that remain postoperatively become the only important wrinkles that existed preoperatively.

References

1. Parkes M: The pinch technique in blepharoplasty. Arch Ophthamol 89:324, 1973
2. Silver H: A new approach to operation of blepharoplasty. Brit J Plast Surg 22:253, 1969
3. Loeb R: personal communication
4. Rees TD, Wood-Smith D: Cosmetic facial surgery. Philadelphia, W.B. Saunders Co., 1973
5. Lewis JR Jr: The Z-blepharoplasty, Plast Reconstr Surg 44:331, 1969

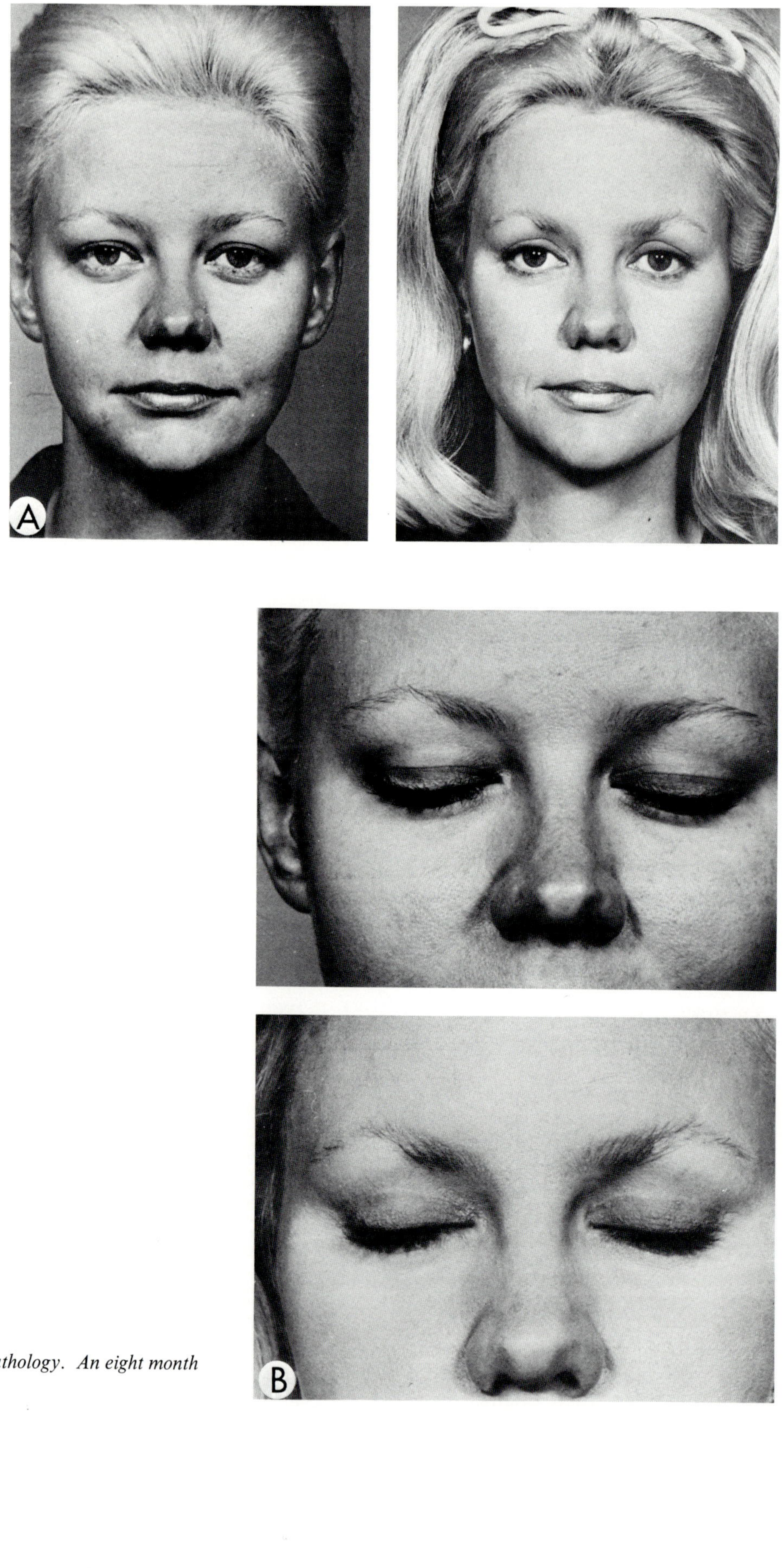

Fig. 6. This case represents minimal pathology. An eight month follow-up photo is shown.

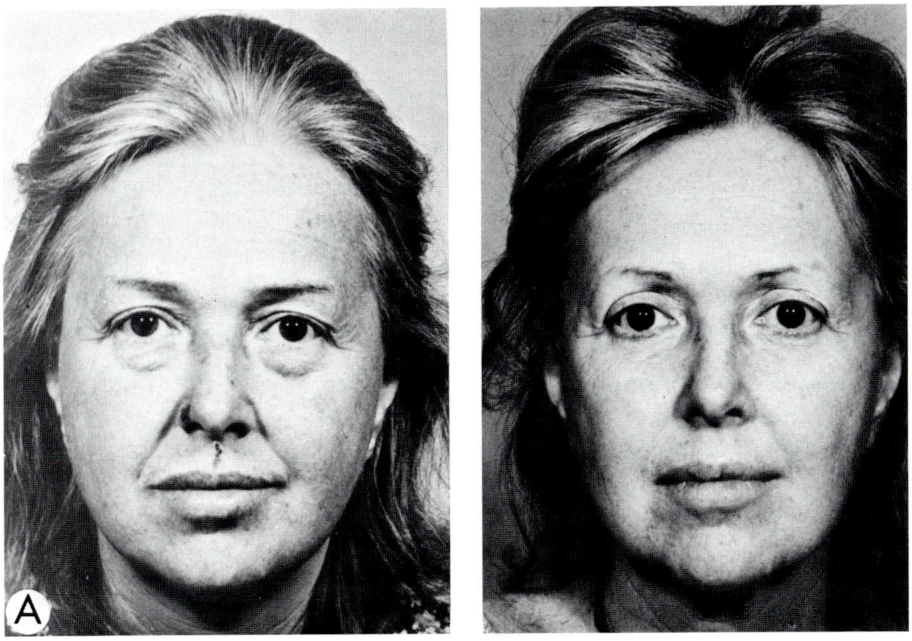

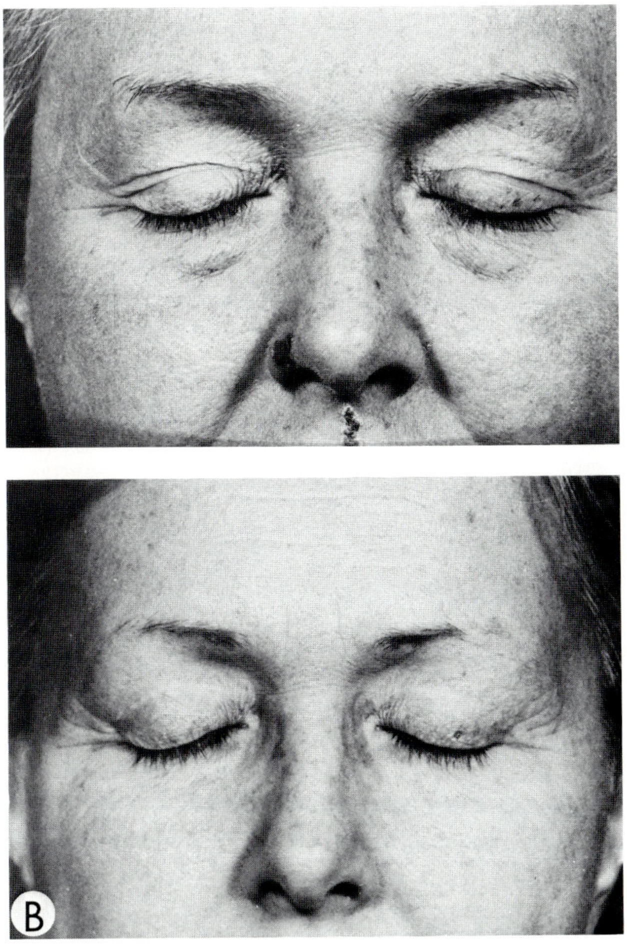

Fig. 7. This case shows moderate pathology of both skin and fat herniations. The postop photos were taken two and one-half years following surgery. Immediately following surgery, there existed a lagophthalmos of 7 mm, which disappeared in one week. The residual fold in the supra tarsal area did not become visible until 20 months after surgery.

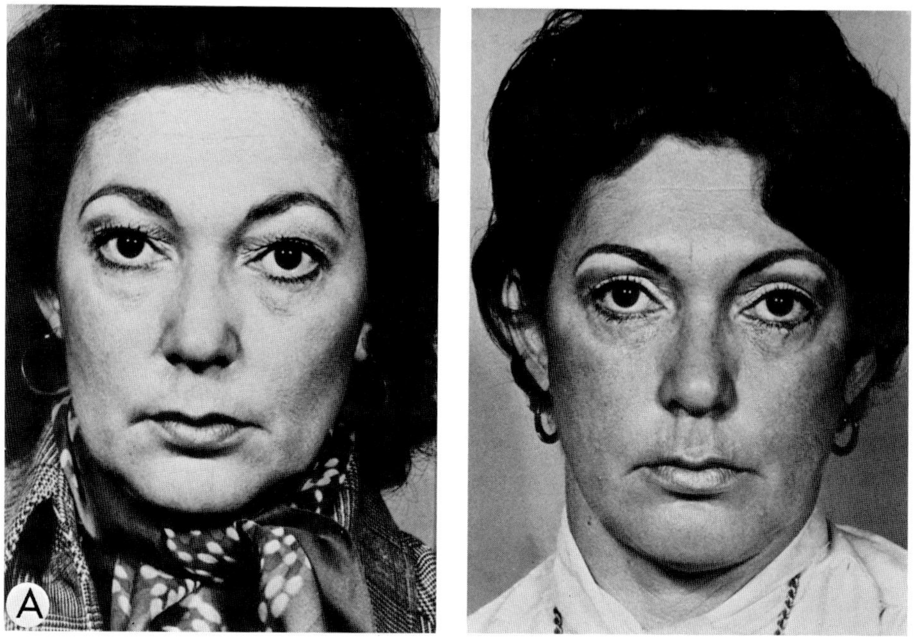

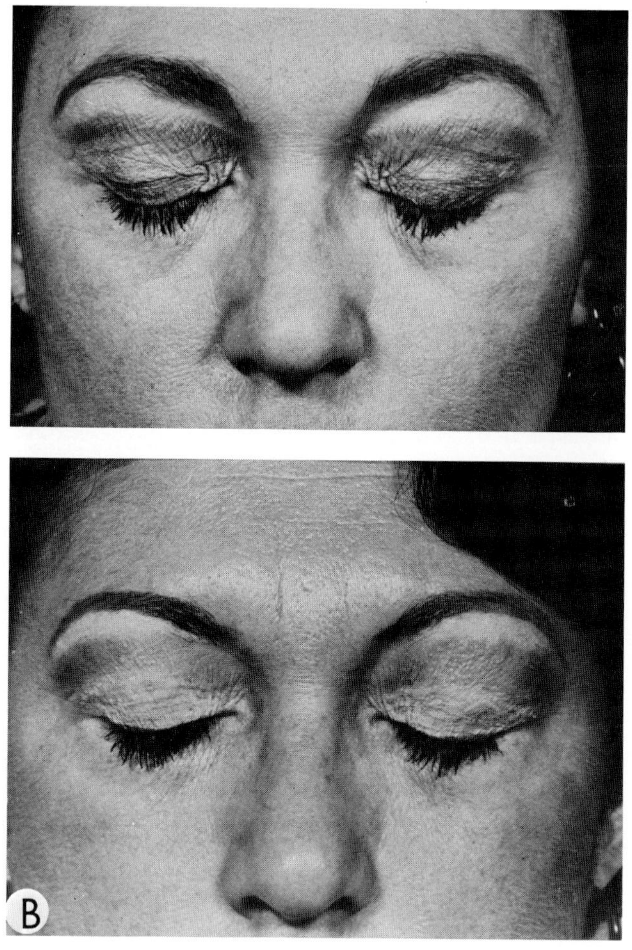

Fig. 8. This case is notable chiefly for the severe chalasis of the upper lid skin, associated with an almost "lizard-like" texture. Surgery was deferred until the recurrent vasomotor swelling of the eyelids was controlled by the appropriate antihistamine. The resection of upper lid skin was very extensive creating a lagophthalmos of 7 to 8 mm at the end of the surgery. This disappeared in five days. Postop photos were taken at eleven months.

Cosmetic Surgery of the Lower Eyelid

G. Jan Beekhuis, Detroit, Mich.

The basic techniques in cosmetic surgery of the lower eyelid are well established and have been described.[1] Minor specific variations of the procedures lead to improvements in cosmetic result, decreased morbidity, and recovery without postoperative complications. The purpose of this report is to describe my technique that has given satisfactory results in over 100 patients.

Technique

In performing lower eyelid cosmetic surgery, the surgeon may remove solely excess skin, solely herniated orbital fat, or some of both these two components. Preoperatively, I evaluate the individual components, while the patient is erect, and estimate roughly the amount necessary to be removed. The amount of orbital fat herniation is further checked by gentle pressure on the globe, to determine how much bulging occurs in the lower eyelid. The patient's skin elasticity is gauged, and the tonus of the tarsal plate. A weak tarsal plate or impending senile ectropion requires that extraordinary care be taken in any skin excision. Excision of skin always is extremely conservative, and no tension must be placed on the lower eyelid margin.

On approximately three of four patients I prefer to use the *skin muscle* flap technique. This procedure is particularly suitable for a minimum to a moderate skin excision, giving direct access to the herniated orbital fat and permitting adequate removal of these tissues. The *skin* flap technique is used only on patients who have relatively thin atrophic loose skin hanging in wrinkles or folds, and when a minimum or no herniated orbital fat is to be removed.

The procedure usually is done with the patient under local infiltration anesthesia combined with intravenous sedation. Usually 0.5 percent Xylocaine with 1 to 200,000 epinephrine is used; it is injected into the subcutaneous tissues of the lower eyelid, in those areas where I anticipate that skin incisions or undermining will be necessary. (Orbital nerve blocks are not done.) The injection does not completely anesthetize the orbital fat, and minor discomfort may be felt by the patient when traction is exerted on the orbital fat pads, but this discomfort is obviated largely by intravenous sedation.

The initial incision is made through the skin from a point immediately adjacent to the lateral canthus, and follows a natural skin fold going directly laterally; this position gives a better cosmetic result than an incision made in a downward direction. The distance from the lateral canthus usually is no more than about 0.5 cm, and is even less when there is only fat herniation and minimal looseness of skin. The distance may be greater in patients with considerable looseness of the skin and a weak tarsal plate, in which case more tension will be placed laterally than along the lower eyelid margin. After the incision is made, sharp pointed iris scissors are inserted and a skin flap is elevated along the lower eyelid margin. Using the same curved scissors, the skin incision is made along the lower eyelid margin (Fig. 1). For the optimum cosmetic result this incision should be as close to the follicles of the lashes as possible without damaging them. To get this close it is essential to use curved scissors that follow the natural curvature of the lower eyelid. The incision is slightly beveled towards the lashes, but should be no more than about 1 mm from the lashes themselves.

Next, the remainder of the lower eyelid flap (skin or skin/muscle) is elevated all the way down to the infraorbital ridge, or further when necessary. This is done with fine Metzenbaum scissors. Hemostasis is obtained with gentle electrocoagulation.

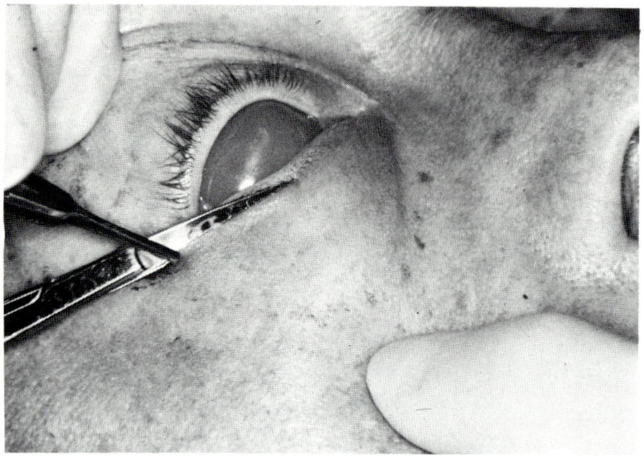

Figure 1.

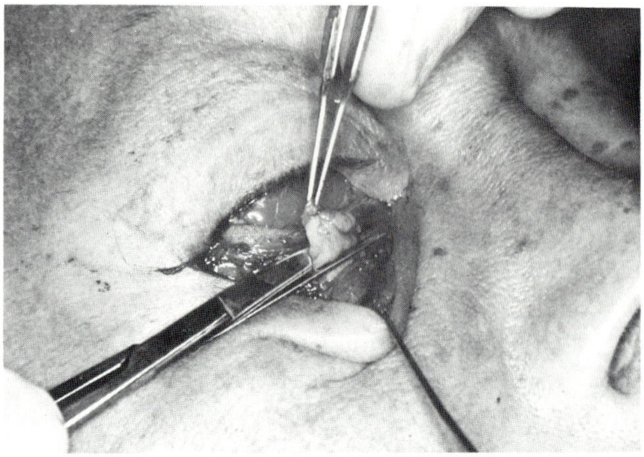

Figure 2.

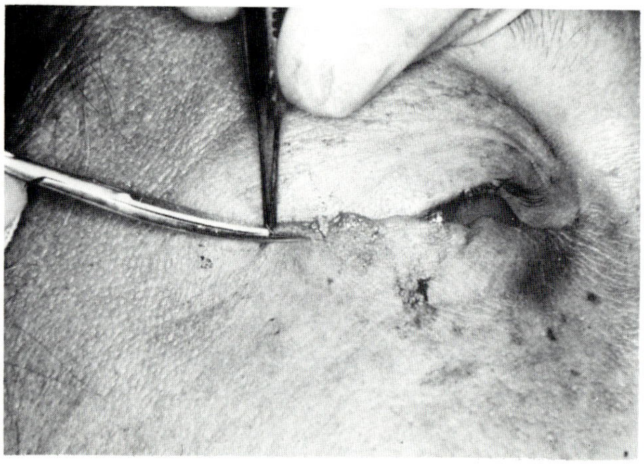

Figure 3.

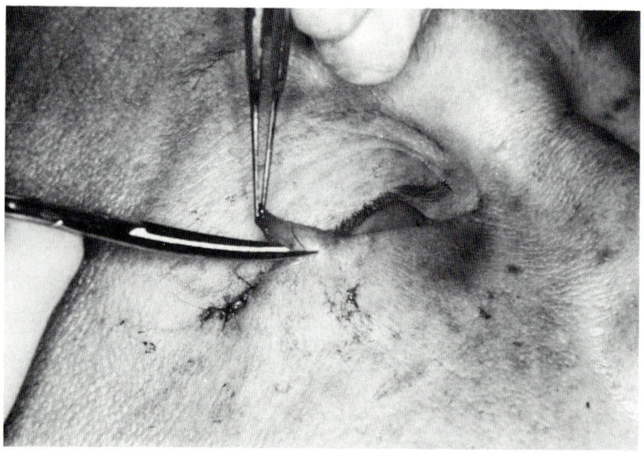

Figure 4.

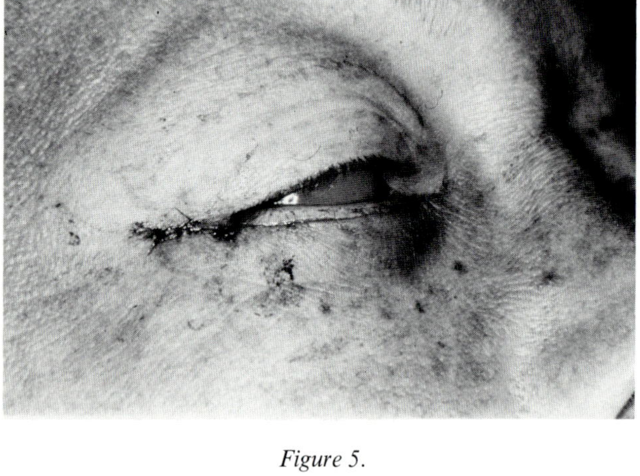

Figure 5.

The flap is retracted, and with gentle pressure on the globe, the area of herniated orbital fat is exposed. The *middle* compartment of fat is the most important, and this is where the orbital septum is opened, and the thin covering of fascia overlying the fatty tissue is opened. These fascial layers should not be excised, because that would cause bleeding. The fatty tissue itself has few blood vessels in it, and can be excised without clamping, ligatures, and/or electrocoagulation. I remove fatty tissue piecemeal, without putting traction on the orbital fat. Each time gentle pressure is exerted on the globe, some excess fat emerges, and this is snipped away with scissors (Fig. 2). By not cutting the fascial layers, bleeding rarely occurs. When there is a small bleeding point, it usually can be readily seen and electrocoagulated with pinpoint cautery.

In the *medial* compartment there frequently is a venous arcade that should be avoided. Only in rare instances is it essential to remove the fatty tissue adjacent to this arcade, and if so, the vessel is electrocoagulated before the fat is removed. I believe that this piecemeal removal of the fatty tissue is a more precise method than the conventional method of exerting pressure on the globe, traction on the orbital fat, clamping an uncertain amount of fat, and then tying it off with a suture.

In the *lateral* compartment, minimal fat is removed; there may be some small vessels that require electrocoagulation.

Next, the flap is advanced superiorly, and a small conservative triangle is excised laterally (Fig. 3). The undersurface of the lower flap is thinned down so that the epithelial edges can be approximated with precision. This part of the incision usually is closed with only two or three fine nonabsorbable interrupted sutures.

After this, the redundancy along the margin of the lower eyelid is resected with curved scissors, again following the contour of the lower eyelid. This is always done conservatively, leaving some excess of skin. It now should be possible to approximate the epithelial edges along the eyelid margin without any tension on the skin flap or the lid. The lower flap is thinned down by excising some of the subcutaneous tissue and muscle along the free border of the flap (Fig. 4). The few bleeding points encountered are cauterized. At this step in the procedure, the thin epithelial flap can be approximated to the eyelid margin. Rarely are any sutures used along the entire margin of the lower eyelid, except beyond the lateral canthus (Fig. 5). The rationale for this is as follows.

1. No sutures are needed since it should not be necessary to pull the epithelial edges together—without tension on the flap and correct trimming there should be sufficient skin to exactly approximate these edges of their own accord.
2. The advancement and position of the lower eyelid flap is maintained by the sutures at the lateral canthus.
3. The initial skin incision along the margin of the lower eyelid is so close to the lashes that it is extremely difficult to suture these flaps together; in any case the incisional wound becomes adherent within several minutes to an hour.
4. This technique, in my experience has led to a better eventual cosmetic result. In addition, there are some *theoretical* advantages to this technique, where there is no suturing along the margin of the lower eyelid.
5. When there is incipient ectropion, the epithelial edges might pull apart slightly without giving rise to a true ectropion.
6. When there is postoperative hemorrhage (which may lead to blindness[2,3]), it seems likely that this blood, rather than accumulating in the retrobulbar space, will drain from the incision line preventing pressure buildup.

Postoperatively no dressings are used, except occasionally a narrow strip of tape is placed from the zygomatic prominence to the forehead lateral to the lateral canthus.

The few sutures lateral to the lateral canthus are removed from 5 to 7 days. By that time the incision line along the margin of the lower eyelid is fixed and well healed. Within a few weeks after the initial surgery, the wound closure along the eyelid margin is hardly noticeable to the naked eye, thus a quick and entirely acceptable cosmetic result is obtained.

References

1. Rees TD, Wood-Smith D: Cosmetic facial surgery. New York, WB Saunders Co., 1973
2. Hueston TJ, Heinze JB: Successful early relief of blindness occurring after blepharoplasty. Plast Reconstr Surg 53:588–592, 1974
3. Hartley JH, Lester JC, Schatten WE: Acute retrobulbar hemorrhage during elective blepharoplasty. Plast Reconstr Surg 52:8–15, 1973

Blepharoplasty as an Office Procedure

F. Mark Rafaty, Palo Alto, Calif. and
Ronald W. Strahan, Los Angeles, California

The ascending spiral of hospital costs in recent years has forced many surgeons to utilize some type of outpatient arrangement, such as an office surgical unit, in performing most of their elective operations. The majority of aesthetic surgical procedures are done under local anesthesia, are performed only on the integumentary system, and are relatively short in duration. Consequently, they can be easily adapted to outpatient surgery.

Modification of aesthetic blepharoplasty to an office procedure has increased its popularity demonstrating its acceptance.

The advantages of performing the operation in the office surgical unit are:

1. The cost to patient is reduced thus making the operation accessible to a greater number of candidates. This is an important factor as most cosmetic operations are not covered by patients' medical insurance policies.
2. Hospital beds are conserved.
3. Significant time is saved for the surgeon in paper work, travelling, hospital visits and rounds thus increasing his productivity.
4. There is greater convenience and privacy for the patients, the majority of whom do not like the hospital environment.
5. There may be possible reduction of hospital-acquired sepsis.

The disadvantages are:

1. Increased initial investment for the purchase of equipment and supplies and greater overhead expenses.
2. Fear of increased medical liability in relation to "the usual and customary practice in the community".[1]

We must draw from the extensive experience of our dental colleagues to show the safety of local procedures in the office. In 1966 the American Society of Oral Surgeons surveyed the experience of 1098 dentists who had reported 3,068,000 office surgical procedures. There was one death per each 1,493,000 patients operated upon under local anesthesia.[2] Williams[1] in 1973 reviewed the literature and reported his own ten-year experience with office plastic surgical procedures performed on 5000 cases. He had no deaths or cardiopulmonary emergencies.

We feel that a qualified surgeon utilizing a well-planned and equipped office surgical unit can perform aesthetic blepharoplasties on properly selected and informed patients and enjoy an efficient and productive practice with few post-operative complications and little or no additional risk of medical liability. This paper describes how!

Preoperative Evaluation of the Patient

The process of patient selection reflects the maturity of the surgeon as a clinician. In the case of office surgery, the surgeon must exercise an even greater degree of discretion. Children and borderline physical and psychological candidates are best done in a hospital operating room.

Patient evaluation begins with the history. The patient's motive for the operation is inquired so that misconceptions are identified and corrected. The patient is questioned regarding any history of cardiopulmonary, renal, hepatic, metabolic, and allergic problems. Particular attention is paid to any history of abnormal bleeding, scarring, and the status of vision.

The physical examination of the patient includes identification of the type of skin, symmetry, status of the periorbital fat pads, extraocular muscles, and the tarsal plates. If the patient has not had an ophthalmological consultation within the preceding six months, one is obtained or, if preferred, visual acuity and fields are checked and recorded by the surgeon using standard eye charts.

Preoperative photographs are important. Anterior full-face, close-up of the eyes, and right and left lateral views are obtained. It is helpful to have the pictures available for reference in the operating room while the patient is in supine position and his preoperative findings are distorted.

A booklet explaining the purpose of the operation with a realistic description of its goals, limitations, and possible complications is given to each patient. The booklet also contains preoperative instructions regarding the method of skin preparation with Phisohex the night before and the morning of surgery, use of medication, time of "NPO," and the need for advance arrangement for patient's transportation after the surgery.

Thirty minutes prior to the operation, five milligrams of diazepam (Valium) is given intramuscularly. An I.V., using a 20 gauge Cathlon IV catheter, is started. During the procedure the patient is titrated with intravenous meperedine in 25 mg increments. Naloxone hydrochloride (Narcan) is drawn up in a syringe to counteract possible untoward effects of meperedine. The patient's pulse is monitored during the surgery. Music is found soothing to the patient and the surgical team.

The availability of emergency equipment is mandatory. The following list contains only the minimum required:

1. Oxygen
2. Suction
3. Ventilation tubes (oral, naso-pharyngeal and endotracheal)
4. Laryngoscope
5. Ambu resuscitation bag and mask
6. Emergency drugs epinephrine, pentobarbital, and naloxone hydrochloride (Narcan)
7. Intravenous fluid (e.g., 5 percent dextrose and lactated Ringer solution)

The Operation

It must be emphasized that only surgeons possessing thorough experience with the procedure should perform the operation in an office set-up.

Any technique of blepharoplasty applicable to the patient's problem may be used. The instruments for blepharoplasty are few and simple. We have found the Concept disposable cautery unit useful. It cuts the herniated fat pads very readily and eliminates the possible danger of retrograde conduction of current to the optic nerve.

The Postoperative Care

At the termination of operation the lids are covered with sterile iced-saline-soaked sponges. Sufficient recovery from the medication is generally noted in one or two hours. A postoperative instruction card for the care of the eyes is given, and the patient is asked to call the office in case of undue pain or swelling. We do not use any postoperative pressure dressing, as we have found them unnecessary. They may also prevent early diagnosis of complications. A companion drives the patient home.

The patient is given an analgesic that does not contain salicylates. The scabs on the incision line are cleaned with hydrogen peroxide twice daily followed by application of an antibiotic eye ointment to the lids. The patient is instructed to keep his head elevated with two pillows for a few days while in bed. Small cellophane sandwich bags filled with ice chips over the lids are comforting and help to reduce edema and ecchymosis. A telephone call to the patient within the first 24 hr after the operation to inquire about pain, swelling, and bleeding reassures him and also strengthens the rapport between the surgeon and the patient. The sutures are removed three or four days later.

Results

In 100 consecutive cases of aesthetic blepharoplasty performed by the authors in their office operating rooms, there were no cardiopulmonary emergencies, major complications or medical liability threats or actions. The following minor complications were observed:

One case of unilateral ectropion secondary to excision of too much skin was discovered in the operating room. It was grafted with excised lid skin with a satisfactory final outcome. A small unilateral hematoma was evacuated by digital pressure after removing several sutures; no secondary repair was necessary. One case of wound dehiscence in the upper lid healed by secondary intention and required revision. Prolonged induration of the lower lids was noted in three cases requiring injection with triamcinolone and produced a satisfactory result. Discoloration was observed in the lower lids bilaterally in one case and lasted over three years. Milia have been encountered frequently in our series probably secondary to our method of skin closure with running locking 6-0 silk suture. The complications of blindness, entropion, misdirection of lashes, permanent epiphora and "dry eye" were not encountered. There were no postoperative infections.

Summary

With proper selection of cases and preoperative counselling, aesthetic blepharoplasty can be performed safely and efficiently by a trained surgeon in an office operating room with less cost and less inconvenience to the patient.

References

1. Williams JE: Plastic surgery in office surgical unit. Plast Reconstr Surg 52:513–519, 1973
2. Driscoll EJ: Anesthesia morbidity and mortality in oral surgery. Amer Soc Oral Surgeons, 48th Annual Meeting, 1966

Postoperative Pressure Dressing Following Blepharoplasty

F. Mark Rafaty and Richard L. Goode, Palo Alto, Calif.

Controversy exists regarding the need for postoperative pressure dressings following comestic blepharoplasty. Recommendations vary from no dressing at all to the use of bulky pressure dressings combined with tarsorrhaphy.[1–10] Proponents of no postoperative bandages maintain that avoidance of pressure on the globes will reduce the likelihood of raising intraorbital pressure, injuring the cornea, plus optimize the early diagnosis of postoperative complications. In addition, some individuals cannot psychologically tolerate coverage of their eyes.

Advocates of postoperative bandages propose that such dressings keep the wounded lids at rest, reducing the amount of discomfort and pain, plus minimize postoperative edema, ecchymosis and bleeding. Basically, it appears that the "non-pressure-dressers" wish to prevent postoperative complications involving vision, while the "pressure-dressers" wish to minimize the trauma of surgery.

Of particular interest in this controversy is the report of DeMere, Wood and Austin in 1974.[11] They sent out 16,000 questionaires to plastic and ophthalmic surgeons and received 3000 replies, representing 98,514 eyelid surgical procedures performed within the preceding year. There were 40 cases of postoperative blindness, an incidence of 0.04 percent. Eighty percent of the surgeons responding used some type of postoperative dressing. The incidence of postoperative blindness did not appear related to the use of dressings. The importance of preoperative ophthalmologic evaluation was stressed to rule out pre-existing visual deficiencies.

Moser, Dippiro, and McCoy[12] sent out questionaires to plastic surgeons in the United States and foreign countries. Twelve cases of blindness following blepharoplasty were reported. They advised the avoidance of pressure dressing which might obscure the early diagnosis of a visual complication.

Jafek and Kreiger[8] describe in detail a case of blindness following blepharoplasty. They used a postoperative pressure dressing of eyepads and Kling roll around the head. When the patient complained of eye pain several hours after surgery, the dressings were removed and periorbital edema, increased intraocular pressure and decreased vision was found. They felt the dressing was noncontributory to the complication.

Hueston and Heinze[6] describe a case of blindness following blepharoplasty using the skin-muscle flap technique under general anesthesia; pressure dressings were used. Postoperatively, the patient complained of pressure without pain in one eye. The bandages were removed 2 hr after surgery and increased intraocular pressure with decreased vision in the one eye was found. This case illustrates that pain is not always present as an early symptom of increased intraocular pressure.

Jarrett and Brockhurst[13] have demonstrated that even a light pressure dressing may cause a transient increase in intraocular pressure up to 50 mm Hg. Whereas, it is difficult to ascertain the role of postoperative pressure dressings in causing visual complications, their use in reducing postoperative edema and ecchymosis should be measurable. This study was undertaken to evaluate the effectiveness of pressure dressings in improving the early postoperative appearance following blepharoplasty.

Materials and Methods

Thirty-three cases of cosmetic blepharoplasty done under local anesthesia (1 percent lidocaine with 1:100,000 epinephrine) were studied. Eighty-five percent of the cases had upper and lower blepharoplasty; fifteen percent had upper blepharoplasty alone. A standard blepharoplasty technique was used[2]; periorbital fat was removed in every case;

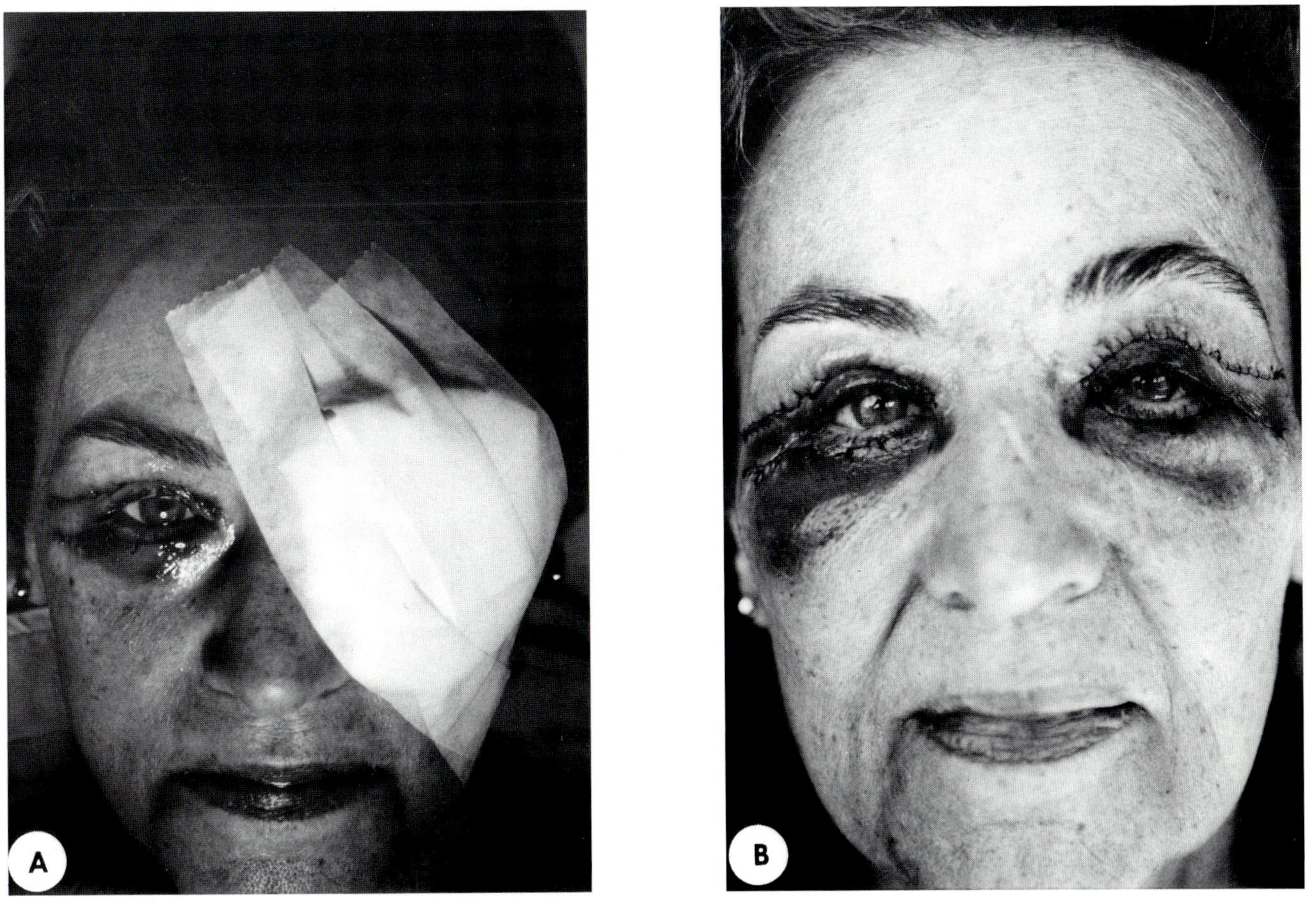

Fig. 1.(A) Immediate postoperative photographs of a patient with a unilateral patch in place. (B) Same patient as Figure 1A immediately after removal of the patch 24 hr following blepharoplasty.

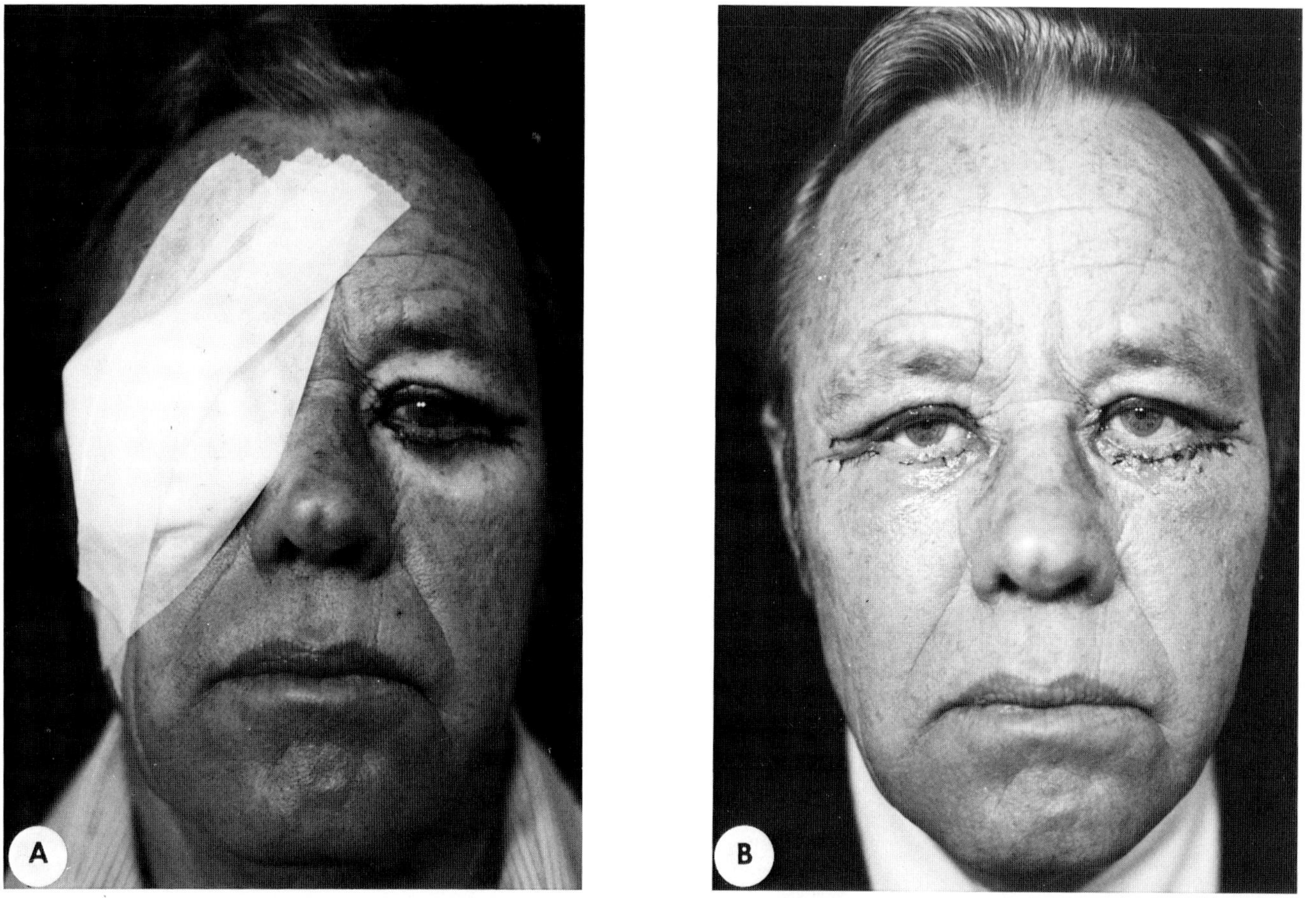

Fig. 2.(A) Immediate postoperative photograph of a patient with a unilateral patch in place. (B) Same patient as Figure 2A 72 hr following blepharoplasty.

the septum orbitale incision was not sutured. Skin incisions were closed with 6-0 silk or nylon and removed 3–4 days later.

At the termination of the operation an antibiotic ophthalmic ointment was applied to the lids of both eyes and a pressure dressing randomly applied to one eye. The dressing consisted of three eyepads placed on the closed lids and held in place with strips of plain or elastic tape stretching from forehead to cheek and exerting mild upward and inward pressure on the globe and periorbital tissues. A closeup color photograph was taken at this time (Figs. 1A and 2A).

The eye dressing was removed 24 hr following surgery and color closeup photographs taken immediately after removal of the dressing (Fig. 1B). Photographs were also taken 48 and 72 hr after the operation (Fig. 2B).

These postoperative photographs were reviewed by two surgeons who had no knowledge of the side of the patch application. They were evaluated as to the amount of edema and ecchymosis present in and around each eye. Three responses were possible in each of the two categories: right eye greater, left eye greater, both eyes equal. Following grading, the code was broken and results tabulated.

Results

The results are summarized in Table 1. In the first 24 hr, edema was *less* in the patched eye in 63 percent of the cases, *more* in the patched eye in 7 percent and equal in 30 percent. Ecchymosis was less in the patched eye in 43 percent, more in the patched eye in 14 percent and equal in 43 percent.

At 48 hr, the patched eye had less edema in 53 percent of cases, more in 10 percent and was equal to the unpatched eye in 55 percent. Ecchymosis in

Table 1. Comparison of the Patched and the Unpatched Eyes for Degree of Edema and Ecchymosis as a function of Time

	Hours Postoperative		
	24 Hr	*48 Hr*	*72 Hr*
Edema			
Patched eye less (% Cases)	63	35	11
Patched eye more (% Cases)	7	10	0
Both eyes equal (% Cases)	30	55	89
Echymosis			
Patched eye less (% Cases)	43	37	22
Patched eye more (% Cases)	14	10	11
Both eyes equal (% Cases)	43	53	67

the patched eye was less in 37 percent, more in 10 percent and equal in 53 percent.

By 72 hr, edema in the patched eye was less in 11 percent and equal in 89 percent. Ecchymosis was less in the patched eye in 22 percent, more in 11 percent and equal in 67 percent. No visual complications occurred.

Discussion

The results of this study imply that the use of a pressure dressing following blepharoplasty reduces edema and ecchymosis for the first 24 hr while the dressing is in place as compared with the unpatched eye. Edema appears more affected than ecchymosis.

At 48 hr, the differences are less marked while by 72 hr the appearance of the two eyes is similar in the majority of cases. The patch appears to have some effectiveness since generally the patched eye looked better than the unpatched eye. However, as can be seen from the data, no difference could be seen between eyes and this percentage increased as a function of postoperative time. The final results appeared unaffected by the use of pressure dressings. The subjective impressions of the patients were quite variable and not analyzed.

The results of this study seem to indicate that the application of a pressure dressing is unnecessary and may prevent early detection of complications.

References

1. Berman WE, Monell CM: Complications in Blepharoplasty and Face-lift Operations, Otolaryng Cl NA 7:87–105, 1974
2. Converse JM: Reconstructive Plastic Surgery, Vol III, W. B. Saunders Co., Philadelphia, 1968
3. Rees TD, Wood-Smith D: Cosmetic Facial Surgery, W. B. Saunders Co., 1973
4. Goldwyn RM: The Unfavorable Results in Plastic Surgery. Little, Brown and Co., Boston, 1972
5. Grabb WC, Smith JW: Plastic Surgery, 2nd Edition, Little, Brown and Co., Boston, 1973
6. Hueston JT, Heinze JB: Successful Early Relief of Blindness Occurring After Blepharoplasty, Plast Reconstr Surg 53:588–592, 1974
7. Lewis JR, Jr: Atlas of Aesthetic Plastic Surgery. Little, Brown and Co., Boston, 1973
8. Jafek BW, Kreiger AE, Morledge D: Blindness following blepharoplasty. Arch Otol 98:366–369, 1973
9. Berry EP: Planning and evaluating blepharoplasty. Plast Reconstr Surg 54:257–262, 1974
10. Farrior RT: Esthetic blepharoplasty. Laryngoscope 81: 848–865, 1971
11. DeMere M, Wood T, Austin W: Eye complications with blepharoplasty and other eyelid surgery. Plast Reconstr Surg 53:634–637, 1974
12. Moser MH, Cipirro E, McCoy FJ: Sudden blindness following blepharoplasty. American Society of Plastic and Reconstructive Surgeons, Las Vegas, Nevada, 1972
13. Jarrett WH, Brockhurst RJ: Unexplained blindness and optic atrophy following retinal detachment surgery. Arch Ophth 73:782–791, 1965

Auricle

Present Day Otoplasty

David Bernstein, New York, N.Y.

Since development of the procedures described in the "ZC Otoplasty Skin Incision"[1] and "Soft Tissue Techniques in Otoplasty"[2] opportunity has been afforded to perform and carefully observe at least an additional one hundred otoplasties for protruding ears and to arrive at more definitive approaches to the operation with particular reference to soft tissue remodeling as well as the very important and customarily emphasized skeletal reconstruction. Historically, once the significance of reconstruction of the antihelix had been realized the next essential step was the concept of antihelical tubing. This led to many questions. By what type of skin incision should we expose the skeletal structures? Are cartilaginous incisions necessary? How much and what type of cartilaginous thinning or cross hatching is necessary to facilitate tubing? What is the best approach to correction of the deep concha and protruding lobule? Shall we use buried nonabsorbable sutures and if so may such vertical or horizontal sutures be depended upon in place of cartilaginous incisions? It appeared for a while that simple buried sutures alone might solve the problem. That more is required is becoming apparent especially in the light of Mustarde's follow-up studies[3] and the experience of others.[4] Most likely any standard technique would be effective in highly expert hands. It would appear necessary, however, to strive for procedures that are more uniformly and generally successful. Perhaps a step by step description of the operation would best illustrate this.

Preliminaries

Age, indications, preoperative photography, premedication, and anesthesia are rather well standardized and require little comment. Preschool age is the optimum time and protrusion of even less than 20 mm may be considered for surgery if the antihelix is poorly formed, conchal depth exceeds one centimeter and the lobule curls outward. Photographs are medical records and should be so treated. They are indispensable, are excellent guides to the needed surgery and to subsequent healing and if sketches are made upon them should not be offered to the patient as an indication of the final result. This, it seems, could constitute a contract which might be difficult to satisfy. In grown patients operated upon under local anesthesia the barbiturates seem to create a greater degree of tractability than the various types of tranquilizers. It has been noted that patients under phenothiazines especially are more often completely out of reach.

Incision

Basically an incision should afford ready exposure and should be amenable to proper closure. A simple ellipse leads to straight line closure in what is essentially a crescentic topography. The bilateral dumb bell incision should produce more flattening above and below but again if the ends are rounded dog ears could be difficult to control. The ZC incision shown in Fig. 1 has therefore been uniformly employed inasmuch as it conforms to the shape of the auricle and its Z ends facilitate uncomplicated closure. It is readily adaptable to any extent of skin excision which may be required, avoids distortion of the occipito-aural sulcus and it is very simple to begin by excising less than appears necessary and to adjust the flap at the end of the operation when finally closing the skin. This type of closure is seen in Fig. 2.

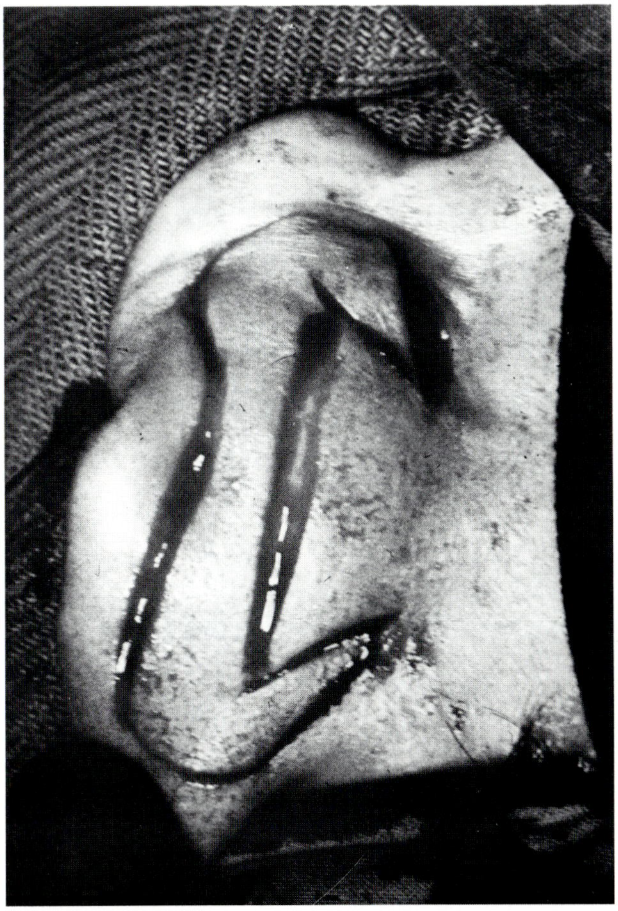

Fig. 1. ZC Otoplasty Skin Incision. Note the terminal Z's and the general C shape corresponding to the pinna.

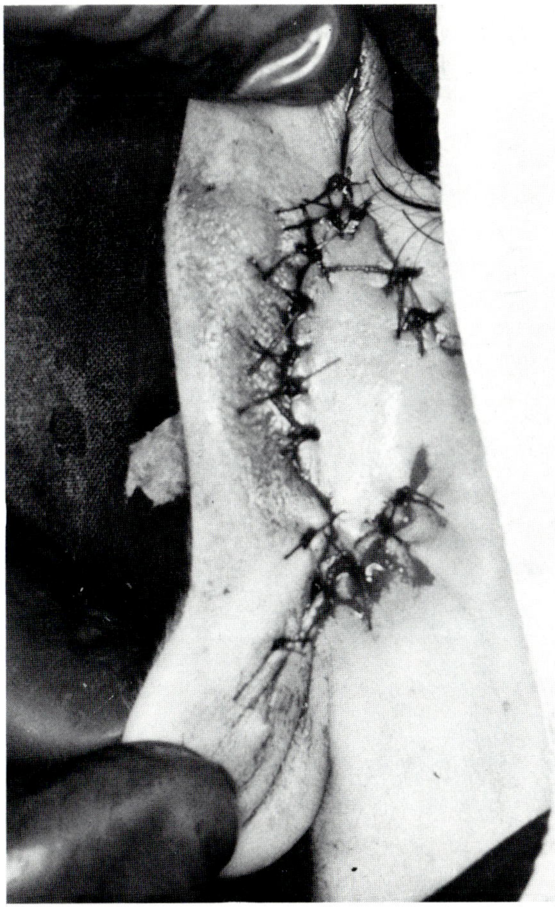

Fig. 2. Skin closure of the ZC incision is shown. Dog ears, puckering and distortion are readily controlled.

Cartilaginous Incisions

Rarely have protruding ears been encountered to my observation in which cartilaginous incisions are not required and even when they would appear to be unnecessary it would still be better to fashion such incisions since they give greater assurance of a permanent result. This incision is basically an inverted U as seen in Fig. 3. Its helical component follows the outline of the skin incision leaving a suitable margin of helical cartilage at the rim. It extends around the superior pole high enough to be covered by the downward curl of the upper part of the helix and then downward just in front of the inferior crus describing a crescent in the concha following the outlines of the new antihelix. Both the anterior and posterior ends of the lower poles of the incision extend parallel to one another. They are not connected below whereas the upper part of the incision is connected as in an upside down U. Once having made the incision its edges are elevated for a distance of two to three millimeters to encourage tubing. The body of the antihelix below may be completely elevated. This is never required in dealing with the superior crus since this region is normally much flatter. Thinning of the cartilage may be done by dermabrasion techniques or by means of a No. 15 blade which would appear to be preferable. Perichondrium along the line of the projected antihelix is readily removed with the scalpel and the underlying cartilage is thinned as much as is necessary. It has been possible by this method to effectively reduce the thickness of even pathologically calcified cartilage encountered in a recent operation.

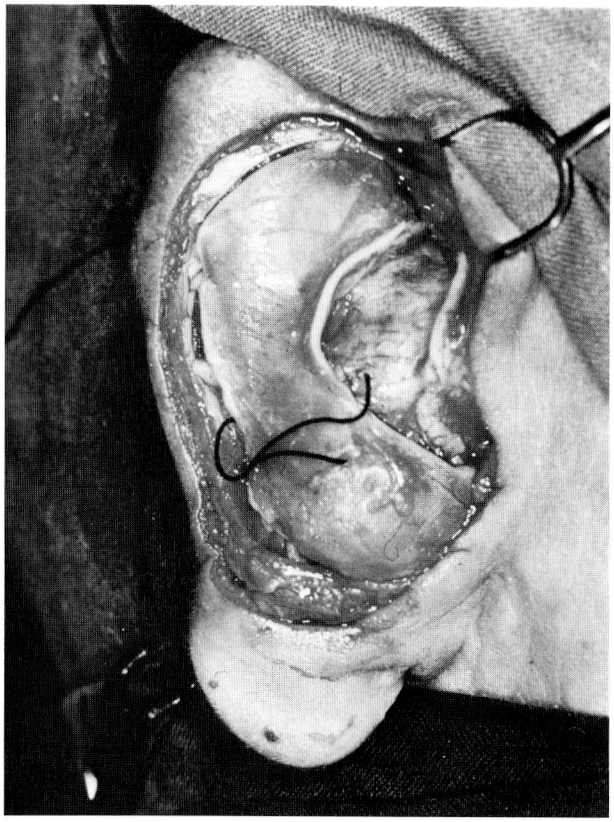

Fig. 3. The inverted U cartilaginous incision, conchal resection and horizontal mattress guide sutures are visualized.

Cartilage Excision

Should cartilage be excised? The answer must be yes based on this experience. Cross-hatching and related procedures have not been satisfactory. It often shows through the skin and does not seem to accomplish what is attainable by a proper resection. This is necessary in at least two areas. A conchal crescent generally very small is removed depending upon the extent of protrusion when the ear is folded back. This reduces conchal depth and gives greater assurance of permanent retroposition. Figure 3 illustrates this type of excision. Partial resection of antitragal cartilage is perhaps the most effective way to correct lobular protrusion. This is a situation not unlike nasal tip reconstruction in rhinoplasty. Once all other areas of the pinna have been repositioned the lobule, unless corrected, becomes very conspicuous. Cutaneous W and similar operations are seldom required and may easily be combined with antitragal resection.

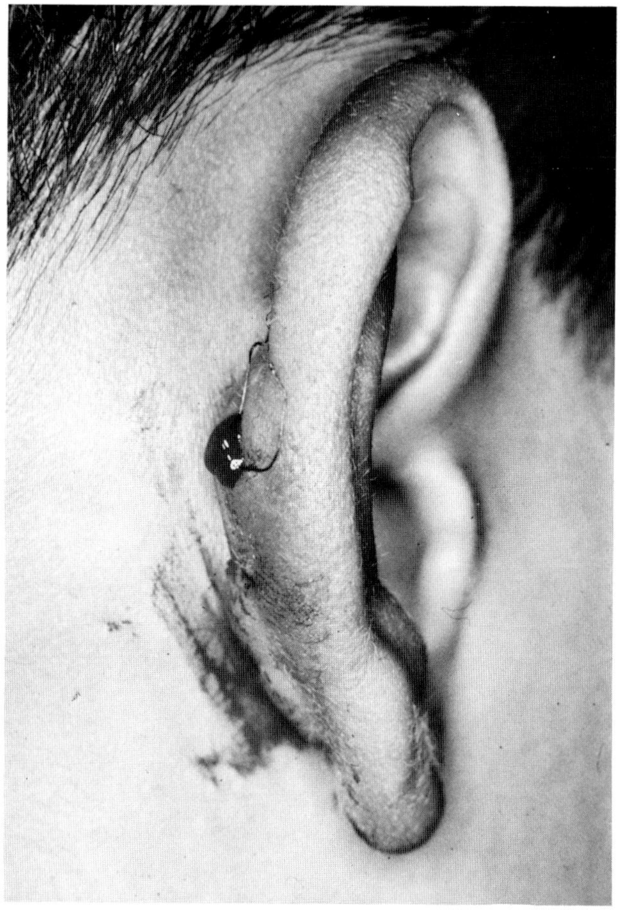

Fig. 4. Extrusion of a non absorbable suture is evident as is recurrence of protrusion. Absorbable vertical cartilaginous mattress sutures reinforced by external horizontal nonabsorbable removable sutures prevent this.

Cartilage Suturing

Once the skeletal structures have been properly fashioned the question of suturing arises. The non absorbable buried suture technique was employed briefly using vertical mattress sutures. In Fig. 3 horizontal mattress sutures are seen. They were often placed as a guide for the vertical sutures. This created a satisfactory tube but sometimes produced the result seen in Fig. 4. The suture after several months is extruding and the ear is protruding. A combined technique has since been employed. Vertical absorbable mattress sutures are placed being sure to encompass the entire thickness of cartilage. No reactions have been noted. As many sutures as are necessary may be employed. The number of sutures is not as important as the

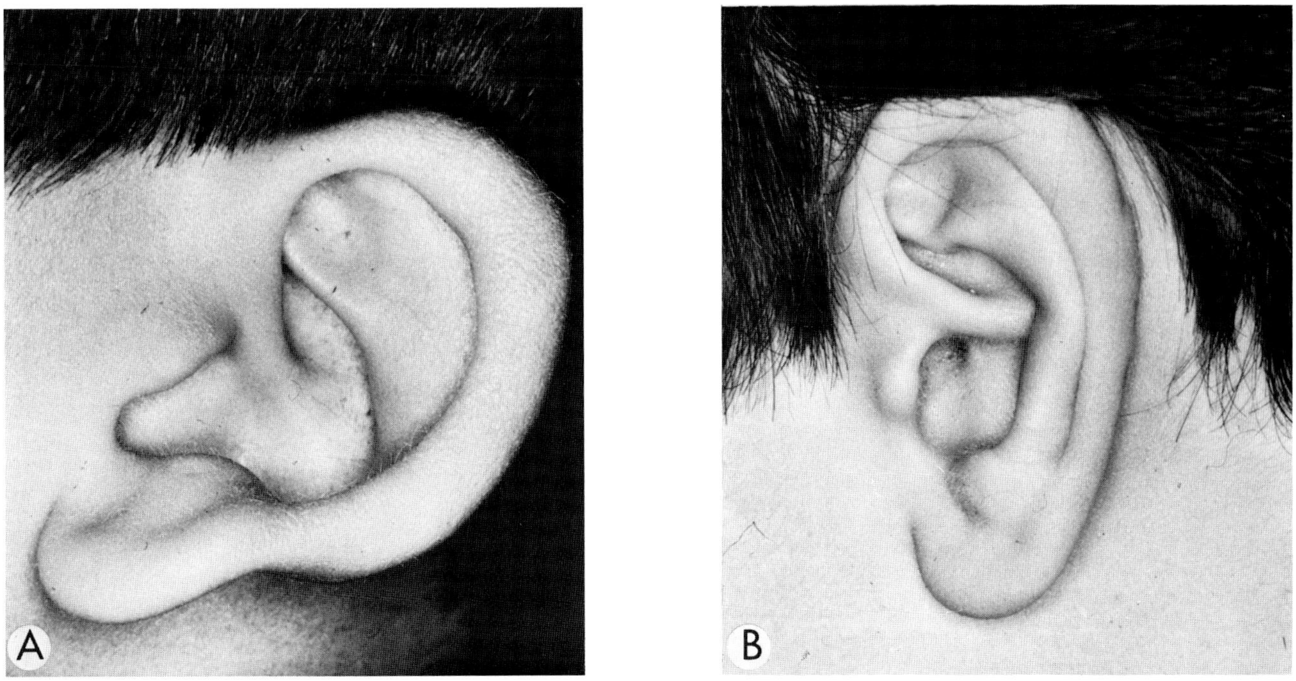

Fig. 5. (A) Severe auricular and lobular protrusion with a poorly formed antihelix is noted preoperatively. (B) Postoperative photograph of the patient in Fig. 5(A) Symmetry has been attained employing the surgical approach described. Conchal depth has been corrected, the ear is properly retropositioned and the lobule is in line with the pinna.

extent to which the cartilage is rolled back. They may be placed as high or as low as is necessary and tied under sufficient tension to create a more prominent tube below than above.

Closure

This is a double procedure. Non absorbable horizontal mattress sutures are placed through skin, cartilaginous tube, and skin again and tied over bolsters. Interrupted postaural sutures are inserted somewhat obliquely being somewhat higher posteriorly than anteriorly in order to keep the pinna from appearing to sag downward and backward. This would be difficult to accomplish with continuous subcuticular sutures. All crevices anteriorly are filled with moist rolled cotton, ample fluffs are used and bandaging should be just firm enough to discourage hematoma formation.

Results

An unusually prominent protruding ear is seen in Fig. 5A. Antihelices are poorly formed and the lobule is badly distorted and protrudes markedly. The method described produced a properly retropositioned ear seen in Fig. 5B, the lobule being placed in a symmetrical position. This is characteristic of the results obtained. There have been no infections, hematomas or unusual postoperative bleeding. Keloids have not been noted. Where one might have been anticipated the operation was done under intralesional steroid and antibiotic coverage. Telephone ears and similar distortions have not been encountered. In an occasional instance the tube if not made wide enough has produced a small degree of sharpness which must be counterbalanced against too wide a tube producing an unduly prominent antihelix.

References

1. Bernstein D: ZC otoplasty skin incision. Arch Otolaryngol 86:87–90, 1967
2. Bernstein D: Soft Tissue techniques in otoplasty. The Eye, Ear, Nose and Throat Monthly. 48:283–288, 1969
3. Mustarde JC: Treatment of prominent ears by buried mattress sutures ten year summary. Plast Reconstr Surg 39: 382–85, 1967
4. Farrior RT: Otoplasty: surgery for protruding ears Chap 30, Vol 3. Otolaryngology, Hagerstown, Maryland New York London, Harper and Row, pp. 1–23, 1974

General

Adjunctive Offerings with Rhinoplasty

Robert L. Simons, N. Miami Beach, Fl.

The patient seeking consultation for rhinoplasty is actually asking "How can I look better?". To fully answer that question the surgeon must consider many facial features besides the nose. Naturally prominent in position, the nose is only beautiful when it does not stand apart from the rest of the face. The nose must agree with the other bony and soft tissue features such as eyes, lips, forehead and chin. For true facial beauty rests in the dynamic harmony of component parts.

It is not difficult to graphically visualize the difference in nasal appearance effected by changing surrounding components. The weakened chin in the center gives a shortened, more projected appearance to the nasal profile (Fig. 1). A long, sloping forehead with a shallow nasofrontal angle adds length and prominence to the nose. A combination of these factors turns a basically attractive nose into the snout of an inferior physiognomy.

And yet, how often does the patient on the right walk into your office requesting that something be done about her nose. It is during moments of truth, such as these, that it is essential to realize that without harmony there is no beauty.

To establish this harmonious relationship the surgeon must frequently go beyond the sole performance of a rhinoplasty. He must concern himself with dentition, the relative position of maxilla to mandible, the aging process of the skin and the proper use of makeup and hairstyling.

Though not necessarily practicing all disciplines, the complete rhinoplastic surgeon is aware and knowledgable of the work of the orthodontist, the oral surgeon, the prosthodontist, the facial cosmetic surgeon, and the cosmetologist. Each of these specialists offers adjunctive aids to rhinoplasty.

Treatment of the patient begins with an honest analysis of the problem. The exercise of rating an entrant's overall appearance has merit. It hopefully quells the surgical fantasy that one can transform a Class IV toad into a Class I princess merely by a simple maneuver with the operative wand. As surgical experience has repeatedly taught, it is difficult enough to assure an orderly advancement up the scale of beauty let alone promise a jump in Class

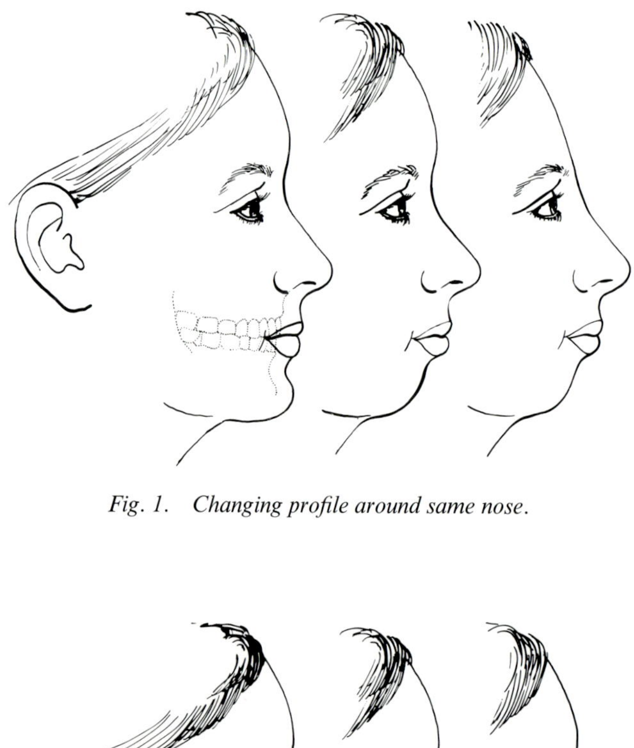

Fig. 1. Changing profile around same nose.

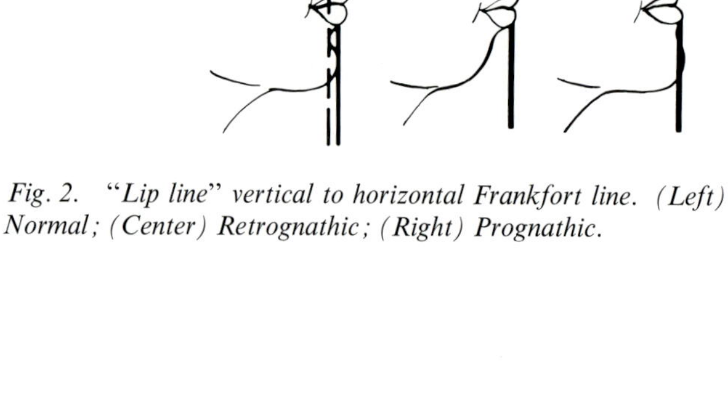

Fig. 2. "Lip line" vertical to horizontal Frankfort line. (Left) Normal; (Center) Retrognathic; (Right) Prognathic.

standing. Indeed, if one is fortunate enough to effect a dramatic change in appearance it is generally not through a rhinoplasty alone.

In our experience approximately 25 percent of the patients presenting for rhinoplasty are in need of chin refinement.

Of more practical interest is the frequency with which patients ignore the chin deficiency. Less than 2 percent of all potential candidates request chin correction and therefore, the procedure must often be suggested and "sold" to the patient. To successfully cope with this imbalance between need and patient awareness or demand, the procedure offered must not measurably increase the operative time, the postoperative morbidity or financial cost of the primary rhinoplasty.

Many determinants have been employed for evaluating the need for chin augmentation. We have found the method recommended by Rish, the simplest and most effective. On profile photography with the Frankfort horizontal line properly parallel to the floor, drop a vertical line from the lower lip. If the chin does not reach the "lip line" consider the need for chin augmentation (Fig. 2).

The best method of correction is still unsettled. The variety of presentations at this meeting alone provides evidence of the continuing circle of controversy over this subject.

For the past 10 years we have been generally satisfied using the preformed Safian silastic chin implants placed extraorally.

With the patient in the supine position the chin is marked in the following manner (Fig. 3A–D).

A small submental incision is made, the periosteum incised, the subperiosteal pocket created and with guide sutures to lead the way the implant positioned. Proper centering is aided by visualization of the implant notch in the midline.

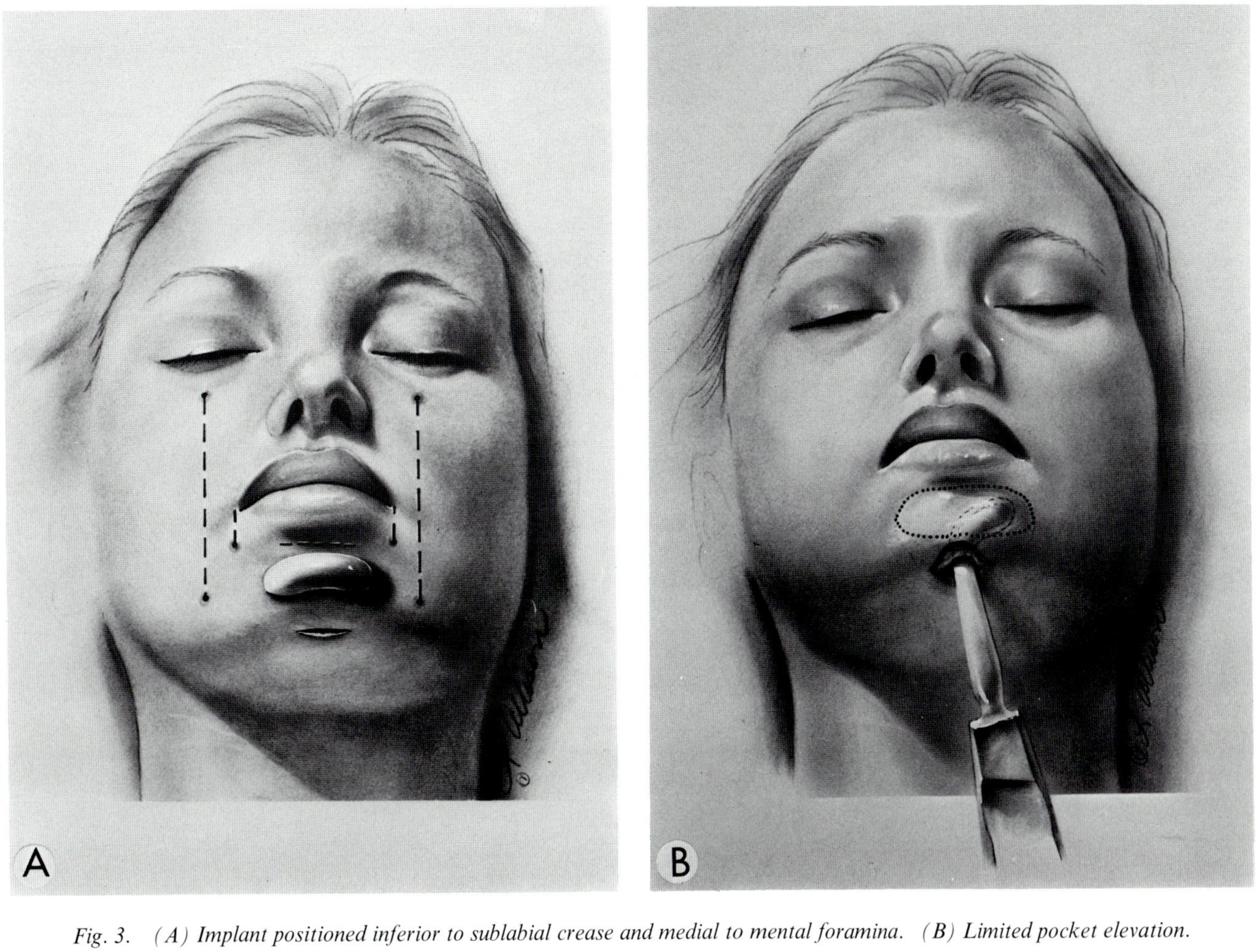

Fig. 3. (A) Implant positioned inferior to sublabial crease and medial to mental foramina. (B) Limited pocket elevation.

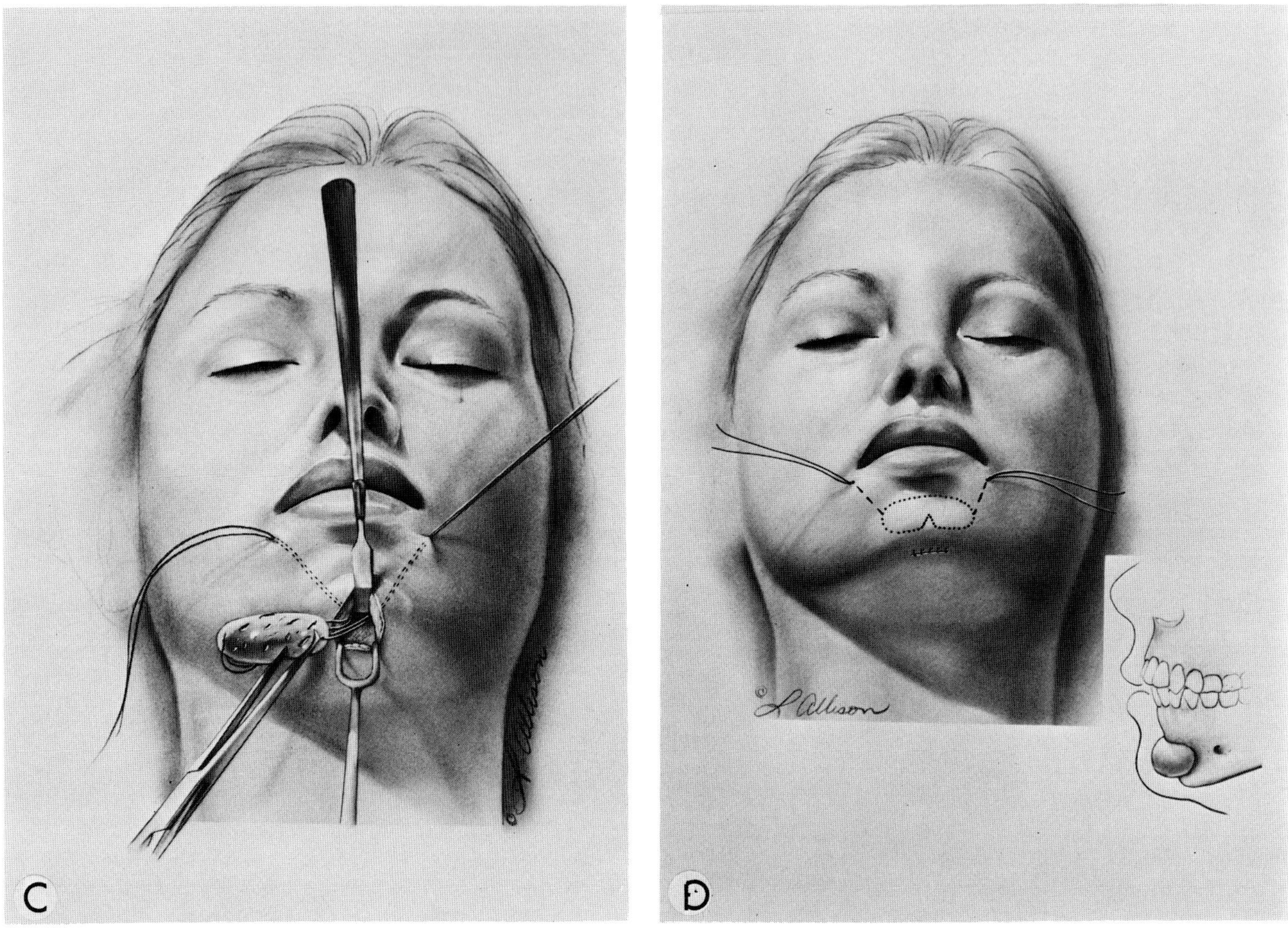

Fig. 3. (C) Positioning of implant with guide sutures. (D) Centering of notched implant.

We prefer performing the mentoplasty prior to the rhinoplasty for reasons of sterility as well as aesthetic planning. The value of this combined procedure is a repeated phenomenon (Fig. 4A–D).

In less frequent instances, our concern with mentoplasty involves the reduction rather than augmentation of the chin.

The majority of patients with prominence of the chin have total overgrowth of the mandible with an occlusion characterized by an anterior or mesial positioning of the lower dentition relative to the upper and are truly prognathic. This group, in order to gain better masticatory function and cosmetic appearance is best treated by mandibular osteotomies and repositioning of the mandible.

However, a small number of these patients in whom overgrowth has not progressed sufficiently to produce marked forward displacement of the mandibular arch are amenable to symphysical surgery for aesthetic improvement.

In these cases a degloving incision is used to expose the mandibular prominence. With Striker saws the anterior third of the mandible is removed as shown in the following manner (Fig. 5A–E).

This operation can be performed in conjunction with a rhinoplasty or staged in separate procedures. The fact that it adds little to the postoperative morbidity makes it a worthwhile adjunctive offering with rhinoplasty.

In the treatment of patients with facial disharmony, evaluation of the dental occlusion is of primary importance in the selection of the appropriate mode of therapy.

If occlusion is unacceptable one must consider the need for either conservative or surgical orthodontics.

When the patient recognizes and agrees with the need for extensive orthodontia with the prospect of orthodonic appliances for 12 to 24 months, defer the nasal surgery until the teeth have been aligned.

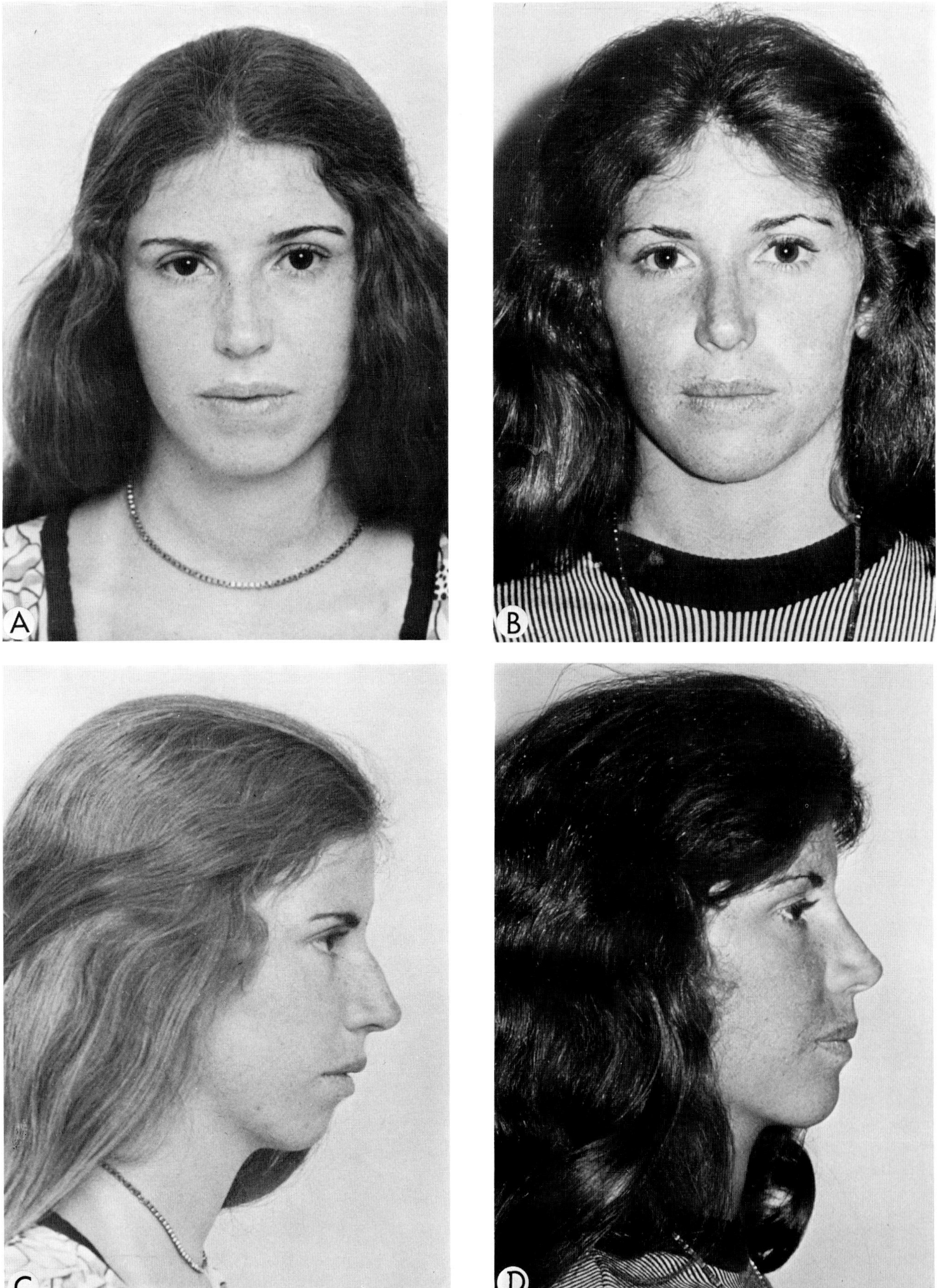

Fig. 4. (A) Preoperative frontal view. (B) Postoperative frontal view combined procedure. (C) Preoperative lateral view. (D) Postoperative lateral view combined procedure.

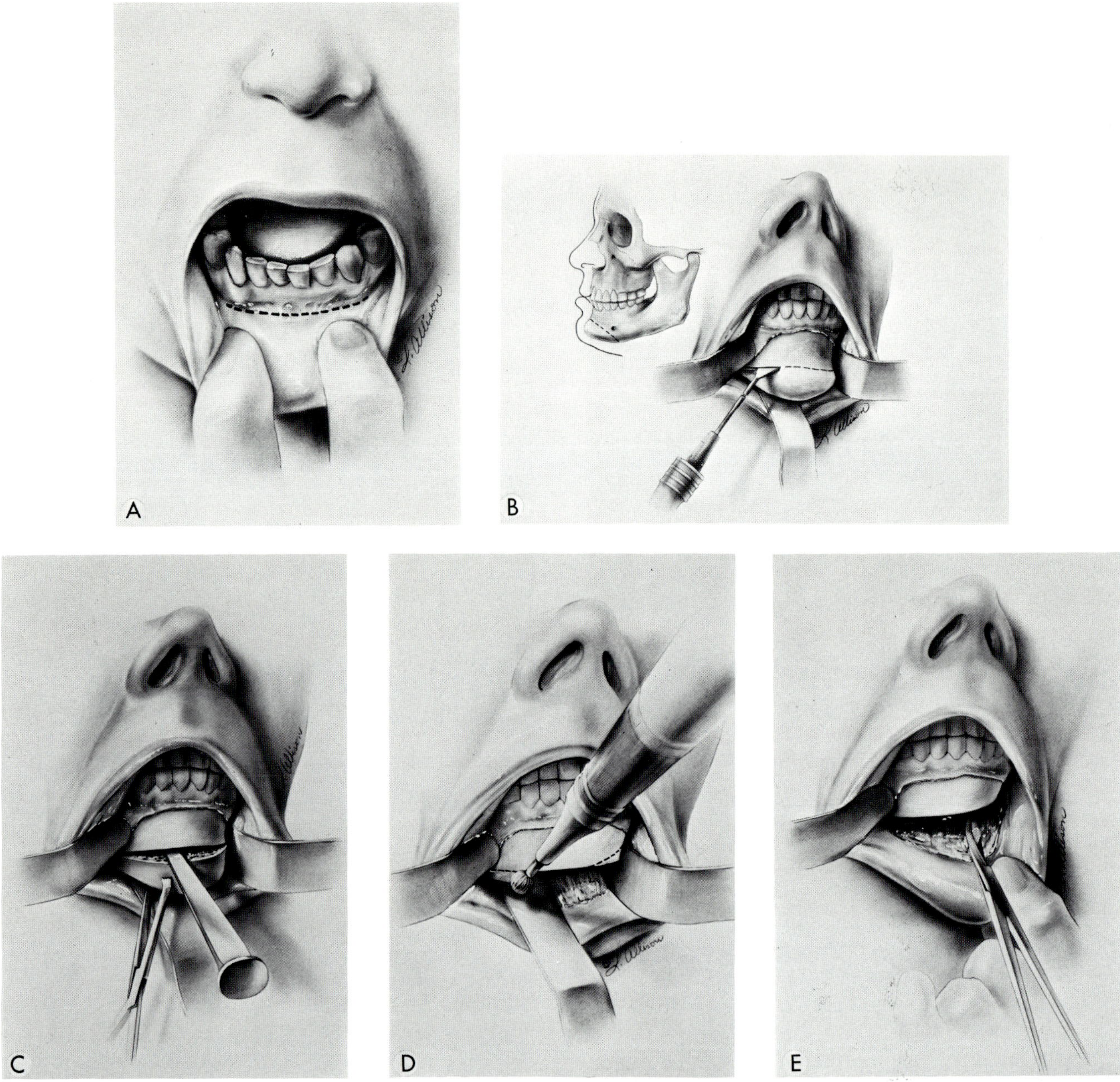

Fig. 5. (A) Buccal incision extending from canine teeth. (B) Ostectomy started with Stryker saw. (C) Ostectomy completed with osteotomies. (D) Rounding of square edges. (E) Trimming hypertrophied mentalis muscle.

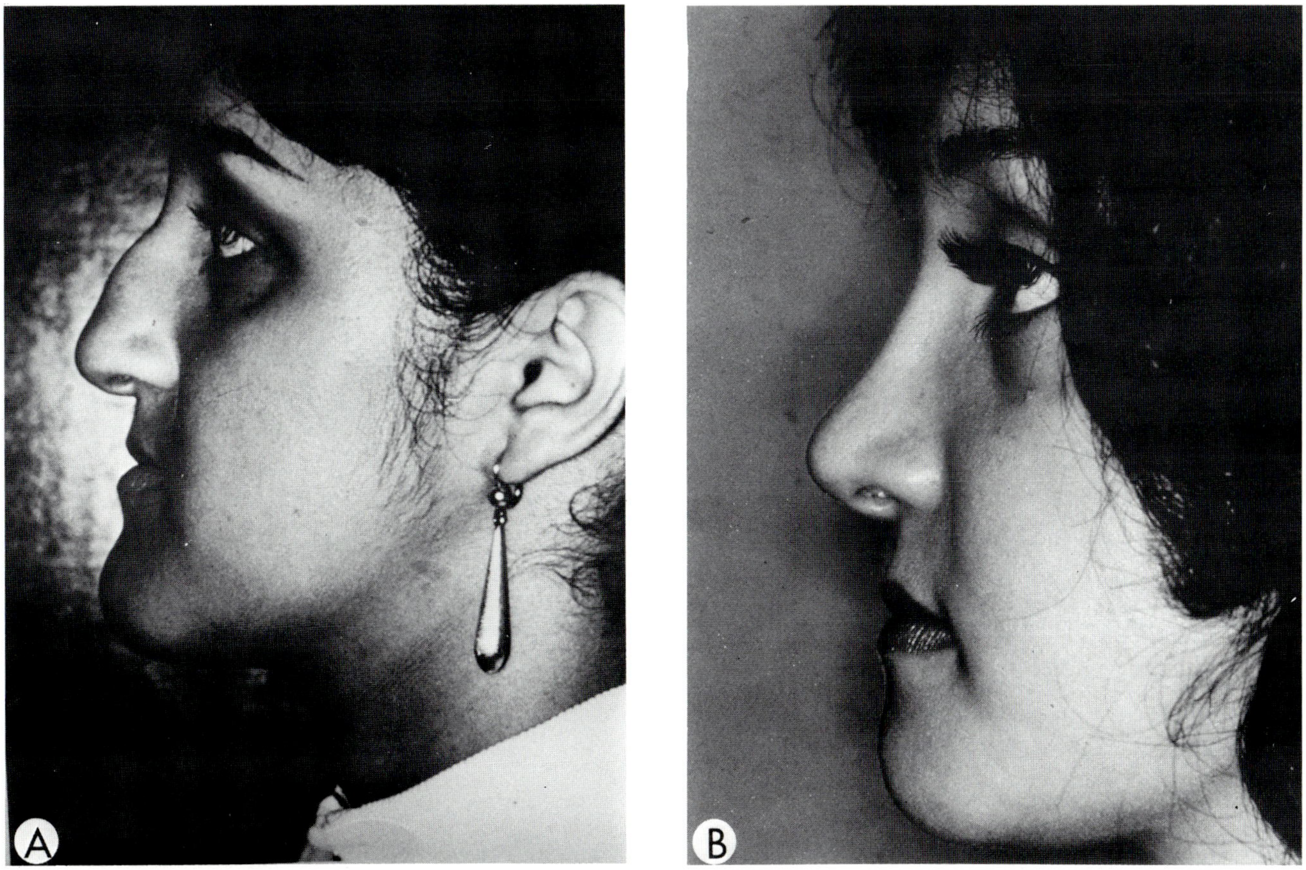

Fig. 6. (A) Preoperative lateral view. (B) Postoperative lateral view.

This will allow for a more accurate judgment for positioning of the nose in relationship to the lower third of the face.

When significant skeletal disharmony exists with unacceptable occlusion, then oral surgical intervention is required.

The extent of the procedure and postoperative morbidity attendant with a LaFort I or II correction of a hypoplastic maxilla or a parasagital osteotomy repair of a prognathic mandible is beyond the criteria of true adjunctive offerings in rhinoplasty.

Yet, we should familiarize ourselves with the aims and abilities of the orthognathic surgeon for interdisciplinary teamwork is often the correct answer to the patients' problems.

In this patient a correct reading of the preopcephlagram revealed maxillary hypoplasia with a relative pseudoprognathism accentuated by the focal hypertrophy of the symphysis (Fig. 6 A & B).

Proper correction required a LaFort I procedure for maxillary advancement to correct the mid-third weakness prior to rhinoplasty and a subapical horizontal mandibular ostectomy.

Nasal projection depends upon good maxillary support. In the elderly individual with loss of teeth and alveolar resorption, nasal support is lost and the nose "lengthens." Replacement of absent or defective teeth with proper dentures will improve lip posture and help to combat the drooping, elongated nasal profile in the elderly.

The prosthedontist can further help to overcome poor nasal projection due to maxillary hypoplasia by creating removable prosthetic devices to augment deficient malar, pyriform aperture or premaxillary areas.

As most rhinoplastic surgeons have learned, the illusion of tip projection is further achieved by augmenting an acute nasal labial angle or retracted columella with cartilage or bone grafts (Fig. 7A–D).

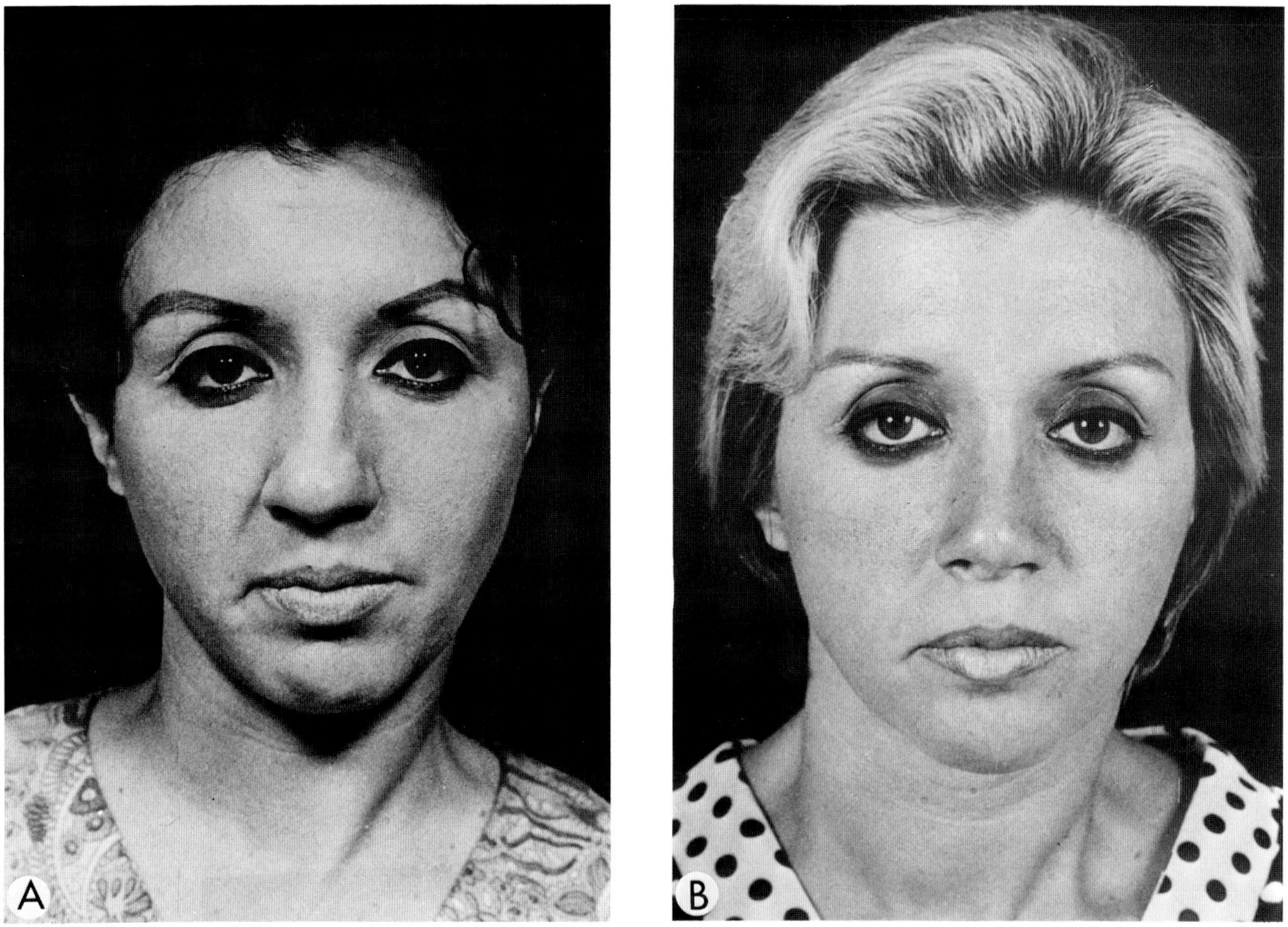

Fig. 7. (A) Preoperative frontal view. (B) Postoperative frontal view combined procedure with columella batten.

Not infrequently the woman who undergoes a rhinoplasty returns a month later with a new hairstyle or coloring. Sudden attention to hair, makeup and dress seem appropriate with the patients recent investment in facial appearance.

A successful rhinoplasty is generally hidden from surgical appraisal, allowing the patient to smile comfortably over friendly compliments about her new hairdo, eye shadow, or weight loss. Cosmetics provide the means for enhancing beauty. They are not a substitute for good surgery or intended to camouflage poor operative work. A knowledge of their use however, can frequently embellish a good job, cheer an unreasonably depressed recent postoperative patient, and go beyond the surgical limits in providing aesthetic facial improvement.

Proper hairstyling or wigs can hide foreheads with shallow nasal frontal angles. A new length or shape of the hair can transform square, triangular or round facial form into the more desirable oval configuration. For men, beards and moustaches provide relief from weak chins and recessed middle third and facial features.

Beauty is frequently an illusion of highlights and shadows tastefully created with makeup. Dark colors will subtly shadow to create a hollowing effect. Lighter shades will highlight or offset recessed features.

Thus, a wide, flat nose may be "narrowed" and "heightened" by darkening the nasofacial grooves, a shallow naso-frontal angle "deepened" with shadowing, and a crooked nose "straightened" with a highlight down the center of the dorsum.

Most cosmetologists believe the major focus in facial beauty rests within the eyes. Attention must be given to proper shadowing, the use of artificial lashes, eyeliner, and mascara.

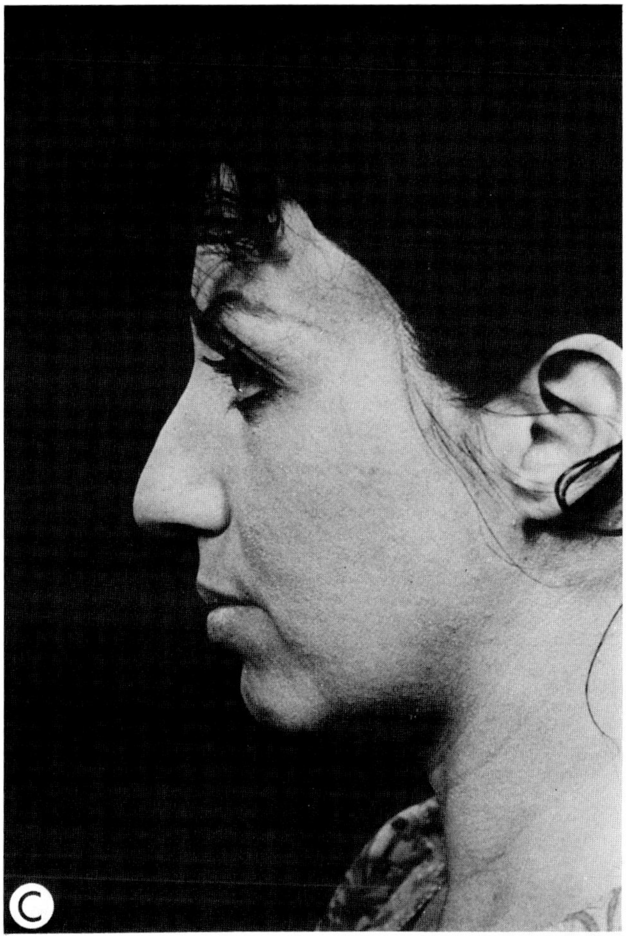

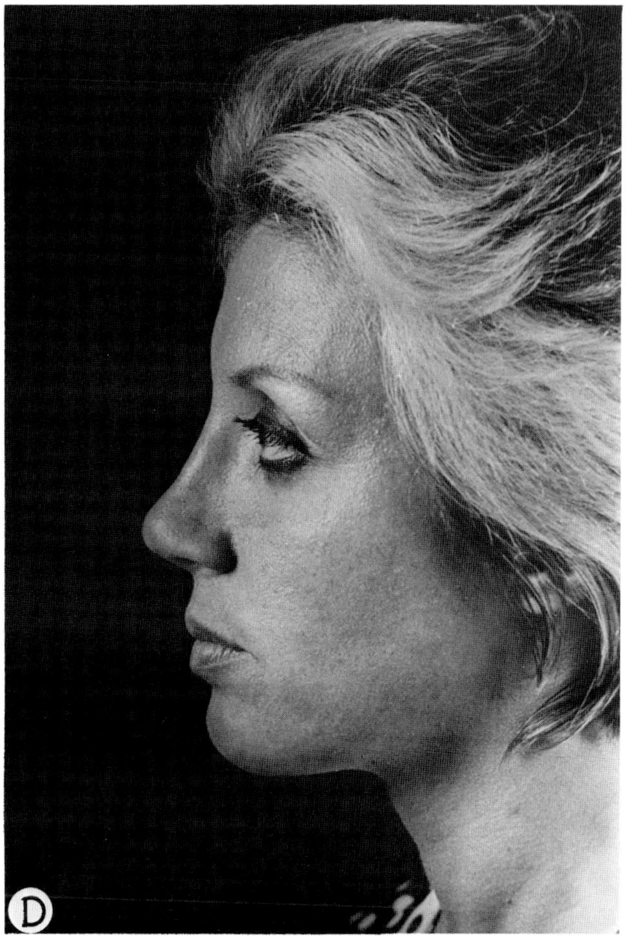

Fig. 7. (C) Preoperative lateral view. (D) Postoperative lateral view combined procedure with columella batten.

The cosmetic needs of each patient will vary as greatly as their backgrounds of involvement or interest with the subject. Few, however, will not appreciate or benefit from a postoperative consultation with a reliable beautician or cosmetologist.

When cosmetics fail to hide their wrinkles or their application becomes increasingly difficult, the patient may first consider the need for some form of rhytidectomy.

It is well recognized that a modified rhinoplasty or mere shortening of the nose along with the face lift will enhance the total effect of facial rejuvenation in the elderly patient. Conversely, the rhinoplasty patient will often benefit from revitalization of the eyes through blepharoplasty or brow lift procedures. Deep nasal labial folds that add to nasal length can be ameliorated with rhytidoplasty.

The rhinoplasty may be performed in conjunction with the blepharoplasty, brow lift and/or face lift.

Summary

Modern day rhinoplasty demands more than a plan for a new nose. It requires consideration of the individual in terms of a new facial image.

Frequently facial disharmonies can be corrected with relatively simple procedures that will be readily accepted by the patient and in the long run aid that person in attaining a happier and more satisfying rhinoplastic experience.

Wound Healing—A Brief Review

Bernard H. Cohen, Leonard A. Lewis, and Sorrel S. Resnik, Miami, Fla.

The skin of a normal adult is about eight pounds and twenty square feet of activity and complexity. It is a mechanical, chemical and thermal protective device. It contains a complete immunologic and microbial defense system; and, can regulate body temperature through an integrated system of sweat glands and blood vessels as complex as the kidney. Amazingly, about one square inch of each fingertip is the basis of an international identification system of which no two individuals are exactly alike. Not only is the skin simultaneously stretchable and shrink resistant; but it is waterproof, shockproof, and antimagnetic.

This paper will describe the skin's response to surgical manipulation. It is not intended to be innovative in context, nor totally comprehensive in scope. It is, rather, a brief review intended to remind and perhaps reeducate the practicing cutaneous surgeon about the basic principles of wound healing.

The Phases of Wound Healing

When the skin is cut to its full depth, the edges separate, blood vessels spill their contents into the defect, cellular elements along the margins are either traumatized or destroyed, and the base of the wound is opened wide to contamination. At this juncture, Phase No. 1 (The Substrate or Lag Phase) becomes operative. A vascular system of arterioles and venules after initial vasoconstriction, vasodilates and becomes permeable with resultant exudation. Platelets aggregate on the vessel with the formation of fibrin and subsequent clot. Simultaneously, a cellular system of leukocyts and erythrocyts adheres to the vessel wall. Mast cells elaborate histamine while factors such as chemotaxin and leukotaxin are already present at the site of damage. As evaporation follows, a fibrin clot forms. This clot will serve to seal off the vessels, protect against further microbial contamination and provide the framework for future activity.

As the clot retracts, the fibrin becomes oriented and mesenchymal undifferentiated cells become migratory fibroblasts. By the end of the second day, the histiocytes have removed much of the necrotic debris and particulate elements in the fresh clot.

Two major events now happen as Phase No. 2 (The Proliferative Phase) commences: (1) In the depths of the wound, contraction. (2) On the surface of the wound, migration of epithelium. About the fourth day, fibroblasts migrate out along the fibrin scaffold and deposit collagen. The endothelium of the cut vessels begins to bud and form granulation tissue, elaborating plasmogen which dissolves fibrin in its path. The wound, if its edges are agape, begins to contract and continues to decrease in size at the rate of approximately 0.5 to 1.0 mm per day. At the same time, surface epithelium has already advanced from both edges as well as from cut hair follicles. This epidermis methodically cleaves a path beneath the dried crust by elaborating enzymes. By the end of Phase No. 2, the wound has completely epithelized, the scab has been shed, and fresh collagen is well on its way to developing.

By the 21st day, Phase No. 3 (The Remodeling Phase) begins. Over the next few months, the wound approaches its maximal tensile strength by reshaping and realigning its collagen. The proportion of insoluble to soluble collagen increases while collagen synthesis proceeds. Eventually a mature scar results. This state of "maturity" unfortunately never quite approaches the breaking strength of the original intact skin.

Regeneration and Repair

The type of wound healing that has just been described is called *repair*. However, wound healing in its broadest sense, involves both *regeneration and*

Table 1. Factors Influencing the Healing Process

1. Mechanical
2. Humidity and Climate
3. Oxygen Tension
4. Injection
5. Health, Age, Nutrition
6. Steroids and Toxins

repair. The basis of their difference is that of damage depth. Regeneration is the result of superficial damage and results in complete restitution of appearance and function. Surgical wounds that heal by regeneration are classically dermabrasion, acid peeling, superficial freezing and superficial burning. Repair is the result of deeper damage. It results in scar formation and a basic architectural distortion from the original. The surgical wounds which heal by repair are classically primary, secondary, and tertiary skin closures, plus skin grafts. In each of the surgical procedures above, the surgeon is still obliged to deal with multiple factors which will influence the rapidity of the healing process and the final cosmetic result. (See Table No. 1.)

Mechanical Factors

The mechanical factors most often considered in wound healing are basically three: (1) The placement and direction of the scar. (2) The concept of tensile and breaking strength. (3) Wound contraction and remodeling.

Incision lines are designed to create minimal tension on the wound edge and are placed in locations to render them as cosmetically inconspicuous as possible. Wrinkle lines and Langer's lines, for practical purposes, are essentially the same; their direction being at right angles to the underlying muscle. Landmark lines or contour lines such as lip margins, eyebrow margins, angle of jaw, etc. are also successfully used.

Tensile strength and breaking strength are terms which often create more confusion than they do enlightenment. *Tensile strength* is the force or load applied on both wound edges expressed in weight/square area (length of interface × depth of interface). On the contrary, *breaking strength* is simply the force needed to separate a wound, without consideration of cross-sectional area. It should become obvious that variations in skin thickness and length of incision can account for the discrepancy in tensile versus breaking strength of any particular wound. In addition, the speed at which the force is applied to the wound edge will determine the amount of stretch that preceeds the final measurement of tensile and/or breaking strength. This ability of the skin to stretch is called *extensibility* and varies with anatomic location, age, and many other obscure factors. This property (extensibility) must also be considered when characterizing the mechanical properties of a wound.

Wound contraction, as seen in healing by secondary intention, is not the result of *new* tissue formation, but rather the movement of *existing* tissue. If a full-thickness square defect is cut into a large expanse of skin; the square, in a month or two, will contract down to the shape of a four pointed star. This configuration, as defined by tattoo marks, relaxes and eventually matures to a shape somewhat square again but significantly smaller in area that the original defect.[1] This remodeling process of simultaneous collagen lysis and synthesis can continue for as long as two years.

Humidity and Climate

Humidity will significantly influence the process of epithelization. If a plastic occlusive dressing is used to cover a fresh wound, not only will the epithelium migrate twice as fast, but no crust will form. A similar response is seen when an occlusive ointment is used. The disadvantage of occlusion, at least in theory, is that an abscess roof is created, and the inability of the wound to drain may promote infection. Crusts or scabs form when the surface is allowed to dehydrate. They have the advantage of acting as an excellent dressing and a vehicle for carrying necrotic debris to the surface to be shed.

High humidity may be the result of geographic variations. In comparison studies performed in Miami, Yuma, and Fairbanks, the inflammatory index of identical wounds was lowered more quickly in the hot, humid Florida environment.[2]

Oxygen Tension

Oxygen tension has been shown to have an optimal saturation at which maximal tensile strength will develop.[3] Clinically, the oxygen tension can be lowered by ischemia, venous stasis, hematoma, and compressed vessels.

Infection

Of all factors, infection is probably the most common cause of wound healing failure. Years ago it was shown by Dunphy that the presence of foreign or necrotic material in the depth of a wound increased its vulnerability to infection by a factor of more than a thousand fold.[4] In fact, precise technique with minimal tissue trauma often results in perfectly fine healing, in spite of gross deliberate bacterial contamination. Systemmic antibiotics appear to be significantly effective only if started preoperatively.[5] Meanwhile, the search for a nonabsorbable suture which handles easily and causes no tissue reaction relentlessly continues.

Health, Age, and Nutrition

As the skin ages, it sags and generally "fits" more loosely. For this reason, wound edges can be closed under less tension and a minimal amount of remodeling and contraction becomes necessary. With advancing age however, diseases such as diabetes, arteriosclerosis, etc. all adversely affect the healing capacities of the surgically wounded skin. Nutrition, in the sense of vitamin C, as related to scurvy; vitamin K, as related to clotting; vitamins A and E, as related to their effects on collagen synthesis and epithelization; zinc, as related to some poorly understood enzyme system; and amino acids such as methionine all have some role in wound healing.[6–8]

Steroids and Toxins

Steroids, toxins, immunosuppresants, and antimetabolites all slow down wound healing through various pathways. On the frontier, experimental lathyrism with beta aminoproprionitrile has been used successfully to slow down the scarring of flexor tendon repairs.[9] Various wound accelerators have also been described which may show promise in the future.[10]

Summary

The biology of wound healing is indeed a complex process. From Phase 1 to Phase 3, an orderly progression of events takes place in the repair process. Various factors influence the rapidity and cosmetic appearance of this phenomenon. Physical, microbial, nutritional, and environmental factors all have some role in the end result.

Perhaps this brief review will stimulate the practicing cutaneous surgeon to reevaluate his techniques and be more critical of his results.

References

1. James DW, Newcombe JF: Granulation tissue resorption during the free and limited contraction of skin wounds. J Anat 95:247, 1961
2. Bothwell JW, Rovee DT: Effect of climate in the repair of cutaneous wounds in humans, in Maibach HI, Rovee DT (ed), Epidermal wound healing, Yearbook Medical Publishers, Chicago, 1972
3. Chase RA: Oxygen tension and wound healing. Surgery 71:150–151, 1972
4. Dunphy JE: Wound healing. Medcom Press, New York, 1974
5. Waterman NG, Pollard NT: Local antibiotic treatment of wounds, in Maibach HI, Rovee DT (ed), Epidermal wound healing, Yearbook Medical Publishers, Chicago, 1972
6. Herrman JB, Woodward SC: Stimulation of fibroplasia by vitamin A. Surg Forum 20:500, 1969
7. Ehlich PH, Hunt TK: Effects of cortisone and vitamin A in wound healing. Ann Surg 167:324–330, 1968
8. Fulghum DD: Zinc, zealots and zetetics. Arch Derm 104: 210–211, 1971
9. Peacock EE Jr, Maddin JW: Some studies in the effect of beta-aminoproprionitrile in patients with injured flexor tendons. Surgery 66:215–220, 1969
10. Herrman JB, Woodward SC: An experimental study of wound healing accelerators. Am Surg 38:26–34, 1972

Updating Hair Transplantation

D. Bluford Stough, III, Hot Springs, Ark.

Facial Evaluation

The primary purpose of hair transplantation is an improvement in appearance. Initially, the etiology of hair loss is determined, after which the amount and type of donor hair is evaluated.[2] Motivation of the patient is also an important consideration. While analyzing the patient's physiognomy, the surgeon assesses the symmetry of the features and contour of the head, especially the prominence of the forehead. Proper framing of the face is paramount for enhancement of the appearance.

A hairline compatible with the patient's features and age should be predetermined in order to adequately frame the face.[3] Factors to be considered are anticipated future hair loss, quality of donor grafts, and intended hair style. The artistry and imagination of the surgeon will be reflected in construction of the frontal area,[4] although adherence to established principles of harmonious proportions is also essential.[5] One suggestion for roughly determining an appropriate frontal configuration is the use of the curvature formed by the web between the index finger and thumb. When the hand opposite the part side is placed on the forehead with the tip of the index finger in the part area and the apex of the outstretched thumb over the opposite base, a proportionately suitable frontal margin is usually outlined. The resultant hairline will be lopsided to the part side; when the hair is combed, it will then fall naturally away from the part. A deep lateral recession should be avoided. We endeavor to design a contemporary hairline with an oval configuration in contrast to the previously popular widow's peak (Fig. 1).

Since initial grafts are usually the best grafts they are utilized in the most advantageous manner, routinely in the anterior margin of the frontal region. Concentration on the first 2.0 to 3.0 cm in depth of this frontal margin is advocated. If the patient is to receive maximum benefit, this area is treated at every opportunity as the frontal area is the "corner stone" or "building block" for proper contemporary grooming.[6] If there is extensive baldness, it is even more important to concentrate the better grafts in the frontal area near the part side with fewer placements on the opposite side (Fig. 2). The acquisition of as much hair as possible should be the first and most important attainment, followed by the achievement of a natural look.

Donor Grafts

In organizing the sequence of donor graft extraction, the initial grafts are usually taken from the mid-occipital region opposite the part side. Since the part area must be avoided, the occipital region opposite the part side will normally yield a greater number of grafts. Later, blender grafts will be taken from the lower occipital area. By following this sequence, usually a sufficient number of desirable grafts is assured for placement along the critical frontal margin.

Blender Grafts

To attain a natural effect, 2.0 to 4.0 mm blender grafts are taken from the lower occipital area where finer hair is found and placed no deeper than 1.0 cm into the frontal region. These small blender grafts are also inserted into skip areas, anterior acute angles between larger grafts, and in any place of clumping or marked contrast along the anterior margin.

Whenever the patient is exceptionally tenacious in seeking the most natural appearance, 2.0 to 2.5 mm hair-bearing grafts are extracted from

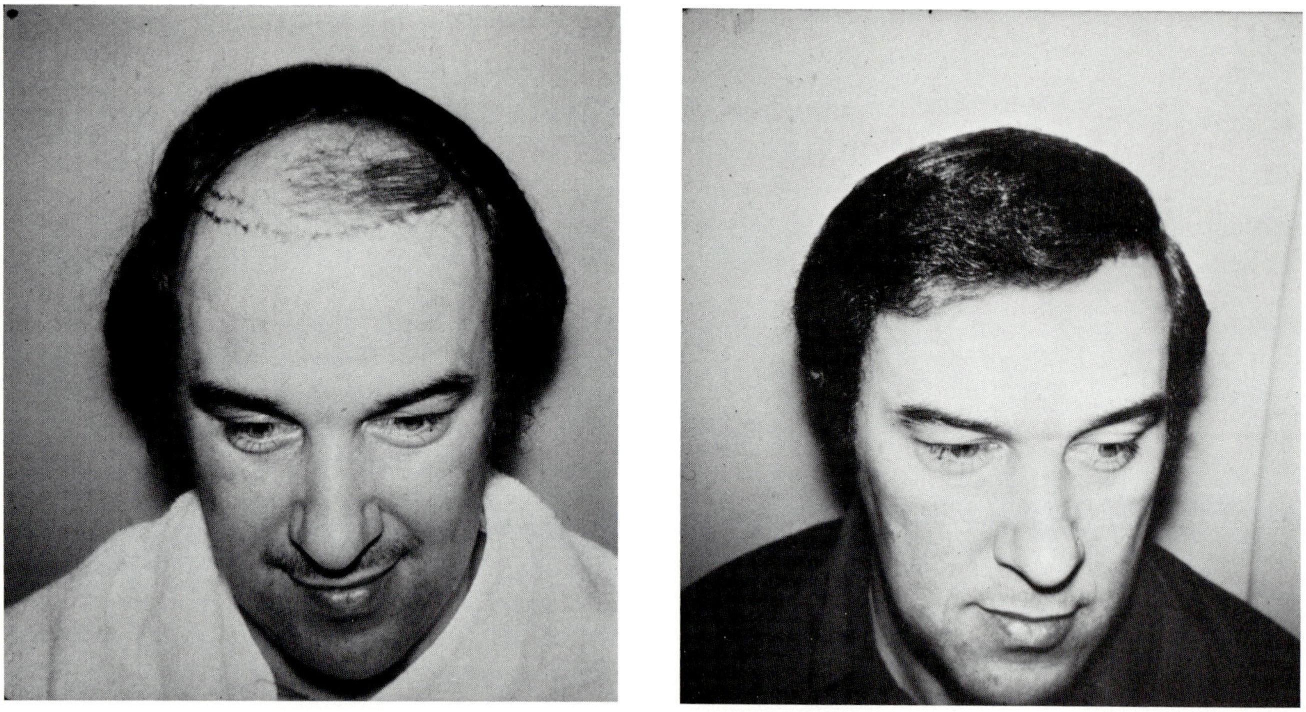

Fig. 1. (A) A 34-yr-old male with male pattern baldness (after initial hair transplantation session). Note: oval configuration. (B) One year after hair transplants.

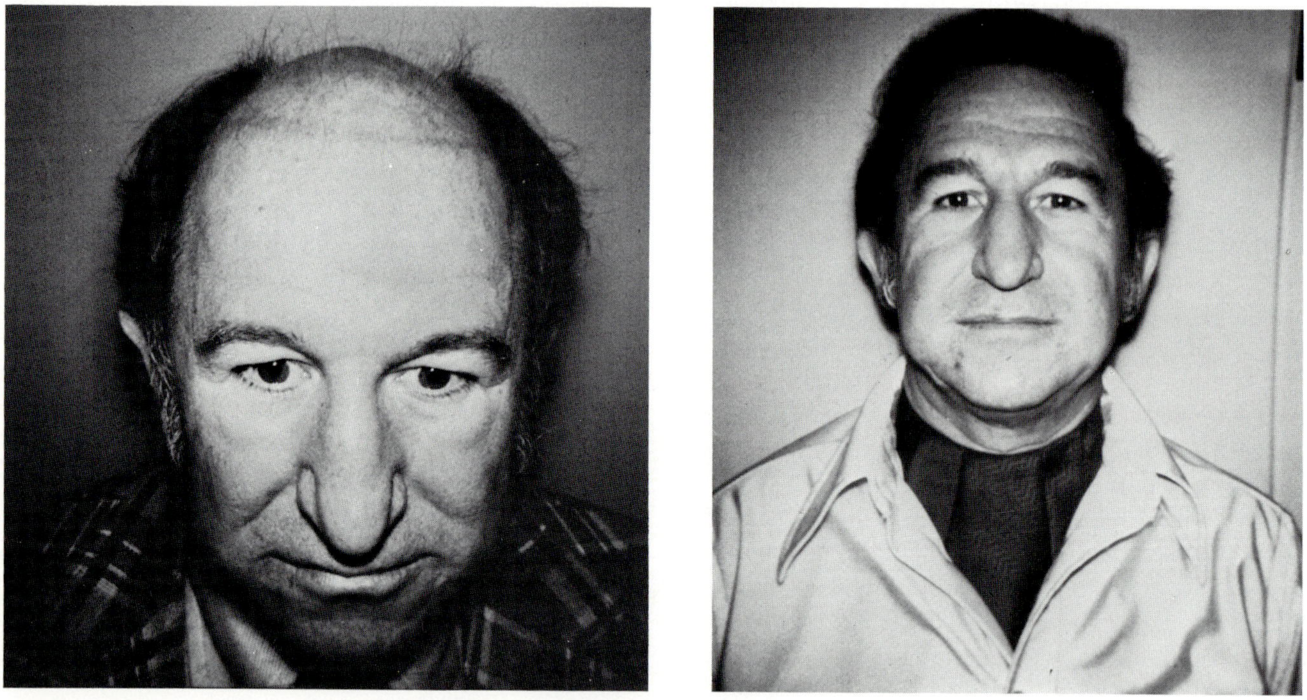

Fig. 2. (A) A 49-yr-old male before hair transplantation. (B) Nine months after punch grafts.

the lower occipital region, hand-trimmed to a slightly smaller size and placed in small slits along this frontal margin. Blending, when properly performed, eliminates a "moth-eaten" or abrupt artificial appearance.

Strip Punching

"Strip punching" is the placement of 4.5 or 5.0 mm grafts less than 1.0 mm apart along the frontal margin.[4] At the first session these larger 5.0 mm grafts are placed continuously in Row 1 but spaced 5.0 mm apart in Row 3. During the second session, Row 2 is established, again with the continuous placement of 4.5 or 5.0 mm grafts less than 1.0 mm apart.

In recipient plug extraction a punch 1/2 mm smaller than the one used for the donor graft is advocated. Angling the incision may reduce visible scarring. However, it is essential that the angle be uniform and restricted to prevent the possibility of transecting previously transplanted hair or disturbing the original surviving hair.

Donor Graft Instrumentation

Extreme sharpness of a punch is essential whether it is a manual punch that requires varying degrees of pressure or one which is motor driven with pressure restricted to a minimum.

The use of a power-driven Bell 5B hand instrument to excise donor grafts has recently been employed in our clinic. This machine with a small handle affords a delicate and smooth sensation to the touch. The precision handling often enables the surgeon to obtain superior quality grafts compared to those extracted by a manual punch. The crunching sound (a frequent complaint when hand punches are used) is minimized and, with experience, procedure time is often reduced. Its speed varies from 800 to 18000 RPM but, when excising grafts, it is used on low RPM (about 1500) with minimal pressure. Only slight pressure is recommended as it is important to avoid distortion of the hair shaft with resultant transection of the hair. To date, the use of this instrument in our clinic has been confined to donor graft extraction.

As previously mentioned, it is mandatory that both manual and power-driven punches be exceptionally sharp.

Saline Injections

The injection of approximately 10–30 ml of saline into the donor area (according to the number of grafts extracted) is especially recommended for the patient with fine sparse delicate hair. The subsequent distension of the donor area provides increased donor substance which extends tissue stability for the attainment of better quality grafts. Saline injections may enhance hemostasis and consequently, facilitate cleaning of the grafts.

Marcaine Injections and Cooling of Grafts

We have found that 1:200,000 epinephrine in 1/2 percent Xylocaine produces an adequate anesthesia and has a wide margin of safety. However, if the procedure is prolonged, the use of 1/10 percent solution of Marcaine may be administered. Due to the excessive burning sensation which occurs upon injection of Marcaine, the patient is initially anesthetized with Xylocaine.

In our experience, cooling of grafts afforded very little advantage. Apparently, the majority of those who perform hair transplants also concur with this opinion.

Proper Grooming Techniques

Proper grooming advice and the recommendation of certain grooming aids cannot be overemphasized. A hair stylist may determine the most suitable length to which the hair should be trimmed, as well as the proper style for an individual according to features and age. Sometimes, a patient may be advised to grow a beard, side-burns or a mustache to add emphasis, or complement the hair style.

There are many reliable grooming aids on the market which increase the texture of the hair and give a semblance of greater thickness. An electric hand-styling dryer is most essential for creating this effect. Good grooming demands clean, manageable hair and frequent, even daily shampooing.

Summary

The principal factors in the updating of hair transplantation are the use of newer techniques and instruments, and the achievement of anatomical and artistic compatibility by properly assessing the patient's physiognomy. Stressing the importance of skillful concentration in the frontal area has also contributed to the current success of hair transplantation.

References

1. Hair Transplantation Comes of Age: Medical World News, July 19, 1974
2. Norwood O'Tar: Hair Transplant Surgery, published by Charles C Thomas, Springfield, I11, 1973, 49
3. Stough DB: Current trends in hair transplantation. Arch Otolaryngol 98:1973
4. Stough DB: Surgeon and Narrator, Video Tape, 1st Annual Hair Transplant Symposium and Workshop, co-sponsored by The American Academy of Facial and Plastic Reconstructive Surgery, and The American Academy for Dermatologic Surgery, Feb 1974, produced by the University of Arkansas Medical Center, Div of Bio-Medical Communications, Little Rock, Ark
5. Patterson CN, Powell DG: Facial analysis in patient evaluation for physiologic and cosmetic surgery. The Laryngoscope, 84: 1, 1974
6. Stough DB: Advancements in hair transplantation and skin allotransplantation. CUTIS: 8: 1971

Surgical Reduction of the Laryngeal Eminence

Richard W. Babin, Rinaldo F. Canalis and Mark E. Krugman, Los Angeles, Calif.

The laryngeal eminence or Adam's apple is the single prominent landmark in the neck. A large or projecting Adam's apple is a male characteristic. It can add to or detract from the overall appearance of the facial profile.[1,2] The presentation to the head and neck clinic of a patient with an inappropriately prominent Adam's apple, and the procedure subsequently undertaken to reduce this prominence prompted this report.

Anatomy

The laryngeal eminence is formed by the leading edges of the two fused thyroid cartilages. It is covered by skin, subcutaneous fat, fascia and to some extent by the strap muscles. It is usually most prominent just at the base of the thyroid nodule. The infantile larynx is of equal size in both sexes and it lies relatively high in the neck. At birth the inferior edge of the cricoid is at the level of the upper border of the fourth cervical vertebra and the epiglottis is opposite the first cervical vertebra. During early childhood and then strikingly after puberty the larynx descends to its adult position. The tip of the epiglottis will then be opposite the third cervical vertebra while the cricoid will be at the level of the sixth or seventh cervical vertebrae. As the larynx descends the thyroid cartilage elongates, and the thyrohyoid membrane becomes a more distinct feature.

After puberty, the development of the male and female thyroid cartilage differs (Fig. 1). The female larynx continues to grow in proportion to other neck structures. The resultant relative prominence is due to its overall anterior-posterior dimension. Its prominence is tempered by the close midline approximations of the strap muscles, and the amount of subcutaneous fat overlying these structures, especially over the thyrohyoid membrane.

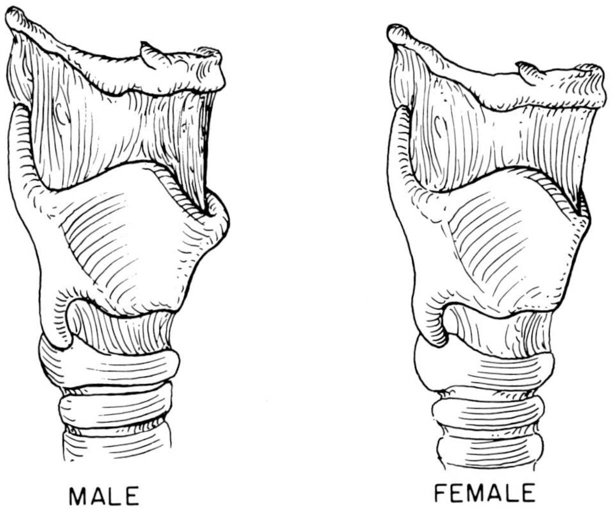

Fig. 1. Line drawing demonstrating the increased projection of the male laryngeal eminence as compared to the female.

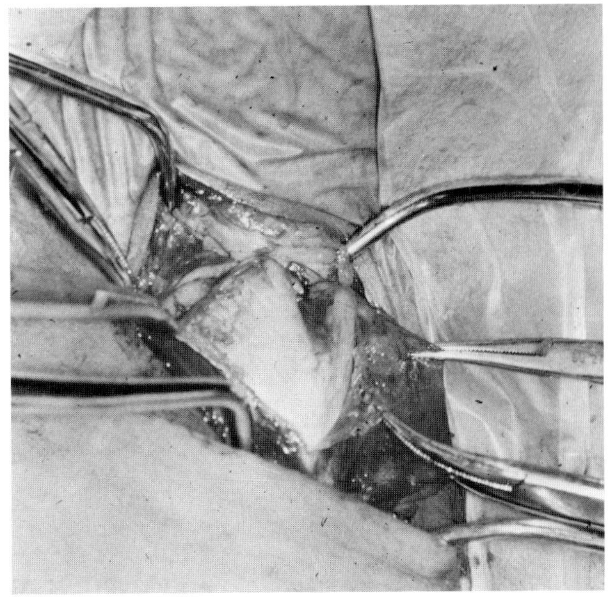

Fig. 2. Exposure of the thyroid ala by vertical excision of the investing layer of cervical facial and lateral retraction of strap musculature.

The male thyroid cartilage after puberty undergoes a differential growth pattern with a more rapidly growing and eventually flaring superior edge. This outward flaring is superimposed on the overall anterior-posterior dimension of the thyroid cartilage and further increases the projection and definition of the Adam's apple. The relative projection is also enhanced by a diastasis of the sternohyoid muscles, and the resultant loss of bulk immediately adjacent to the anterior thyroid cartilage and over the thyrohyoid membrane. This may result in a hollow on profile just above the thyroid cartilage. Thus the relative projection of the male Adam's apple may be decreased by reducing the overall anterior-posterior dimension, reducing the flare, or increasing the surrounding tissue bulk laterally, and especially superiorly over the thyrohyoid membrane.

Procedure

The procedure is performed under local anesthesia with the patient in a supine position, and the head extended. A horizontal incision is made over the thyroid cartilage through the platysma muscle and extending not quite to the border of the sternomastoid muscle bilaterally. Flaps are raised to the hyoid bone above and to just past the cricoid cartilage below. The investing layer of the middle cervical fascia is incised vertically from hyoid to cricoid and the fascia and sternohyoid muscles are retracted laterally (Fig. 2). The perichondrium is then incised along the most superior aspect of the thyroid cartilage similar to the technique utilized for a supraglottic partial laryngectomy. An ink or bovie mark is placed below the thyroid notch at the junction of the middle and superior one-third of the thyroid cartilage. This represents the approximate position of the anterior commissure, and serves as a guide to perichondrial and cartilage removal. The perichondrium is then stripped inferiorly to this mark. The inner perichondrium is then carefully stripped from the medial aspect of the thyroid cartilage approximately 4–5 mm from the superior edge. The superior border of the thyroid cartilage is then removed in parallel strips until the desired reduction is accomplished (Fig. 3). The excision is not carried all the way laterally, to prevent disconnecting the superior cornu. Care is taken not to extend the excision as far as the safety mark (Fig. 4). No attempt is made to deepen the foreshortened thyroid notch (Fig. 5). The new superior border is then externally beveled to gain even more reduction, without approaching the level of endolaryngeal musculature (Fig. 6). The perichondrium is trimmed, and approximated over the bevel. The

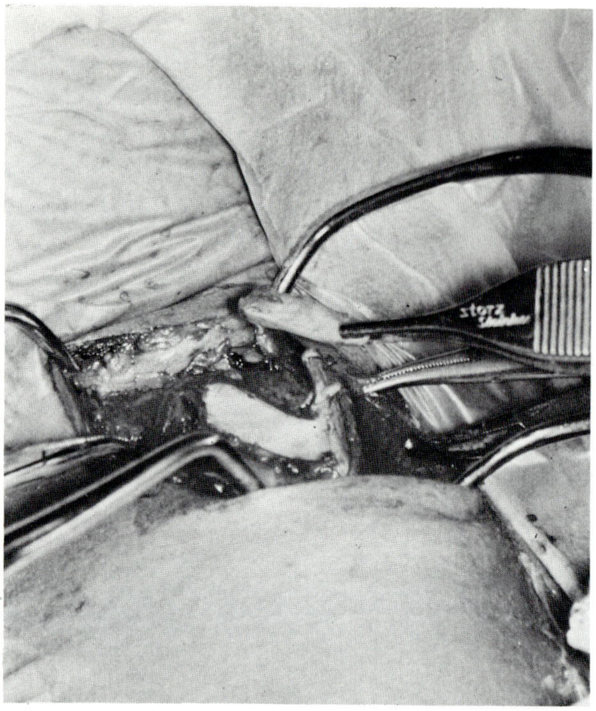

Fig. 3. Excision of the superior edge of thyroid cartilage after stripping the perichondrium.

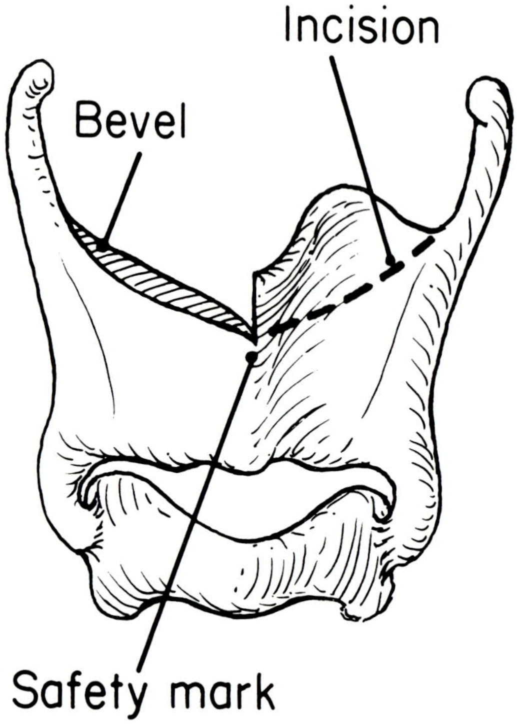

Fig. 4. Line drawing of the thyroid cartilage showing area excised and beveled.

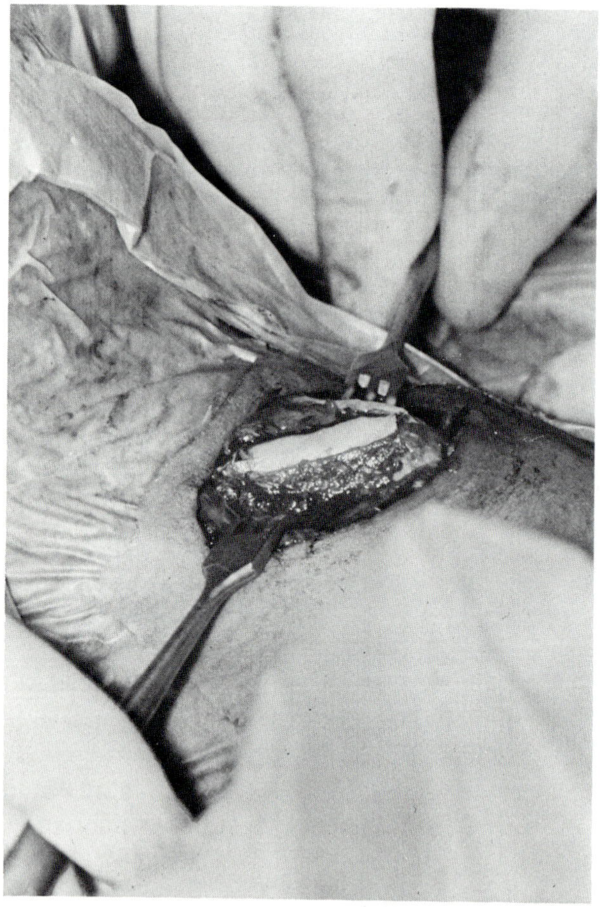

Fig. 5. Thyroid cartilage after excision.

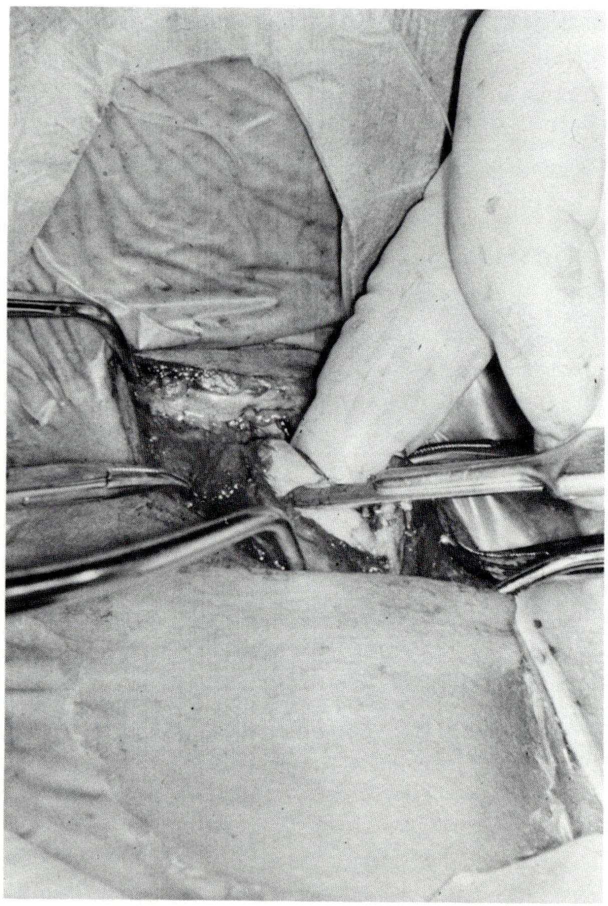

Fig. 6. Beveling anterior edge of superior thyroid cartilage after excision.

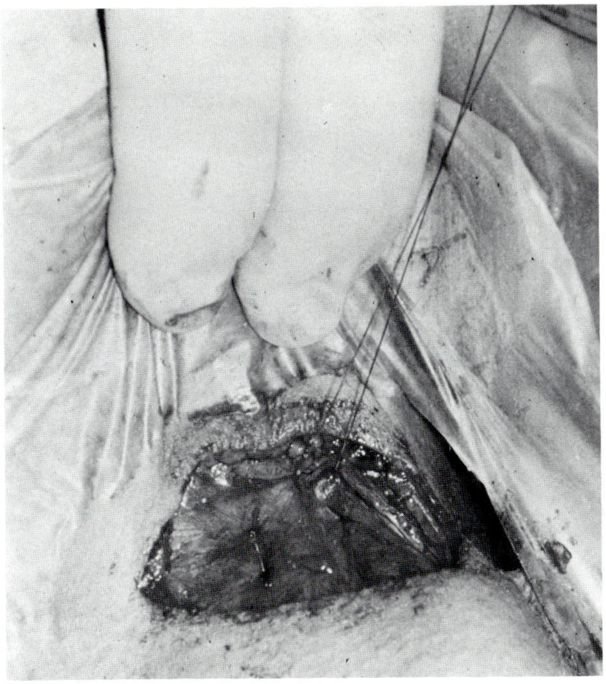

Fig. 7. Imbrication of sternohyoid muscles above the newly formed laryngeal eminence.

anterior borders of the sternohyoid muscle are freed up to the hyoid, and the two muscles are imbricated over the midline from the hyoid to just above the newly placed Adam's apple, filling in any hollow remaining in this area (Fig. 7). The subcutaneous tissues and skin are closed over a small hemovac suction catheter.

Case Presentation

L.J. is a 26-year-old black individual who underwent a several stage male to female sex change by the division of Urology. The patient's facial features were sufficiently feminine that no cosmetic surgery was desired or indicated. The patient's Adam's apple, however, was particularly prominent, even by male standards (Figs. 8, 9). This appeared to be due to a pronounced flaring of the superior aspect of the thyroid cartilage, diastasis of the strap muscles, and lack of subcutaneous fat.

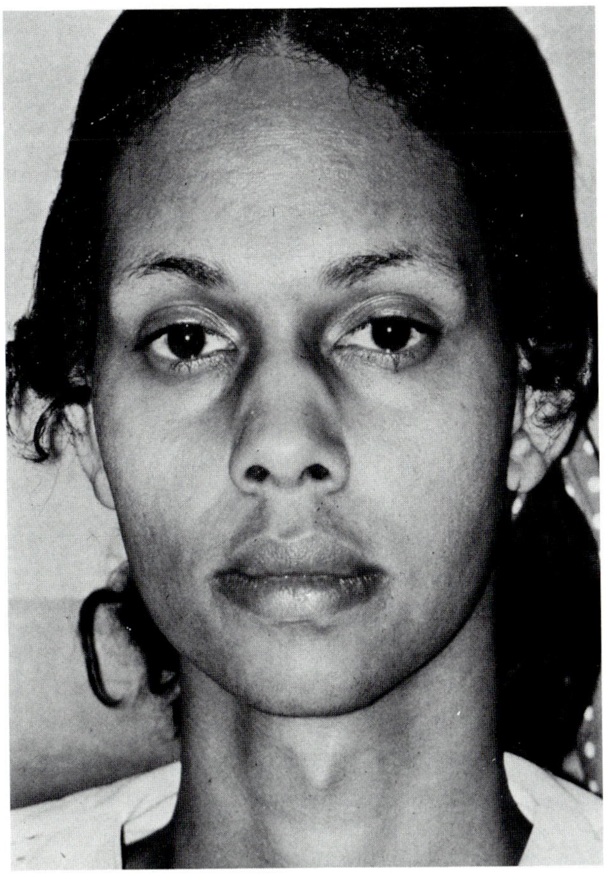

Fig. 8. Preoperative anterior-posterior view of patient.

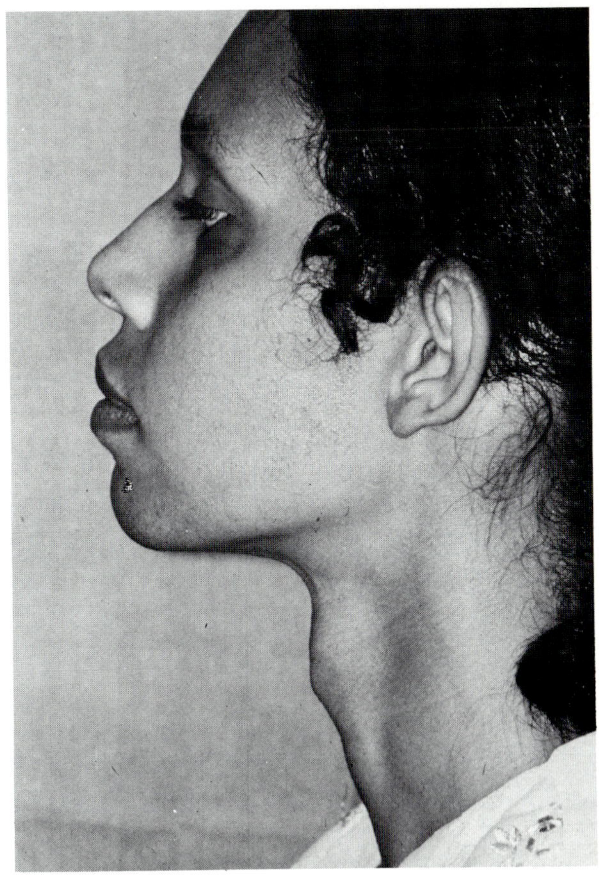

Fig. 9. Preoperative lateral view of patient.

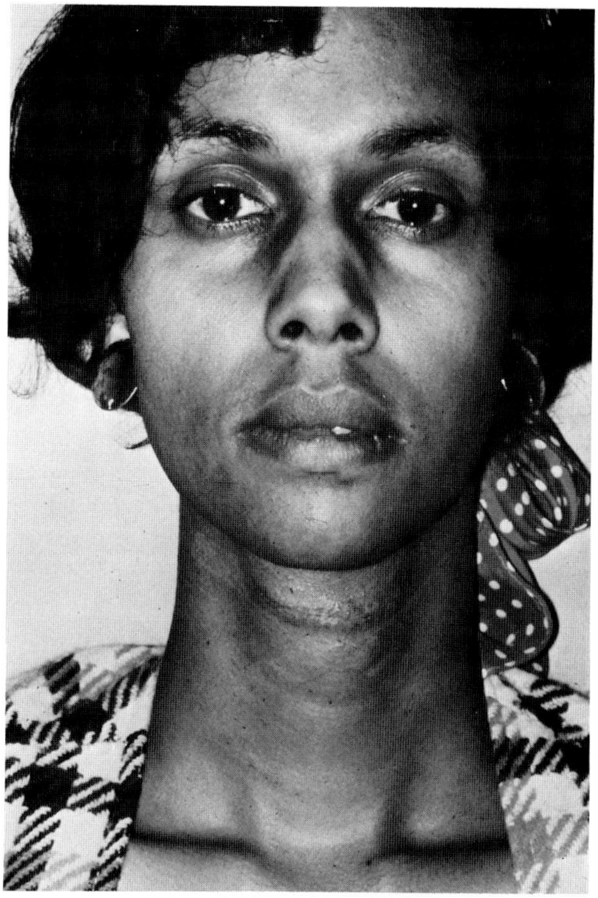

Fig. 10. Anterior-posterior view 10 days postoperatively.

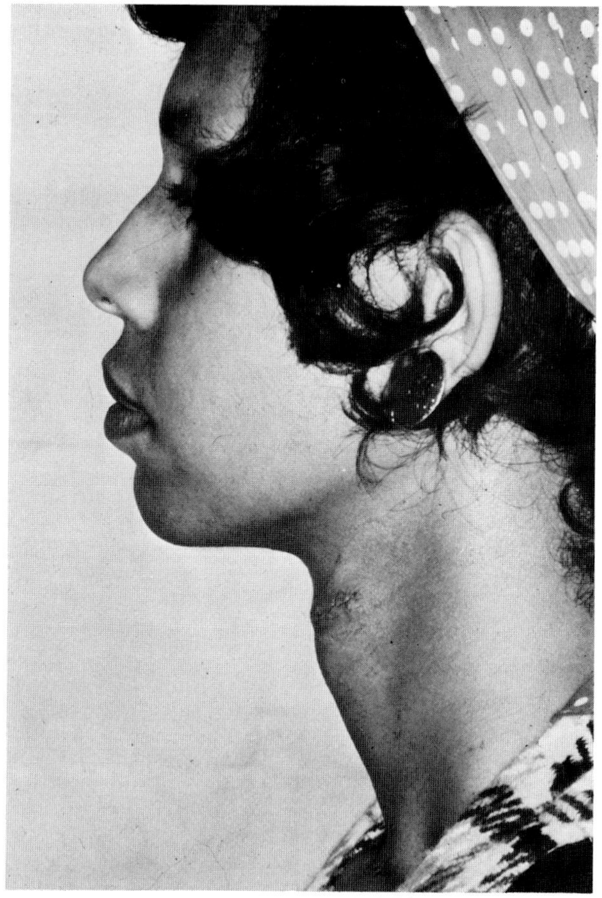

Fig. 11. Lateral views of patient 10 days postoperatively.

Vocal cord function was normal. The patient underwent a thyroid cartilage shave under local anesthesia as described above. There was no transient or permanent change in vocal quality, respiration, or deglutination. The hemovac drain was removed on the second postoperative day and the skin sutures the seventh postoperative day. The end result was a marked reduction of the impact of the laryngeal eminence on an elongated neck profile (Figs. 10, 11).

Comment

Theoretically, it may seem that a more anatomic approach might result by wedging out the anterior commissure with the anterior borders of both thyroid ala, shortening the vocal cords, and reconstructing the thyroid notch. This would reduce the entire anterior-posterior dimension of the larynx without lowering the position of it's most prominent point. The inherent dangers of a general anesthetic as well as the increased morbidity and especially the uncertain effect on the airway and vocal mechanism of such a procedure contraindicate it on purely cosmetic grounds. Our patient demonstrated that a satisfactory cosmetic result could be obtained by a simple local procedure which did not enter the endolarynx.

References

1. Edgerton MT: The surgical treatment of male transsexuals clinics Plast Surg 1:285, 1974
2. Goode RL: The thyroid cartilage shave, in Laub DR, Gardy P (eds) Proceedings of the Second Interdisciplinary Symposium on Transsexualism, 1974

Surgical Treatment of Baldness

José Juri, Carlos Juri, Jorge de Autueno, and
Alberto González Otharán, Buenos Aires, Argentina

We would like to present a technique which we have developed for the surgical treatment of baldness. Our technique consists in the use of parieto-occipital and occipito-parietal flaps which vary in number and design according to the distribution and size of the bald area. The bald and hairbearing areas are studied and, with the cooperation of the patient, one, two or three flaps are planned, depending on the case. We classify baldness in three degrees (Fig. 1).

In degree I, a flap with an anterior parietal pedicle is planned. In degree II a similar flap is traced on the opposite side of the head and then placed behind the first flap. In degree III a third flap is brought up to the crown of the head. This last described flap may have either an occipital pedicle (placed sagitally) or a retroaural pedicle (placed transversely from side to side), depending on the distribution of the bald area (Fig. 2).

Procedure

Design

The superficial temporal artery is palpated and marked. This is the center of the flap base (Point L). The borders of the flap are traced 2 cm above and 2 cm below this point, making a total width of 4 cm (Fig. 3). From here the flap is marked back and down without crossing the occipital midline. A hairbearing area is maintained above the upper border of the flap so that the final scar may be concealed.

Delay

Two delays are made using local anesthesia. The first delay is for the two lines of the parietal area (Fig. 4A), and the second delay is made one week later for the occipital portion (Fig. 4B).

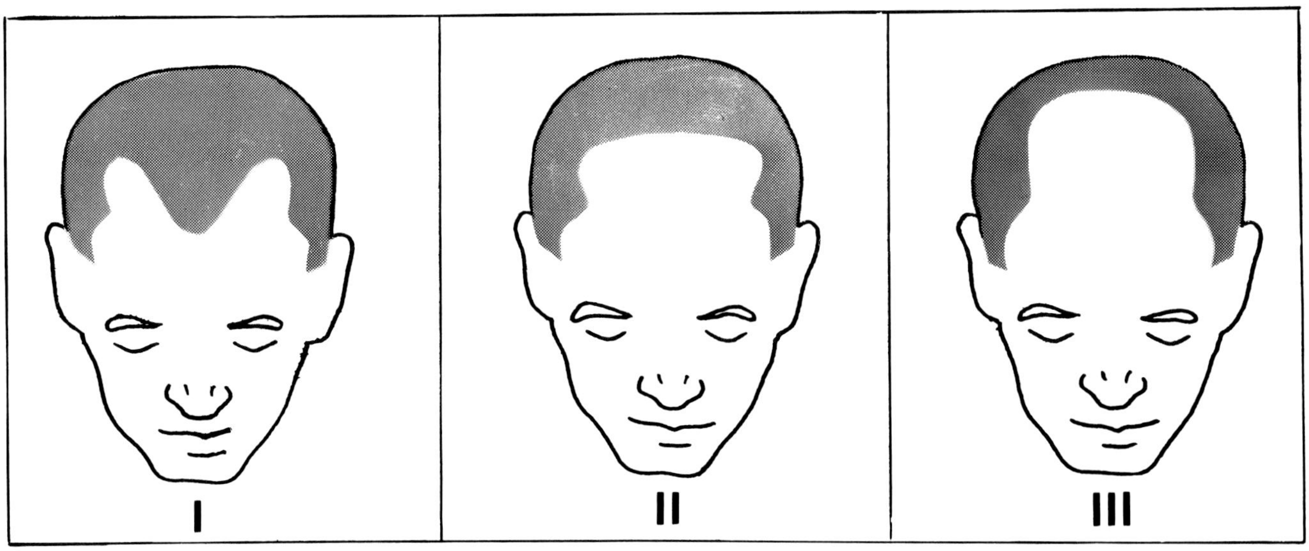

Fig. 1. Baldness classification.

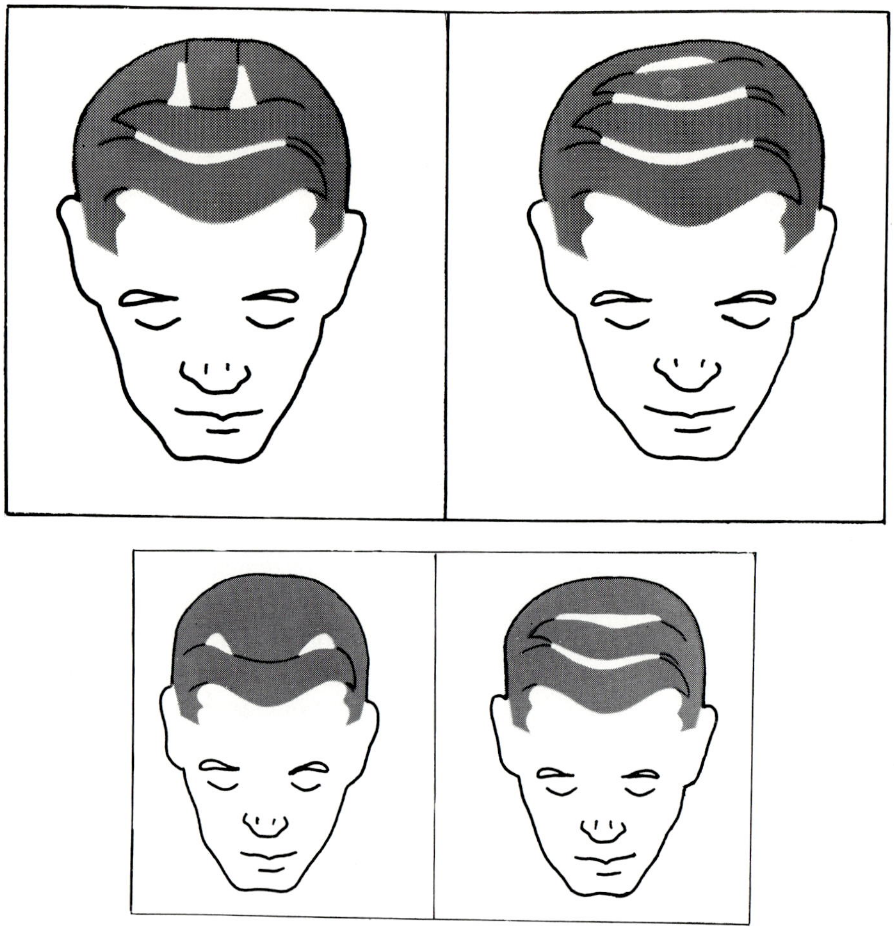

Fig. 2. Number and distribution of flaps according to degree of baldness.

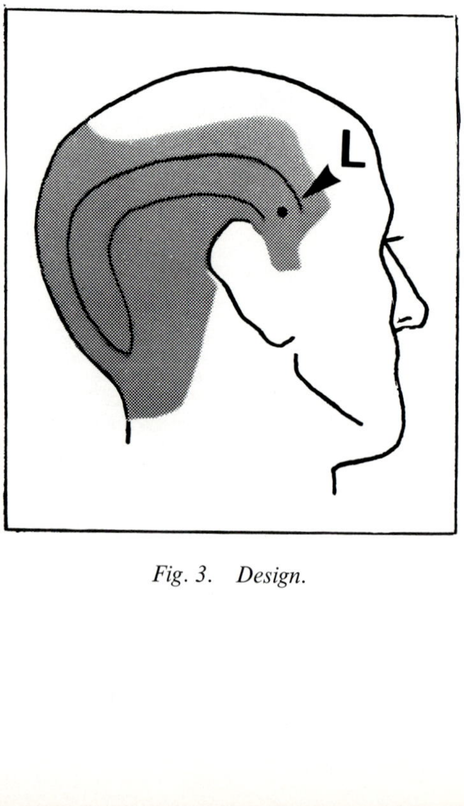

Fig. 3. Design.

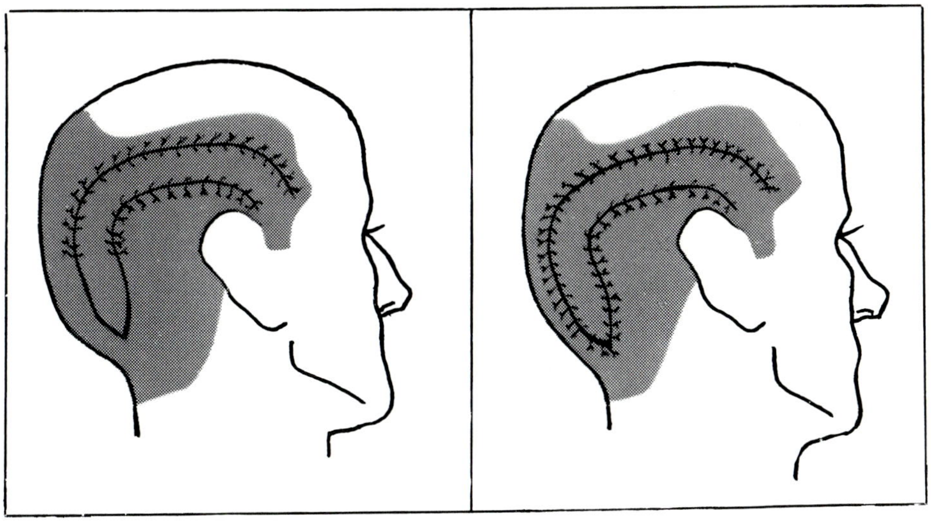

Fig. 4 (left) First delay. (right) Second delay.

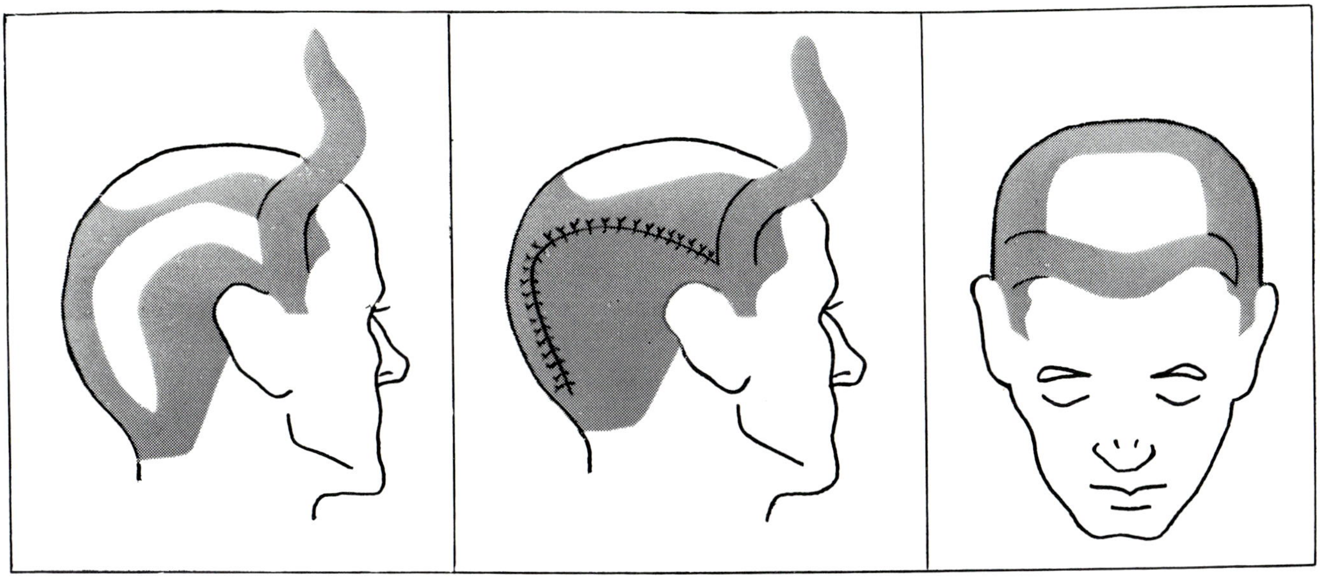

Fig. 5. Transposition of the first flap.

Transposition

One week after the second delay, using general anesthesia, the entire flap is lifted, rotated forward, and transposed to its final position. The donor wound is closed by deep undermining of the lower border, including all the retroaural area and reaching to the neck. The undermining allows the wound of the donor area to be closed without tension, thus avoiding secondary alopecia.

Once the flap has been placed in the desired position on the forehead, the bald scalp is marked and then excised so the flap can fit into place (Fig. 5).

Transposition of the second flap

After a period of no less than 30 days, a similar procedure is carried out on the other side of the head, and this second flap is placed behind the first. If the bald area is large, these flaps should not be in contact with one another, but 2 cm left between them (Fig. 6). This alopecic area between the flaps can be excised two months later, and the flaps advanced towards each other. The aponeurosis is removed to aid this advancement. Residual small alopecia scars can finally be corrected with Z-plasties.

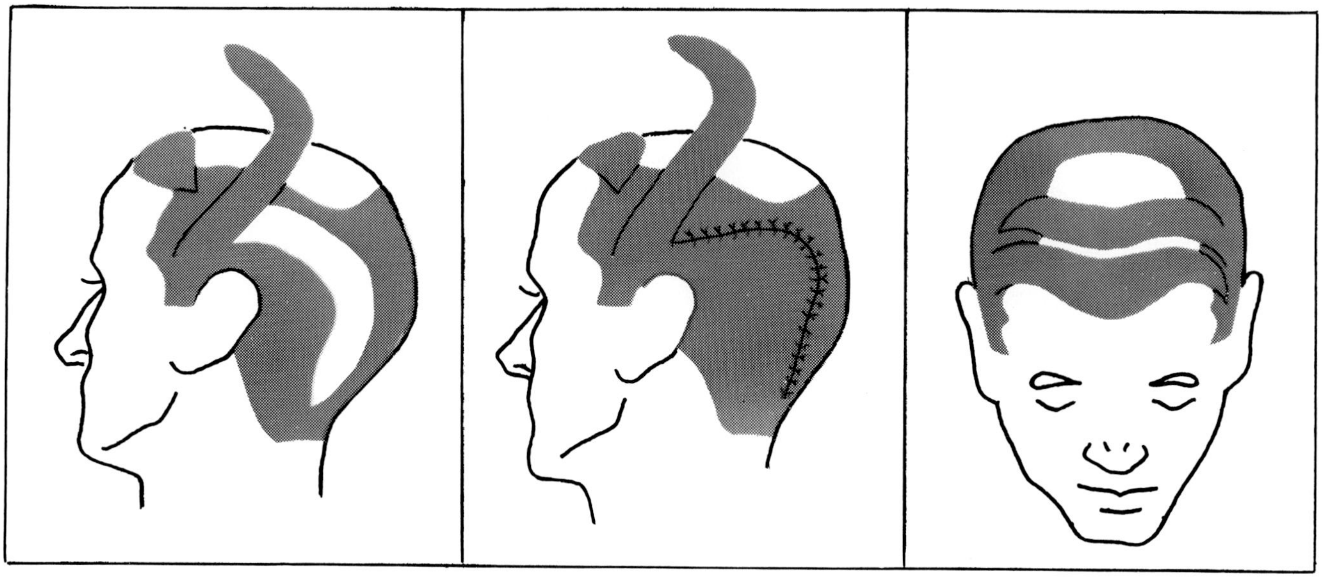

Fig. 6. Transposition of the second flap.

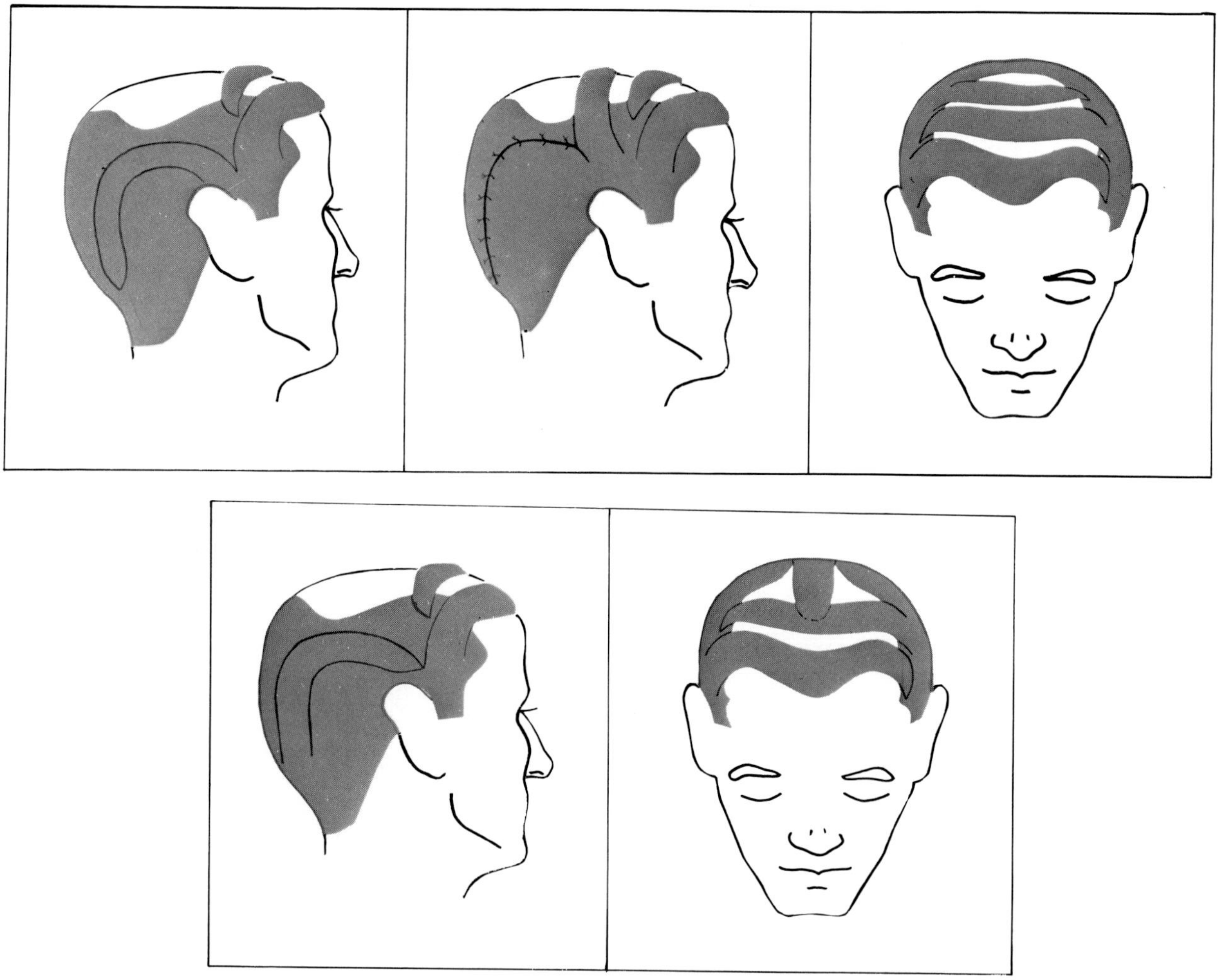

Fig. 7. Transposition of the third flap. (top) Using occipital pedicle. (bottom) Using retroaural pedicle.

Transposition of the third flap

In third degree baldness, a third flap can be made using a similar procedure. An occipital or a retroaural pedicle may be planned, depending on the distribution of the remaining bald area (Fig. 7).

Summary

The authors present a surgical procedure for the treatment of baldness using parieto-occipital and occipito-parietal flaps. The number and distribution of the flaps depend on the degree of baldness, the donor area, and the wishes of the patient. We have a total experience of 400 cases. The overall results have been excellent. Our only complications have been dehiscence of the donor wound at the beginning of this series, when the wound was under tension (15 cases), and necrosis of the distal 2 cm of the flap (10 cases) was also observed in our first cases.

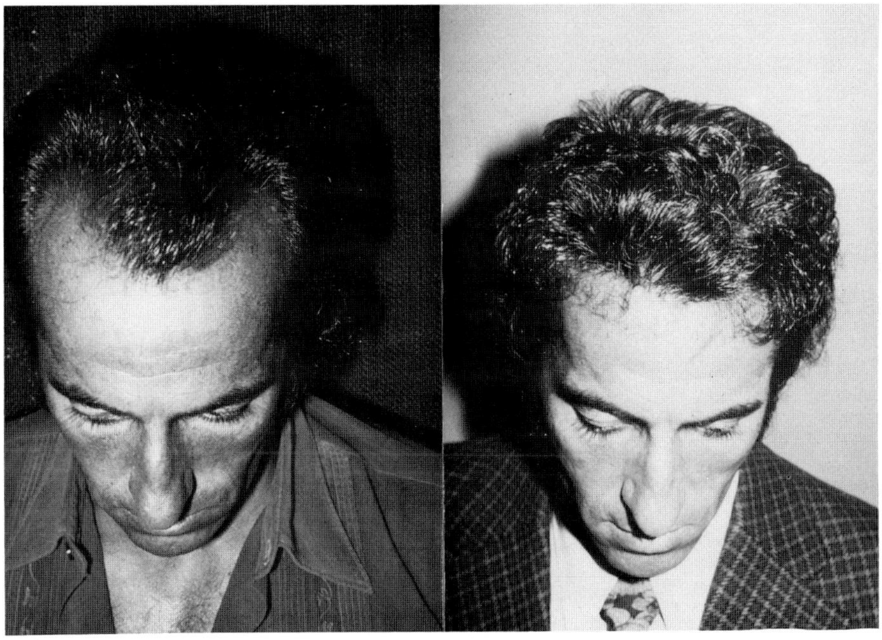

Fig. 8. (left) Degree I Baldness. (right) Result using one parieto-occipital flap.

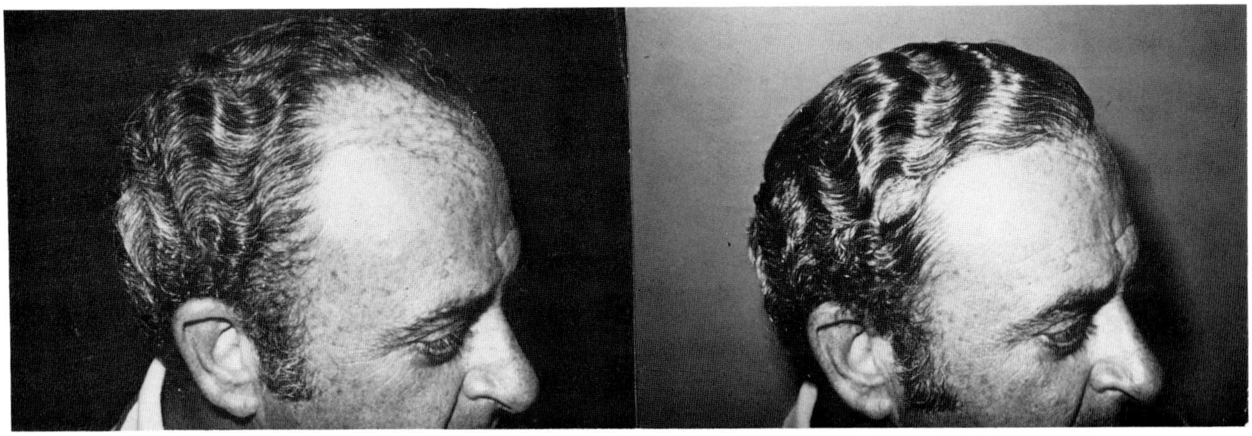

Fig. 9. (left) Degree I Baldness. (right) Result using one parieto-occipital flap.

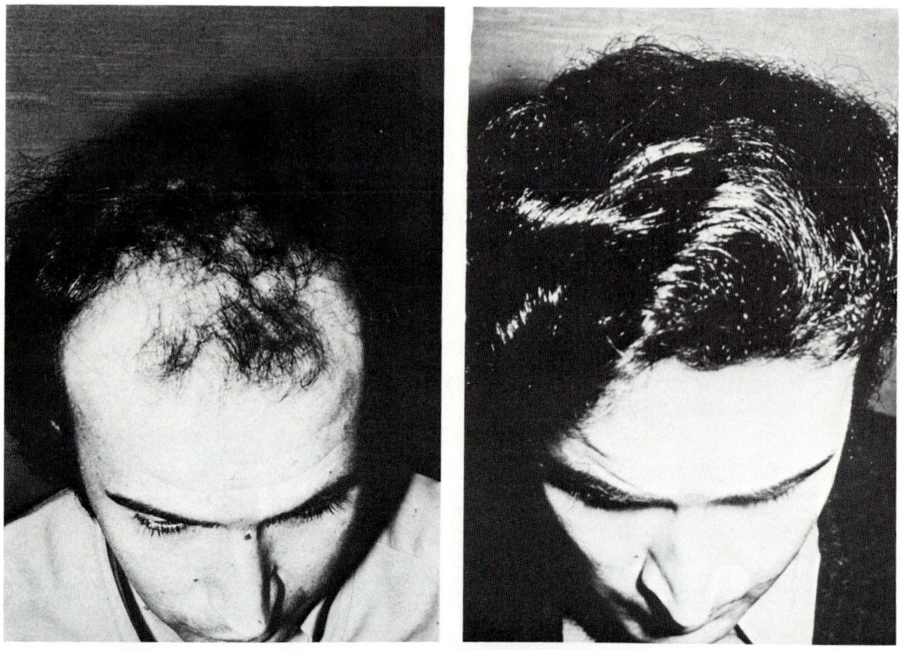

Fig. 10. (left) Degree II Baldness. (right) Result using two parieto-occipital flaps.

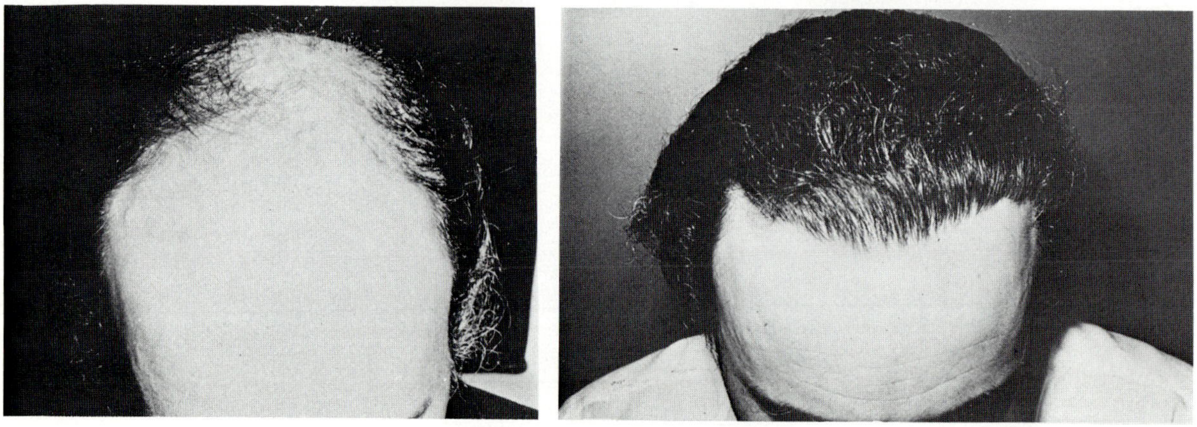

Fig. 11. (left) Degree II Baldness. (right) Result using two parieto-occipital flaps.

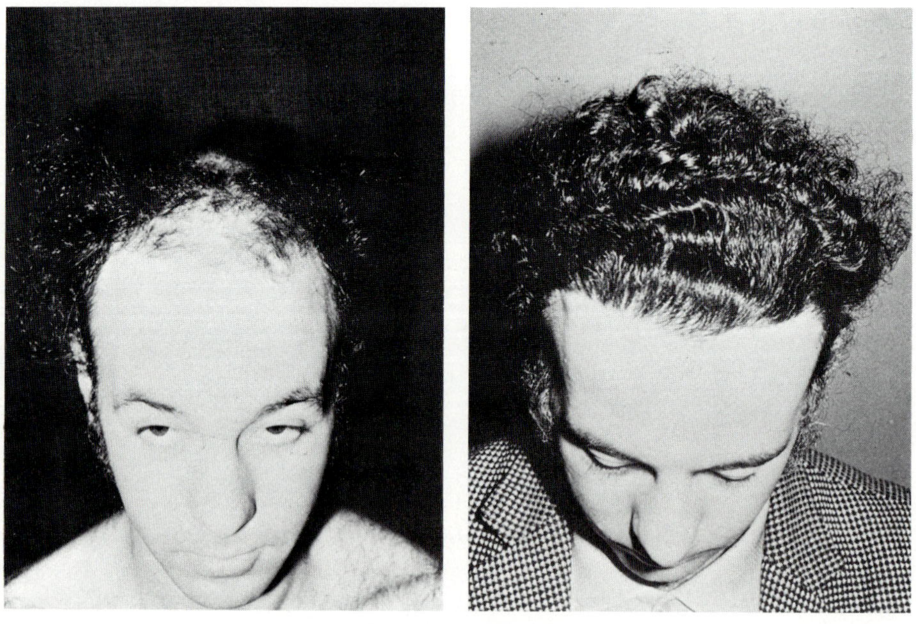

Fig. 12. (left) Degree III Baldness. (right) Result using two parieto-occipital flaps and one occipito-parietal flap.

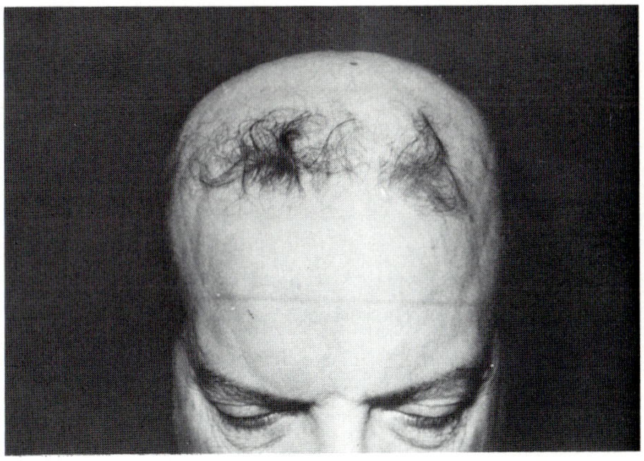

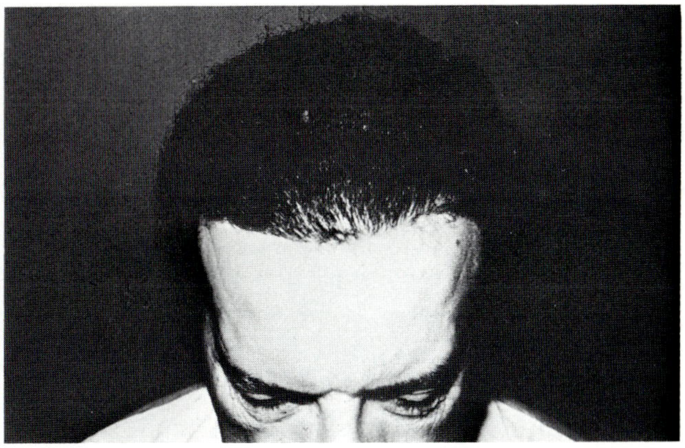

Fig. 13. (left) Degree III Baldness. (right) Result using two parieto-occipital flaps and one retroaural flap.

References

1. Correa M, Arufe HN: La cirugía plástica en las alopecías parciales definitivas del cuero cabelludo. Bol trab Soc cir Buenos Aires 41:10, 1957
2. Orentreich N: Autografts in alopecia and other selected dermatological conditions. Ann NY Acad Sci 83:463, 1959
3. Passot R: Chirurgie Esthétique Pure. G Doin et Cie, Paris, 1931
4. Vallis CP: Hair transplantation for male pattern baldness. Surg Clin N Am 51:519, 1971
5. Lamont ES: A plastic surgical transformation. Report of a case. West J Surg 65:164, 1957

Essentials in Molding a Facial Plastic Surgical Practice

E. Gaylon McCollough, Birmingham, Ala.

In today's society there appears to be an increased emphasis on youth and beauty. Each year over one-half million people in the United States have surgery to improve their appearance. The principal of supply and demand prevails in medicine as well as in other aspects of the business world and patients have become more sophisticated in their pursuit of perfection, therefore, the responsibility of training physicians to provide these services is more complex. Once a small group of physicians attempted to keep the "secrets of plastic surgery" under lock and key; as a result, the specialty was hampered. The current trend seemingly leans toward the sharing of knowledge with one's colleagues and encouraging more young men to become interested in the field of aesthetic surgery. Whether we adopt the term "cosmetic facial surgery, facial plastic surgery, aesthetic surgery, etc," the ultimate goal is to improve the patient's appearance either by correcting congenital and acquired defects or by reversing the signs of aging. Stemming from the growing demand for services, many surgical specialties provide training in aesthetic surgery, but beyond residency, fellowships and workshops are available for the individual interested in pursuing such a career. Following the completion of his technical training, the physician is faced with the question "now, how do I get started in practice?" The author has recently experienced those problems common to the young surgeon trying to establish himself in practice and the following are suggestions that might prove helpful.

Providing one possesses the technical skills to perform the surgery and the ability to analyze the psychological nature of each patient's problem, there are many ethical ways to "mold" a practice in aesthetic surgery. Waiting until the office is open may be too late; the ground work should be laid even while still in training.

Probably the first thing anyone should do when interested in achieving a specific goal is to associate himself with other individuals interested in the same goal. The American Academy of Facial Plastic and Reconstructive Surgery offers membership and training to physicians in residency programs of many specialties providing they demonstrate an interest in aesthetic, reconstructive, or facial plastic surgery. Junior membership in this organization entitles one to participate in its activities and helps simplify the transition to the status of Associate Fellow after residency. By attending the workshops and meetings provided by this and other organizations, one demonstrates to his colleagues and other individuals in his community that he possesses a special interest in a career of this nature. Whenever possible, he should visit and observe the work of other men in his community who perform facial surgery. By planning vacations wisely, it should be possible to visit individuals in other cities who have already established reputations as "cosmetic" or "facial surgeons." During residency training it is beneficial to spend as much time as possible in the accident or emergency room performing and teaching others plastic surgical techniques in the management of soft tissue trauma. Equally as important is the development of close interpersonal relationships with other physicians who perform general and regional plastic surgery. This includes the general plastic surgeons, the otorhinolaryngologists, opthalmologists, dermatologists, orthopedists, urologists, and others. Many specialties have overlapping interests and in some institutions more than one specialty performs the same surgical procedure. A healthy working relationship should be advantageous to all since the more good surgery that is performed, the greater will be the public's demand for this type of surgery. During the training period one should keep accurate records and photographs of the cases performed for they will prove to be valuable for future references and applications to medical societies and to hospital staffs.

Poor surgical instruments compromise the results of surgery, therefore, each resident should obtain his own set of surgical instruments while in training so that all possible conditions are optimal during those critical moments at the operating table. Many surgical supply houses provide special arrangements and deferred payment programs for residents.

In order to improve upon technical skills, skin surgery may be practiced in the animal laboratories or on pigs' feet purchased in the super markets. Frequent visits to the anatomy laboratory for review of the anatomy and dynamics of facial tissues should cultivate technical skills and solidify a working knowledge of the surgical anatomy. Medical students studying in the laboratory usually are delighted when someone demonstrates practical applications of anatomy to them. These students are our professional colleagues of the future.

Since good public relations with patients is advantageous, it is our policy to provide them with preoperative and postoperative instructions in booklet or pamphlet form so that they have a referral source for answering questions that might arise before or after consultation and/or surgery.

Even in residency training the physician must spend ample time in preoperative consultation with the patient and in addition to the routine hospital consent form should have a separate consent form signed for cosmetic and plastic surgical procedures. Especially in facial surgery, accurate records and good photographs are an absolute necessity, whether one is involved in private practice, a teaching program, or in training. Medicolegally these records and photographs may prove to be invaluable at a later date.

Following the completion of residency training, some physicians desire additional experience. Fellowship programs sponsored in association with the American Academy of Facial Plastic and Reconstructive Surgery and other organizations offer "exposure" and development of new ideas which may enhance the surgeon's versatility.

While the training period has been completed the physician must decide upon the location of his "new practice." If he has adhered to the suggestions outlined, establishing his practice in the area where he trained should prove to be a relatively smooth transition since he should have already confirmed himself as a physician with special interests and skills in facial surgery. When moving into a new community, he should consider an affiliation with a physician who is already established as a "facial surgeon," or with a clinic who needs someone to concentrate on this particular aspect of surgery.

The office must be carefully planned with comfortable, artistic surroundings. Professional advice with interior decoration is helpful. Every medical office requires certain essentials: waiting room, business office, nurses station, diagnostic rooms or laboratory, examination, and treatment rooms; but in addition to these, the aesthetic surgeon's office should include a consultation room, minor surgery room, and photography room. The decor of the office displays the surgeon's application of beauty, continuity, and artistic judgment. First impressions are important; patients usually have their doctor pictured in their mind's eye prior to meeting him face to face. The atmosphere of the office must be professional, yet warm and friendly so that each patient leaves with a feeling that their confidence in the physician by requesting an appointment has been appreciated.

In the beginning the physician developing a practice in facial surgery should select patients carefully and perform the procedures for which he is best qualified. An otolaryngologist might use the nose as his lead item, an ophthalmologist might use the eyelids, and a dermatologist might use dermabrasion, chemical peeling, or removal of facial lesions. There are ways to tactfully instill a nidus of thought or plant a seed with patients who come into the office for reasons other than for cosmetic surgery. One must be careful, however, not to appear to criticize the patient's appearance or seem overly aggressive in such suggestions or in the examination of deformities of the face and skin. Pamphlets obtained from the Medical Society or organizations such as the American Academy of Facial Plastic and Reconstructive Surgery have been written for patient information and education. When used with tact and discretion they are helpful.

A physician must work toward good relationships with other physicians in his community by using consultants when indicated and being available to assist other specialists with problem cases. Most physicians appreciate copies of preoperative and postoperative photographs of patients they have referred to another physician. Maintain an open-door policy in the operating room and always send patients back to the physicians who have referred them for treatment of a specific problem.

Once established in practice, it is a good policy to send letters of thanks to patients and physicians who refer patients to you. One should join and participate in the activities of his local, state, and national medical societies, as well as those organizations with special interests in the field in which he has chosen to pursue. One might become actively involved in teaching programs in his area and must be willing to share his knowledge, skills, and experience with every physician and student who expresses a desire to learn.

Cultivate the reputation of an ethical, capable, and nonaggressive physician and strive to maintain the highest moral conduct, but most importantly, develop an obsession about doing good work.

Index